8 July 2002

For Willo:

To a wonderful scientist, colleague, & friend.

We appreciate all that you do each & every day.

Continued health & success.

Ralph

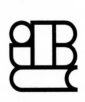

EMERGING THEORIES IN HEALTH PROMOTION PRACTICE AND RESEARCH

EMERGING THEORIES IN HEALTH PROMOTION PRACTICE AND RESEARCH

Strategies for Improving Public Health

Ralph J. DiClemente
Richard A. Crosby
Michelle C. Kegler
Editors

Foreword by Lawrence W. Green

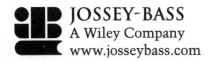

JOSSEY-BASS
A Wiley Company
www.josseybass.com

Published by

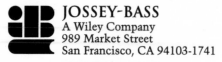

JOSSEY-BASS
A Wiley Company
989 Market Street
San Francisco, CA 94103-1741

www.josseybass.com

Jossey-Bass books and products are available through most bookstores. To contact Jossey-Bass directly, call (888) 378-2537, fax to (800) 605-2665, or visit our website at www.josseybass.com.

Substantial discounts on bulk quantities of Jossey-Bass books are available to corporations, professional associations, and other organizations. For details and discount information, contact the special sales department at Jossey-Bass.

We at Jossey-Bass strive to use the most environmentally sensitive paper stocks available to us. Our publications are printed on acid-free recycled stock whenever possible, and our paper always meets or exceeds minimum GPO and EPA requirements.

Jossey-Bass also publishes its books in a variety of electronic formats. Some content that appears in print may not be available in electronic books.

Library of Congress Cataloging-in-Publication Data
Emerging theories in health promotion practice and research :
strategies for improving public health / Ralph J. DiClemente,
Richard A. Crosby, Michelle C. Kegler, editors.
   p. ; cm.
Includes bibliographical references and index.
   ISBN 0-7879-5566-3 (alk. paper)
   1. Health promotion—United States. 2. Health
promotion—Research—United States. 3. Community health
services—United States. 4. Public health—United States.
   [DNLM: 1. Community Health Services—United States. 2. Health
Promotion—United States. 3. Health Behavior—United States. 4.
Models, Organizational—United States. WA 546 AA1 E48 2002] I.
DiClemente, Ralph J. II. Crosby, Richard A., date III. Kegler,
Michelle C., date
   RA427.8 .E447 2002
   613'.0973—dc21
                                                              2001008667

FIRST EDITION
HB Printing 10 9 8 7 6 5 4 3 2 1

CONTENTS

FOREWORD

What emerges as interesting theory in any particular era to health promotion practitioners usually reflects the most compelling demands on them by governmental imperatives, economic and epidemiological pressures, technological opportunities, and community or public expectations. Behavioral theories in the 1950s, for example, addressed why people seek diagnostic examinations and immunizations (see for example Hochbaum, 1956), as these were the compelling epidemiological issues and the technological opportunities presented by new diagnostic tests and new vaccines. In the 1960s, theories of mass media (Griffiths & Knutsen, 1960) and social change (Steuart, 1965) responded to technological advances in communications, especially television, and legislative initiatives. In the United States, the legislative initiatives came with the New Frontier of President John F. Kennedy and the New Society of President Lyndon Johnson, culminating with Medicare and Medicaid laws in 1966. The escalating costs of medical care that followed these initiatives produced an emphasis on cost containment and self-care in the late 1960s and early 1970s (Green, 1974; Levin, Katz, & Holst, 1976).

From then, beginning with the 1974 Lalonde Report in Canada and Public Law 94-317 in the United States (the Health Information and Health Promotion Act in 1975), the remaining decades of the twentieth century have seen more specific policy initiatives defining and supporting health promotion. The policies, then, have driven the demand for specific types of theoretical guidance of health promotion practice. The 1979 *Healthy People* initiatives in the United States, for example, and the 1986 Ottawa Charter from the First International Conference on Health Promotion have set broad expectations on practitioners for theories that address health behavior and social change as interacting systems of reciprocal causation. These in turn have produced more ecological models of practice, forcing the use of theories in tandem or in combination to encompass the range of causal factors requiring intervention on multiple levels.

Practitioners' interests in theories also tend to gravitate to the biases of their former professors and what leaders in the field seem to be recommending. Because health promotion, as the editors of this book describe it, is transdisciplinary, the biases of practitioners tend to follow the disciplines from which they joined the field. Some lean toward application of psychological theories, some toward sociological, some toward communications theories that blend these two disciplines with technological considerations and the experience of other fields in applying communications in marketing, political campaigning, or advocacy. Similarly, community organization theories emerge from the blending of psychological, sociological, and political theories with the experience of community workers in social welfare, labor organizing, urban development, rural extension, and political mobilization.

When a book such as this steps out ahead of the demand side of practitioner needs, its authors and editors must offer as "emerging theories" for practice and research those that meet additional criteria. They must blend and balance those same practical imperatives, pressures, and demands with their own scholarly judgment and wisdom on several considerations.

The most obvious consideration is whether the bodies of theoretical literature that are competing for attention and application hold promise for the immediate problem-solving guidance of the field. A second is whether a given theoretical front should be considered a fad or a durable response to genuine trends; whether it is more than a flash in the academic pan, with real potential for contributing to the development of the field. These two criteria require the use of bifocal lenses, one viewing proximal needs for problem solving, the other taking a longer view of changing and projected needs.

The health promotion theorists in the new generation represented in this book are grounded in research *and* practice, more so than most of those in earlier generations of social and behavioral science who brought their theories to public health. The latter-day emerging theories are better informed by a range of social and behavioral science theories and constructs, not just those of the single disciplines from which the earlier generation of theorists graduated. This group of authors comes largely from applied sociobehavioral, health education, and health promotion programs in schools of public health and other professional schools. In such incubators, they were required to start with problems and look to theory to solve them, rather than starting with theories and looking for problems on which to test them.

Sharp contrasts and false dichotomies of old debates in health education and health promotion have given way in this representation of emerging theories to more subtle, more nuanced, more balanced understanding of the necessary duality, complementarity, and reciprocal determinism of forces in health behavior and social change. Nevertheless, the chapters of this book compete with each other in ways that should enliven and enrich old debates and stimulate new ones. For example, Petty, Barden, and Wheeler, in Chapter Four, offer two types of information processing and attitude change that would seem to suggest that the notions of social marketing (Kennedy and Crosby, Chapter Ten) might tend to lead to the less enduring, more superficial type of change.

Some of the "emerging theories" reflected here attempt to give a twenty-first-century theoretical reality test to complex interpretations of community cohesion, to "unpack the complexities" of community trust and cooperations (Kreuter and Lezin, Chapter Nine). Some seek "to step back from the *practice* of building coalitions and forge a comprehensive *theory* of community coalitions" (Butterfoss and Kegler, Chapter Seven). These efforts to recapitulate and to theorize notions that have ascended from practice, rather than the earlier generations of theory applied from the disciplines to prescribe or proscribe practice, suggest that practitioners have a greater role to play in theory building. They open the way for more participatory research in which practitioners can be coresearchers rather than merely subjects or intermediaries in theory building for health promotion.

March 2002

Lawrence W. Green
Public Health Practice Program Office
Centers for Disease Control and Prevention
Atlanta

References

Green, L. W. (1974). Toward cost-benefit evaluations of health education: Some concepts, methods, and examples. *Health Education Monographs 2* (Suppl. 1), 34–64.

Griffiths, W., & Knutson, A. L. (1960). The role of mass media in public health. *American Journal of Public Health, 73*, 18–24.

Hochbaum, G. M. (1956). Why people seek diagnostic X-rays. *Public Health Reports, 71*, 377–380.

Levin, L. S., Katz, A., & Holst, E. (1976). *Self-care: Lay initiatives in health.* New York: Prodist.

Steuart, G. W. (1965). Health behavior and planned change: An approach to the professional preparation of the health education specialist. *Health Education Monographs, 1*(20), 3–26.

ACKNOWLEDGMENTS

We are deeply indebted to Linda Brockman, our editorial assistant at Emory University, for her relentless dedication, attention to detail with every chapter, and masterful editorial skills, which have allowed us to shape this book into the desired form.

We express our enormous gratitude to our good friends at Jossey-Bass. In particular, we express our heartfelt appreciation to Andy Pasternack, Amy Scott, and Justine Villanueva for their incomparable expertise, patience, and willingness to share their wealth of knowledge that was critical throughout the development of this book and the editorial process. We also acknowledge our friends from Jossey-Bass for making this a pleasant and rewarding experience.

We thank all of the women and men in our families: our grandparents, parents, siblings, and in-laws who have given us the historical inspiration, motivation, and support to write this book. In particular, we express our love for our spouses, who have supported and nurtured our development as health educators and researchers. We are blessed by their love and support.

Finally, we thank all of the contributors to the book. It is through their hard work, dedication, and commitment that this book has come to fruition. We have had the privilege of working with many outstanding health promotion scientists in diverse fields. The field of health promotion practice and research has benefited enormously from their contributions to the professional literature.

ABOUT THE EDITORS

Ralph J. DiClemente is Charles Howard Candler Professor of Public Health and associate director, Emory Center for AIDS Research. He holds concurrent appointments as professor in the School of Medicine, Department of Pediatrics, Division of Infectious Diseases, Epidemiology, and Immunology; in the Department of Medicine, Division of Infectious Diseases; and in the Department of Psychiatry. He was recently chair of the Department of Behavioral Sciences and Health Education at the Rollins School of Public Health, Emory University. Dr. DiClemente was trained as a health psychologist at the University of California, San Francisco, where he received his Ph.D. degree (1984) after completing an S.M. degree (1978) in behavioral sciences at the Harvard School of Public Health and his B.A. degree (1973) at the City University of New York (CCNY).

DiClemente's research interests include developing decision-making models of adolescents' risk and protective behaviors. He has a particular interest in the development and evaluation of theory-driven HIV/STD-prevention programs for adolescents and young adult women. He has published numerous books and journal articles in the fields of adolescent health and HIV/STD prevention. He currently teaches a course on adolescent health and serves on numerous editorial boards and national prevention organizations.

Richard A. Crosby is an assistant professor in the Department of Behavioral Sciences and Health Education in the Rollins School of Public Health at Emory University.

Crosby received his B.A. degree (1981) from the University of Kentucky in school health education and his M.A. degree (1984) in health education from Central Michigan University. His Ph.D. degree (1998) is in health behavior and is from Indiana University.

Before coming to Emory, Dr. Crosby was a fellow of the Association of Teachers of Preventive Medicine, serving in the Division of STD Prevention at the Centers for Disease Control and Prevention. Dr. Crosby currently teaches graduate courses in behavioral theory, statistics, and research methods at the Rollins School of Public Health. Crosby's research interests include development and application of behavioral theory to health promotion, particularly in adolescent and young adult populations. He is primarily involved in health promotion practice and research that contributes to reducing the incidence of sexually transmitted diseases, particularly infection with human immunodeficiency virus. Currently affiliated with the Emory Center for AIDS Research, Crosby has published numerous journal articles that report empirical findings relevant to the sexual risk behaviors of adolescents and adults.

Michelle C. Kegler is an assistant professor in the Department of Behavioral Sciences and Health Education in the Rollins School of Public Health at Emory University. Kegler is also affiliated with the Office on Smoking and Health, Centers for Disease Control and Prevention. Kegler received her B.A. degree (1983) in psychology from the University of Minnesota and her M.P.H degree (1985) in health behavior and health education from the University of Michigan. Her Dr.P.H. degree (1995) is in health behavior and health education and is from the University of North Carolina at Chapel Hill.

Kegler's research focuses on community approaches to health promotion, including coalitions, community partnerships, community capacity, healthy communities, and evaluation of community-level initiatives. Additional interests include tobacco control and environmental justice. She teaches graduate courses in community assessment and evaluation.

ABOUT THE CONTRIBUTORS

Jamie Barden, M.A., is a doctoral candidate in the Department of Psychology at Ohio State University in Columbus, Ohio.

James N. Burdine, Dr.P.H., is an associate professor in the Department of Social and Behavioral Health, School of Rural Public Health, Texas A & M University System Health Sciences Center.

Frances D. Butterfoss, Ph.D., M.Ed., is an associate professor at the Center for Pediatric Research, a joint program of Eastern Virginia Medical School and Children's Hospital of the King's Daughters.

Alicia M. Dorsey, Ph.D., is an associate professor in the Department of Social and Behavioral Health, School of Rural Public Health, Texas A & M University System Health Science Center.

Eugenia Eng, Dr.P.H., is associate professor in the Department of Health Behavior and Health Education, School of Public Health, University of North Carolina in Chapel Hill.

Michael R. J. Felix is Distinguished Lecturer in the Department of Social and Behavioral Health, School of Rural Public Health, Texas A & M University System Health Science Center.

Jeffrey D. Fisher, Ph.D., is a professor in the Department of Psychology, University of Connecticut in Storrs, Connecticut.

William A. Fisher, Ph.D., is professor, Social Science Center, University of Western Ontario in London, Ontario, Canada.

Christine A. Gehrman, M.A., is a research associate with the Center for Behavioral Epidemiology and Community Health, School of Public Health, and is also in the SDSU/UCSD Joint Doctoral Program in Clinical Psychology, San Diego State University in San Diego.

Jessica Hartos, Ph.D., is a research fellow with the Prevention Research Branch in the Division of Epidemiology, Statistics and Prevention Research at the National Institute of Child Health and Human Development in Bethesda, Maryland.

Stevan E. Hobfoll, Ph.D., is professor and director of the SUMMA-KSU Center for the Treatment and Study of Traumatic Stress at Kent State University in Kent, Ohio.

Melbourne F. Hovell, Ph.D., M.P.H., is professor and director of the Center for Behavioral Epidemiology and Community Health, Graduate School of Public Health, San Diego State University in San Diego.

May G. Kennedy, Ph.D., M.P.H., is a behavioral scientist in the Behavioral Interventions and Research Branch in the Division of HIV/AIDS Prevention at the Centers for Disease Control and Prevention in Atlanta.

Marshall W. Kreuter, Ph.D. (retired), was formerly with the National Center for Chronic Disease Prevention and Health Promotion at the Centers for Disease Control and Prevention in Atlanta.

Nicole Lezin, M.P.P.M., is president of Cole Communications, Inc., in Aptos, California. She received her master's degree in public and private management from Yale University.

Kenneth R. McLeroy, Ph.D., is professor and associate dean in the School of Rural Public Health, Texas A & M University in College Station, Texas.

Barbara L. Norton, M.B.A., M.P.H., is a doctoral candidate and instructor in the Department of Health Promotion Sciences, College of Public Health, University of Oklahoma Health Sciences Center in Oklahoma City.

Edith Parker, Dr.P.H., is an assistant professor in the Department of Health Behavior and Health Education, School of Public Health, University of Michigan in Ann Arbor.

Richard E. Petty, Ph.D., is Distinguished University Professor in the Department of Psychology, Ohio State University in Columbus, Ohio.

Peter M. Sandman, Ph.D., formerly a Rutgers University professor, is now a risk communication consultant based in Princeton, New Jersey.

Jeremiah A. Schumm is with the Department of Psychology, Kent State University, in Kent, Ohio.

Bruce Simons-Morton, Ed.D., is chief of the Prevention Research Branch in the Division of Epidemiology, Statistics and Prevention Research at the National Institute of Child Health and Human Development in Bethesda, Maryland.

Dennis R. Wahlgren, M.A., is a research associate with the Center for Behavioral Epidemiology and Community Health, Graduate School of Public Health, San Diego State University in San Diego.

Neil D. Weinstein, Ph.D., is a professor in the Department of Human Ecology, Rutgers University in New Brunswick, New Jersey.

S. Christian Wheeler, Ph.D., is an assistant professor in the Department of Marketing, Graduate School of Business, Stanford University in Stanford, California.

Gina M. Wingood, Sc.D., M.P.H., is an associate professor in the Department of Behavioral Sciences and Health Education, Rollins School of Public Health, Emory University in Atlanta.

CHAPTER ONE

UNDERSTANDING AND APPLYING THEORY IN HEALTH PROMOTION PRACTICE AND RESEARCH

Richard A. Crosby
Michelle C. Kegler
Ralph J. DiClemente

Health promotion has become integral to our efforts to improve public health. Goals of health promotion include the primary and secondary prevention of disease and health-compromising conditions. Many nations have embraced health promotion as an approach to extending and enriching the lives of their people. For example, in the United States, the U.S. Department of Health and Human Services (2000) established two overarching goals: to increase the quality and years of healthy life and to eliminate health disparities. The broad scope of objectives designed to achieve these ambitious goals presents an enormous challenge to the discipline of health promotion. Fortunately, the past few decades have witnessed rapid advances in the development of behavioral and social science theory designed to enhance our ability to achieve the health promotion objectives for the nation.

Behavioral and social science theory provides a platform for understanding why people engage in health-risk or health-compromising behavior and why (as well as how) they adopt health-protective behavior. Understanding the diverse individual, familial, social, and cultural factors that influence an individual's adoption or maintenance of health-compromising behavior can be extremely useful when applied to planning, implementing, and evaluating health promotion programs (de Zoysa, Habicht, Pelto, & Martines, 1998; Hochbaum, Sorenson, & Lorig, 1992). Thus, theory development and application in the behavioral and social sciences can effectively contribute to improved public health (Smedley & Syme, 2000).

Unfortunately, the full potential of the behavioral and social sciences to promote health-protective behaviors has only been partially realized (Smedley & Syme, 2000). One reason for this may be found in the observation that behavioral and social science theory has yet to reach a pinnacle of utility. Indeed, theories are seldom static; instead, they are often evolving or undergoing modification (Wallander, 1992). Dynamic theories capture the inherent complexity in the interplay of changing factors that influence human behavior.

Theory, research, and practice are interrelated. As theory-guided practice and research unfold, empirical findings subsequently suggest needed refinements in the theory that was applied (Glanz, Lewis, & Rimer, 1997; Jenson, 1999). Although the evolution of theory is an expected and desirable consequence of research and practice, one inherent difficulty is conveying the substance of these emerging theories to the health promotion professionals who will ultimately apply theory in their practice and research and, as a result, contribute to the evolution of a particular theory by testing its utility.

The purpose of this book is to provide readers an understanding of new developments in the field of behavioral and social science theory as applied to health promotion practice and research. We begin with a brief discussion of why theory is important in health promotion practice and research and proceed to describe a trajectory of theory development. We conclude with an overview of the new and emerging theories that will follow in the remainder of the book.

The Role of Behavioral Theory in Health Promotion Practice and Research

Health promotion is newly emerging and transdisciplinary, with a singular focus: enhancing health and preventing disease. As a relatively fledgling field, health promotion does not have a long legacy of scientific theory, principles, and axioms to provide a foundation for informing research. Indeed, one measure of the growing strength and multidisciplinary nature of health promotion is the degree to which other social and behavioral sciences and medical disciplines participate and are engaged in the development of theories, research methodologies, and application techniques in health promotion.

The range of theoretical approaches in health promotion practice is eclectic and diverse, a reflection of the discipline itself. Theoretical approaches from a broad spectrum of disciplines have been used. Indeed, health promotion is currently a highly diverse and multidisciplinary field of practice and research. This diversity is important because advances in health promotion are most readily made through the use of interdisciplinary approaches. In a sense, theory can be viewed as a focal point that brings this diversity into a unified set of propositions about people and their health behaviors.

Behavioral theories are composed of interrelated propositions, based on stated assumptions, that tie selected constructs together and create a parsimonious system for explaining and predicting human behavior (Babbie, 2001; Kerlinger, 1986; Wallace & Wolf, 1986). Generalizability and testability are paramount properties of theory (van Ryn & Heaney, 1992). Generalizability implies that good theory is robust and therefore may be applicable across diverse venues, populations, and social environments, and testability dictates that theory must be open to falsification through directly derived testable hypotheses.

Behavioral and social science theory provides a bridge between biomedical technology (for example, vaccines, screening tests, and identification of risk-reduction practices) and the application of these advances to improving public health. For example, the development of a vaccine and Food and Drug Administration approval of it may not necessarily be followed by widespread acceptance of this vaccine among people at risk of a particular disease (an example is hepatitis B vaccine; see Centers for Disease Control and Prevention, 1995; Francis, 1995). In response, theory-guided interventions may serve as catalysts to promote voluntary use of biomedical advances, such as zidovudine therapy to prevent perinatal transmission of human immunodeficiency virus (HIV) among HIV-seropositive pregnant women (see Curran,

Although theory is not a panacea, it does provide a conceptual framework for selecting key constructs hypothesized to influence health behavior.

1996), or epidemiological information, such as evidence from the Framingham study that established primary and secondary risk factors for coronary vascular disease. Theory also provides insight into diverse psychosocial factors that contribute to and maintain health risk behaviors (McLeroy et al., 1993). Although theory is not a panacea, it does provide a conceptual framework for selecting key constructs hypothesized to influence health behavior and thus provides a foundation for empirical investigations, intervention development, implementation, monitoring, and evaluation (Glanz et al., 1997). Theory also aids the complex process of organizing and understanding information obtained from these efforts. In addition, theory provides a useful reference point to help keep research and implementation activities clearly focused.

Although behavioral and social science theory offers numerous advantages for health promotion practice and research, it is important to recognize that theories that are instrumental in focusing empirical investigations or guiding the design and implementation of health promotion programs can be a double-edged sword. On the one hand, the reason for theory is to help guide the selection of important constructs thought to exert impact on health behavior. On the other hand, by targeting a specific range of theoretically important constructs for examination or as a foundation for designing health promotion programs, theory limits the breadth of observations and investigations and the scope of intervention efforts. Wallander (1992) succinctly captured this paradox when he noted, "Obviously being a way of seeing, a theory can also be a way of not seeing, a potential drawback of theory-driven research. Theory can clearly bias or even blind the researcher" (p. 530).

In the discipline of physics, for example, the influence and current paradigm of the observer (a scientist) is acknowledged as a potential source of bias (Briggs & Peat, 1984). In the discipline of public health, the practice of deductively testing theory in the context of interventions applied to specific health problems may also bias our observations (see Buchanan, 1994, and McLeroy et al., 1993, for elaboration of this concept). This bias may be inevitable given that health behaviors are typically influenced by a diverse array of individual, cultural, and contextual factors that may not be amenable to explanation by any single theory (McLeroy et al., 1993). Yet from a logical positivist perspective, theory should be able to explain parsimoniously and predict even the most complex human behaviors—for example, tobacco addiction, substance abuse, and sexual risk taking. Thus, one issue previously debated in the field of health promotion is whether theory should be specific to given health behaviors and their corresponding interventions or more broadly applicable across multiple health behaviors and interventions (Buchanan, 1994; Green et al., 1994; McLeroy et al., 1993).

With increasing recognition that morbidity and mortality for both adolescents and adults is predominantly linked to behavioral and social factors (McKinlay & McKinlay, 1977; McGinnis & Foege, 1993; Murray & Lopez, 1996; DiClemente, Hansen, & Ponton, 1996; Smedley & Syme, 2000), the role of behavioral and social science theory in public health becomes more prominent. In the coming years, noncommunicable disease, such as tobacco-associated coronary heart and pulmonary disease and malignancies, is expected to account for an increasingly larger proportion of the global disease burden (Murray & Lopez, 1996). These diseases are typically amenable to behavioral and social interventions. Communicable diseases, such as HIV and tuberculosis, and emerging communicable diseases, such as Lyme disease and pulmonary hantavirus, may also require solutions that include modification of behavioral and social factors. The HIV epidemic is a primary example (Garrett, 1994). Thus, there is a continual need to expand and refine theories that may ultimately prove invaluable in informing and guiding the design and implementation of health promotion programs. Theory expansion and refinement is occurring in response to accumulating empirical evidence obtained through research and evaluation in combination with the iterative process of theory development and testing.

A Trajectory of Theory Development

Theory development is a dynamic process. Systematic and consistent use of theory across a range of behaviors, settings, and cultures is necessary to advance the science of health promotion. Robust theories are flexible, accommodating a wide range of populations with different cultural perspectives. Constantly reevaluating the explanatory and predictive capacity of theory allows the discipline of health promotion to grow and mature. By definition, any maturational process involves change. Thus, as theories become less useful (that is, they explain an insufficient amount of variance in particular risk behaviors) or are found wanting as a foundation for guiding the design and implementation of behavior change interventions, they are modified or even discarded in favor of potentially more useful theories. This process of development, elimination, and replacement is gradual. As new theories are synthesized and embraced, they too are subject to empirical validation, and if they are found lacking, they are similarly discarded.

Systematic and consistent use of theory across a range of behaviors, settings, and cultures is necessary to advance the science of health promotion.

Traditionally, behavioral and social science theories tended to focus on identifying, quantifying, and understanding the impact of individual-level determinants of specific health behaviors. For example, the Health Belief Model, the theory of reasoned action, and the theory of planned behavior have been widely applied to health issues such as vaccine acceptance (Armstrong, Berlin, Sanford-Schwartz, Propert, & Ubel, 2001; Liau & Zimet 2000; Zimet, Blythe, & Fortenberry 2000), understanding why people do not adopt HIV-protective behaviors (see Fisher & Fisher, 2000, for a review), and what psychosocial factors predict mammography use (Michels, Taplin, Carter, & Kugler, 1995; Montano, Kasprzyk, & Taplin, 1997). Theories have also been developed to guide intervention programs that target individual-level determinants of health behavior; an example is the Transtheoretical Model.

In many respects, individual-level theories have dominated health promotion efforts. Waldo and Coates (2000) noted, for example, that "virtually all of the psychological theories that have been applied to explain HIV risk behavior locate it at the individual level" (p. S24). Possible reasons for the widespread use of individual-level theories may be that (1) they tacitly posit the individual as the key decision maker responsible for his or her health and, as a corollary, they posit that individuals can implement changes to enhance their health; (2) they assume that people value good health and will make the necessary changes to reduce behaviors associated with adverse outcomes of poor health; (3) they assume that behavior is under volitional control; (4) they assume that cognitive predisposition, such as beliefs, attitudes, and perceptions, drives health behavior; (5) they entail relatively manageable study and analytic designs (for example, the randomized, controlled clinical trial design can be used to test the efficacy of interventions delivered to individuals and small groups); (6) a substantial proportion of health promotion researchers are trained in psychology, a discipline that traditionally focuses on cognitive processes as a cornerstone of individual-level change; and (7) the accumulating empirical evidence suggests that theory-based, individual-level approaches to changing health behaviors can be effective. Given the popularity of this approach and the wealth of associated theories, researchers have continued the quest to develop and improve individual-level behavioral theories.

Many well-established individual-level theories have been refined, and others have been newly created, based largely on the lessons learned from application of the established theories. At the same time, researchers have questioned the wisdom of relying exclusively on individual-level approaches to achieve substantive changes in health behavior and sustain these changes over time in the face of countervailing social influences and pressures (McLeroy, Bibeau, Steckler, & Glanz, 1988; Rutten, 1995; Salis & Owen, 1997; Smedley & Syme, 2000).

Researchers have questioned the wisdom of relying exclusively on individual-level approaches to achieve substantive changes in health behavior.

One sequel to individual-level approaches is delivering interventions at the community level. For example, substantial resources have been allocated to conduct community-level intervention trials designed to reduce coronary vascular disease by influencing community members to adopt protective behaviors; examples are the Stanford Five-City Project (Farquhar et al., 1990; Fortmann et al., 1995), the Pawtucket Heart Health Program (Carleton et al., 1995), and the Minnesota Heart Health Program (Luepker et al., 1994). A similar large-scale demonstration program designed to prevent tobacco use (the Community Intervention Trial for Smoking Cessation) was also delivered at the community level (COMMIT Research Group, 1995). Although one clear advantage of this approach is that interventions reach large numbers of the target community, it is important to note that community-level approaches are often targeting the individual as the primary agent of behavior change; thus, individual-level theories may still be the predominant paradigm, despite application to greater numbers of people.

An important advantage of delivering programs at the community level is that reaching such a large proportion of the community may result in a change of community norms, which themselves may prompt continued diffusion of health-protective attitudes, beliefs, and behaviors (Farquhar, 1978; Rogers, 1983). However, community-level approaches may become particularly effective when they depart from sole reliance on individual-level theory and subsequently adopt theories that address social, cultural, economic, environmental, and policy-related influences on the health behavior of community members. Because of this vastly expanded paradigm, theories that transcend the individual level have been much more difficult to develop, refine, operationalize, and evaluate. Yet they hold great potential to promote and support health behavior change and the long-term maintenance necessary to achieve reductions in morbidity and mortality (McLeroy, Bibeau, Steckler, & Glanz, 1988; Rutten, 1995; Salis & Owen, 1997; Smedley & Syme, 2000).

The trajectory of theory, then, can be viewed as moving from a paradigm that places emphasis on the individual as the primary agent of change to a paradigm that conceptualizes the individual as enmeshed in a complex system of influences that ultimately shape health behavior. It is important to note that the latter paradigm embodies the former, in that individual-level theories are conceived as being an integral part of the larger theoretical approach. This observation clearly implies that theories may be used in a complementary form, therefore suggesting the utility of creating new theory that represents potentially effective combinations of established theory. It should also be noted that some theories essentially shift the entire intervention emphasis to the latter paradigm and exclude efforts based on individual-level theory. These theories typically seek to change policy- and social-level determinants of health. Although the obstacles to achieving these changes are often formidable, the potential for influencing large numbers of people is substantial (Salis & Owen, 1997). Examples of this type of approach include policy-level harm-reduction interventions designed to make clean needles and syringes readily accessible to injection drug users (Des Jarlais, Guydish, Friedman, & Hagan, 2000), condom distribution programs (Guttmacher et al., 1997), and many aspects of the tobacco settlement agreement, such as restrictions in advertising and sales and increases in cigarette taxes (Warner, 2000). Similarly, increasing the age for buying alcohol and lowering the blood-level concentration of alcohol that is considered unlawful when driving are policy-level approaches to achieving public health goals.

This brief description of a trajectory of theory development suggests that the range of theories available to behavioral and social scientists is rapidly expanding. We view this expansion as a positive development in health promotion. Indeed, increasing the range of theories (that is, tools to use) can lead to better theory selection. In turn, improved selection can optimize the ability of any program to identify antecedents of a given health risk behavior and subsequently create efficacious intervention programs that promote protective behavior. Every level of theory has utility. For example, although policy-level interventions may be the most effective approach for promoting the use of clean needles and syringes, the initial determination of reasons that injection drug users reuse their "works" may best be guided by investigations based on individual-level and inter-personal-level theories. Individual-level and interpersonal-level theories are also primary tools for intervention venues such as public schools and clinical settings. Yet in venues that include entire communities, the use of broader-level theories may be preferable to achieving long-term change in health behaviors. In essence, the range of behavioral and social science theories available for both health promotion practice and research affords the practitioner and researcher an opportunity to select the theory that is most appropriate, feasible, and practical for their setting or population.

This book is devoted to describing emerging theories across the continuum of levels of causation. Although it is not an exhaustive review of emerging theories, we believe it represents a well-rounded picture of new thinking and new applications of theory for health promotion practice and research.

A Brief Overview of Emerging Theories

This book is intended to provide researchers, practitioners, and students with an in-depth understanding of selected emerging theories in public health. To facilitate our communication, the term *theory* is used to represent an interrelated set of propositions that serve to explain health behaviors or provide a systematic method of guiding health promotion practice. An excellent related book, *Health Behavior and Health Education: Theory, Research, and Practice* (Glanz et al., 1997), described behavioral theories commonly appearing in the health promotion literature. Adding to the work of Glanz and her colleagues, this book describes theories that have recently evolved from the iterative process of research, practice, and evaluation. Many of the theories described are in the early phases of empirical testing within the realm of public health applications.

This book is intended to provide researchers, practitioners, and students with an in-depth understanding of selected emerging theories in public health.

In Chapter Two, Neil Weinstein and Peter Sandman describe the Precaution Adoption Process Model and its potential applications to health promotion practice. Although this model and the Transtheoretical Model (Prochaska, Norcross, & DiClemente, 1994) share much in common (particularly a stage approach to understanding and promoting long-term behavior change), the Precaution Adoption Process Model differentiates between individuals who are unaware of a given health threat, do not perceive themselves as personally susceptible to the given threat, and are deciding whether to adopt recommended protective behaviors. Progression from stage to stage and the stage of deciding not to act are also distinct features of the model. Supporting data from applications to home radon testing and mammography use are provided.

Just as Weinstein and Sandman provide a theory that adds to the Transtheoretical Model, Jeff Fisher and William Fisher describe in Chapter Three the Information-Motivation-Behavioral Skills Model, a theoretical model that parsimoniously extends elements of the Health Belief Model, the Theory of Reasoned Action, and the Theory of Planned Behavior. Previously applied to understanding HIV and sexually transmitted disease risk behavior, this model has considerable potential for effective applications across a spectrum of health behaviors. One particularly eloquent aspect of it is its ability to explain primarily volitional health behaviors, such as vaccination, and medication adherence, as well as the health behaviors that may be constrained by an individual's social or relational environment, such as condom use among young women. Improved understanding of health behaviors gained through the use of this model may potentially lead to improved intervention strategies.

In Chapter Four, Richard Petty, Jamie Barden, and Christian Wheeler explain how the Elaboration Likelihood Model of persuasion can be an important contribution to the discipline of public health. The purpose of this model is to provide a framework for understanding attitude formation and subsequently facilitating attitude change. Although the model has a rich history in the field of psychology, its application to health promotion is newly emerging. Detailed explanations of central route and peripheral route cognitive processing are provided; these dual routes of persuasion are important to health promotion practice because they can guide widespread health communication efforts. The Elaboration Likelihood Model could also inform the design and content of small-group health promotion curricula. The role of peripheral and central route cognitive processing in achieving short-term and sustained behavior change, respectively, is described in detail. The authors provide multiple examples that collectively support the potential of the model to make a significant contribution to health promotion practice.

In Chapter Five, Bruce Simons-Morton and Jessica Hartos apply theoretical work on authoritative parenting to adolescents' health behavior. They begin with an overview of authoritative parenting style and summarize research linking parenting styles to child and adolescent outcomes. They then present a model for applying authoritative parenting to interventions, conceptualizing authoritative parenting in terms of goals, style, and practices. The implications of the model for health promotion are illustrated through an innovative program designed to increase the safety of teenage drivers through application of authoritative parenting principles.

Several emerging theories address health behavior from the perspective of community-organizing and community-building activities. For example, in

Chapter Six, Eugenia Eng and Edith Parker describe natural helper models and their significance to health promotion practice. They provide a context for understanding how to identify natural helpers and how they can facilitate a host of positive health outcomes. Natural helpers serve as agents who complement the existing services of health professionals. Although a major target of natural helping is individual-level behavior change, the process of helping is described as being intertwined with factors such as community political dynamics and neighborhood attachments. The authors offer a model that illustrates how various functions that natural helpers serve can lead to improved health practices, improved coordination of agency services, and improved community competence. A nutrition and health project, conducted in rural Mississippi, is described to demonstrate how the natural helper intervention model has been successfully applied.

Another common approach to community-based health promotion is the use of community coalitions, which are popular vehicles for bringing diverse organizations and individuals together to address public health problems, but they have been considered largely atheoretical until now. In Chapter Seven, Frances Butterfoss and Michelle Kegler introduce the Community Coalition Action Theory. They integrate what has been learned about coalitions over the past decade through both research and practice and develop a series of practice-proven propositions to explain coalition development and effectiveness. These propositions form the basis of the theory, which emphasizes stages of coalition development, coalition functioning, development of coalition synergy, and creation of community changes that lead to increased community capacity and improved health and social outcomes. The authors illustrate the concepts and propositions with examples from a coalition formed to increase childhood immunizations.

In Chapter Eight, Barbara Norton, Ken McLeroy, James Burdine, Michael Felix, and Alicia Dorsey thoughtfully present contemporary perspectives on community capacity. This ecological approach to health promotion emphasizes relationships that exist within communities and the presence of community factors that may facilitate community mobilization. Community capacity is viewed as both an input and an outcome in the process of developing healthy communities. A series of contrasting theoretical perspectives relevant to community capacity is presented, followed by an in-depth examination of important dimensions that contribute to community capacity. Subsequently, the authors supply a descriptive case study of community capacity development in Hartford, Connecticut. The chapter concludes with a discussion of issues regarding further refinements in the approach to developing and measuring community capacity.

In Chapter Nine, Marshall Kreuter and Nicole Lezin discuss social capital and its implications for community-based health promotion. They review theoretical and empirical contributions to our understanding of social capital and suggest that collective actions through collaboration are mediated by trust, reciprocity, and cooperation. A significant contribution of this chapter is the conceptual framework for understanding two levels of social capital, bonding and bridging, within the context of community-based health initiatives. The chapter also includes illustrations from a study designed to assess the validity of various measures of social capital.

Many of the emerging theories contained in this book embody a multidisciplinary approach to understanding and potentially intervening on health behaviors. For example, in Chapter Ten, May Kennedy and Richard Crosby provide a detailed account of the Prevention Marketing Initiative, an approach to health promotion originally conceived by the Centers for Disease Control and Prevention. The initiative integrates three distinct fields of research: behavioral science, social marketing, and community development. Although applying these fields to health promotion practice is not new, the initiative is the first empirically validated approach to use these three fields synergistically for a health promotion program. Because the Prevention Marketing Initiative relies heavily on community involvement, program sustainability is relatively high. Furthermore, the use of social marketing makes theory-based intervention components accessible to large communities. As an applied example, the authors describe the development and content of an HIV-prevention program developed for youth. While acknowledging the current limitations of this emerging framework, the authors note the vast potential of the Prevention Marketing Initiative to contribute to pubic health practice.

Although the Prevention Marketing Initiative stipulates that changes in a person's environment are needed to achieve lasting improvements in health behavior, the remaining chapters in this book describe theories that provide a much stronger emphasis on environmental changes. For example, in Chapter Eleven, Stevan Hobfoll and Jeremiah Schumm make a significant contribution through their description of Conservation of Resources Theory, which contains a number of propositions that can be useful for understanding and promoting health behaviors. This theory addresses aspects of the objective and perceived environment in relationship to stress and coping. Loss spirals and resource gains are central propositions in the theory; each is associated with personal and environmental resources. The relative importance of protecting from resource loss is emphasized. Conservation of Resources Theory holds that behavior change is resource driven and that resources are interrelated. The authors illustrate applications of this theory to the adoption of HIV-protective behaviors among low-income urban women and to addressing traumatic stress issues such as posttraumatic stress disorder. They also provide a rationale for integrating the theory with a number of other emerging theories described in this book.

Yet another example of an emerging theory that emphasizes key aspects of the environment (in this case, the sociocultural environment) is the Theory of Gender and Power. In Chapter Twelve, Gina Wingood and Ralph DiClemente explain how this theory can be effectively applied to health promotion practice. The theory considers the relationship of sexual inequality and power imbalance to women's health-risk and health-protective behaviors. As such, this theory plays a unique role in health promotion practice because of its applicability to women worldwide. Three structures are hypothesized to influence health behaviors: sexual division of labor, sexual division of power, and the structure of cathexis (the affective component of relationships between men and women). These structures are described at the societal and institutional level. The authors provide illustrations of the theory as applied to women's health issues, particularly sexual risk behavior.

The final emerging theory described in this book emphasizes the role of environmental change in health promotion. In Chapter Thirteen, Melbourne Hovell, Dennis Wahlgren, and Christine Gehrman set out an in-depth description of principles and applications of the Behavioral Ecological Model, which provides a distinct contrast to models that emphasize the role of cognitive mediators of health behavior and self-regulation of these behaviors. The model emphasizes the importance of environmental metacontingencies that can influence behavior change at a population level. Although these authors acknowledge that intervention strategies guided by the model can be logistically complex, they provide substantial evidence supporting the value of this approach in reducing the prevalence of tobacco use and promoting physical activity. This chapter will challenge many readers to think in a different paradigm—one that is based on the psychological tradition of behaviorism and views behavior as rule governed. The model also provides an important rationale for understanding mechanisms that could contribute to sustained behavior change.

The book closes with a chapter that reflects on the utility and application of theory in health promotion practice. It presents issues related to development and testing of emerging theories and concludes by identifying areas of inquiry that may be helpful in the advancement of emerging theories as applied to the evolving nature of health promotion practice. Readers are encouraged to evaluate each of the emerging theoretical frameworks presented and select those that may best apply to their own needs in health promotion practice. Subsequent application and testing of these theories will clearly advance the potential of our discipline to have a positive impact on public health issues.

References

Armstrong, K., Berlin, M., Sanford-Swartz, J., Propert, K., & Ubel, P. A. (2001). Barriers to influenza immunization in a low-income urban population. *American Journal of Preventive Medicine, 20,* 21–25.

Babbie, E. (2001). *The practice of social research* (9th ed.). Belmont, CA: Wadsworth.

Briggs, J. P., & Peat, F. D. (1984). *Looking glass universe.* New York: Simon & Schuster.

Buchanan, D. R. (1994). Reflections on the relationship between theory and practice. *Health Education Research, Theory, and Practice, 9,* 273–283.

Carleton, R. A., Lasater, T. M., Annlouise, A., Feldman, H. A., McKinlay, S., & The Pawtucket Heart Health Writing Group (1995). The Pawtucket Heart Health Program: Community changes in cardiovascular risk factors and projected disease risk. *American Journal of Public Health, 85,* 777–785.

Centers for Disease Control and Prevention. (1995). Recommendations to prevent hepatitis B virus transmission—United States: Recommendations of the Immunization Practices Advisory Committee (ACIP). *Morbidity and Mortality Weekly Report, 44,* 574–575.

COMMIT Research Group. (1995). Community intervention trial for smoking cessation (COMMIT): II. Changes in adult cigarette smoking prevalence. *American Journal of Public Health, 85,* 193–200.

Curran, J. (1996). Bridging the gap between behavioral science and public health for HIV prevention. *Public Health Reports, 3,* 3–4.

de Zoysa, I., Habicht, J. P., Pelto, G., & Martines, J. (1998). Research steps in the development and evaluation of public health interventions. *Bulletin of the World Health Organization, 76,* 127–133.

Des Jarlais, D. C., Guydish, J., Friedman, S. R., & Hagan, H. (2000). HIV/AIDS prevention for drug users in natural settings. In J. L. Peterson & R. J. DiClemente (Eds.), *Handbook of HIV prevention* (pp. 159–178). New York: Plenum Press.

DiClemente, R. J., Hansen, W. B., & Ponton, L. E. (1996). Adolescents at risk: A generation in jeopardy. In R. J. DiClemente, W. B. Hansen, & L. E. Ponton (Eds.), *Handbook of adolescent health risk behavior* (pp. 1–4). New York: Plenum Press.

Farquhar, J. W. (1978). The community-based model of lifestyle intervention trials. *American Journal of Epidemiology, 108,* 103–112.

Farquhar, J. W., Fortmann, S. P., Flora, J. A., Taylor, C. B., Haskell, W. L., Williams, P. T., Maccoby, N., & Wood, P. P. (1990). Effects of communitywide education on cardiovascular disease risk factors: The Stanford Five-City Project. *Journal of the American Medical Association, 264,* 359–365.

Fisher, J. D., & Fisher, W. A. (2000). Theoretical approaches to individual-level change in HIV-risk. In J. L. Peterson & R. J. DiClemente (Eds.), *Handbook of HIV prevention* (pp. 3–56). New York: Plenum Press.

Fortmann, S. P., Flora, J. A., Winkleby, M. A., Schooler, C., Taylor, C. B., & Farquhar, J. W. (1995). Community intervention trials: Reflections on the Stanford Five-City Project experience. *American Journal of Epidemiology, 142,* 576–585.

Francis, D. P. (1995). The public's health unprotected: Reversing a decade of underutilization of hepatitis B vaccine. *Journal of the American Medical Association, 274,* 1201–1208.

Garrett, L. (1994). *The coming plague: Newly emerging diseases in a world out of balance.* New York: Farrar, Straus, & Giroux.

Glanz, K., Lewis, F. M., & Rimer, B. K. (1997). Linking theory, research, and practice. In K. Glanz, F. M. Lewis, & B. K. Rimer (Eds.), *Health behavior and health education: Theory research, and practice* (2nd ed., pp. 19–36). San Francisco: Jossey-Bass.

Green, L. W., Glanz, K., Hochbaum, G. M., Kok, G., Kreuter, M. W., Lewis, F. M., Lorig, K., Morisky, D., Rimer, B. K., & Rosenstock, I. M. (1994). Can we build on, or must we replace, the theories and models in health education? *Health Education Research, Theory, and Practice, 9,* 397–404.

Guttmacher, S., Lieberman, L., Ward, D., Freudenberg, N., Radosh, A., & Des Jarlais, D. (1997). Condom availability in New York City Public High School: Relationships to condom use and sexual behavior. *American Journal of Public Health, 87,* 1427–1433.

Hochbaum, G. M., Sorenson, J. R., & Lorig, K. (1992). Theory in health education practice. *Health Education Quarterly, 19,* 295–313.

Jenson, P. S. (1999). Links among theory, research, and practice: Cornerstones of clinical scientific progress. *Journal of Clinical Child Psychology, 28,* 553–557.

Kerlinger, F. N. (1986). *Foundations of behavioral research* (3rd ed.). Austin, TX: Holt, Rinehart, & Winston.

Luepker, R. V., Murray, D. M., Jacobs, D. R., Mittelmark, M. B., Bracht, N., Carlaw, R., Crow, R., Elmer, P., Finnegan, J., and Folsom, A. R. (1994). Community education for cardiovascular disease prevention: Risk factor changes in the Minnesota Heart Health Program. *American Journal of Public Health, 84,* 1383–1393.

Liau, A., & Zimet, G. D. (2000). Undergraduates' perception of HIV immunization: Attitudes and behaviours as determining factors. *International Journal of STD and AIDS, 11,* 445–450.

McGinnis, J. M., & Foege, W. H. (1993). Actual causes of death in the United States. *Journal of the American Medical Association, 270,* 2207–2211.

McKinlay, J. B., & McKinlay, S. M. (1977). The questionable contribution of medical measures to the decline of mortality in the United States in the twentieth century. *Milbank Memorial Fund Quarterly, 55,* 405–428.

McLeroy, K. R., Bibeau, D., Steckler, A., & Glanz, K. (1988). An ecological perspective on health promotion programs. *Health Education Quarterly, 15,* 351–377.

McLeroy, K. R., Steckler, A. B., Simons-Morton, B., Goodman, R. M., Gottlieb, N., & Burdine, J. N. (1993). Social science theory in health education: Time for a new model? *Health Education Research, Theory, and Practice, 9,* 305–312.

Michels, T. C., Taplin, S. M., Carter, W. B., & Kugler, J. P. (1995). Barriers to screening: The theory of reasoned action applied to mammography use in a military beneficiary population. *Military Medicine, 160,* 431–437.

Montano, D. E., Kasprzyk, D., & Taplin, S. H. (1997). The theory of reasoned action and the theory of planned behavior. In K. Glanz, F. M. Lewis, & B. K. Rimer (Eds.), *Health behavior and health education: Theory, research, and practice* (2nd ed., pp. 85–112). San Francisco: Jossey-Bass.

Murray, C. J. L., & Lopez, A. D. (1996). *The global burden of disease.* Geneva, Switzerland: World Health Organization.

Prochaska, J. O., Norcross, J. C., & DiClemente, C. C. (1994). *Changing for good.* New York: Morrow.

Rogers, E. M. (1983). *Diffusion of innovations* (3rd ed.). New York: Free Press.

Rutten, A. (1995). The implementation of health promotion: A new structural perspective. *Social Science in Medicine, 41,* 1627–1637.

Salis, J. F., & Owen, N. (1997). Ecological models. In K. Glanz, F. M. Lewis, & B. K. Rimer (Eds.), *Health behavior and health education: Theory, research, and practice* (2nd ed., pp. 403–424). San Francisco: Jossey-Bass.

Smedley, B. D., & Syme, S. L. (Eds.). (2000). *Promoting health: Intervention strategies from social and behavioral research.* Washington, DC: National Academy Press.

U.S. Department of Health and Human Services. (2000). *Healthy people 2010.* Washington, DC: U.S. Government Printing Office. Available: www.health.gov/healthypeople.

van Ryn, M., & Heaney, C. A. (1992). What's the use of theory? *Health Education Quarterly, 19,* 315–330.

Waldo, R., & Coates, T. J. (2000). Multiple levels of analysis and intervention in HIV prevention science: Exemplars and directions for new research. *AIDS, 14* (Suppl. 2), S18–S26.

Wallace, R. A., & Wolf, A. (1986). *Contemporary sociological theory: Continuing the classical condition* (2nd ed.). Upper Saddle River, NJ: Prentice Hall.

Wallander, J. L. (1992). Theory-driven research in pediatric psychology: A little bit on why and how. *Journal of Pediatric Psychology, 17,* 521–535.

Warner, K. E. (2000). The need for, and value of, a multi-level approach to disease prevention: The case for tobacco control. In B. D. Smedley & S. L. Syme (Eds.), *Promoting health: Intervention strategies from social and behavioral research* (pp. 417–449). Washington, DC: National Academy Press.

Zimet, G. D, Blythe, M. J., & Fortenberry, J. D. (2000). Vaccine characteristics and acceptability of HIV immunization among adolescents. *International Journal of STD and AIDS, 11,* 143–149.

CHAPTER TWO

THE PRECAUTION ADOPTION PROCESS MODEL AND ITS APPLICATION

Neil D. Weinstein
Peter M. Sandman

Imagine that you are a health educator trying to understand why young adults engage in behaviors that put them at risk for acquired immunodeficiency syndrome (AIDS). You develop a questionnaire to ask them about the likelihood that they will come in contact with someone who is positive for human immunodeficiency virus (HIV); the likelihood of becoming infected by this person; the effectiveness of various precautions, such as condoms and abstinence; the social consequences of taking these precautions; their perceived ability to take these precautions; what others think about the risk of AIDS and about AIDS precautions; and other topics like these that are drawn directly from widely used theories of health behavior. It seems obvious that assessing these beliefs will help you understand why someone is or is not engaging in risky behavior.

This approach seems fine today, but what if the year is 1987, when the public is first learning about AIDS? Young adults might know little more than that

This chapter is a modification of one that originally appeared in D. Rutter and L. Quine (Eds.), *Changing Health Behavior: Intervention and Research with Social Cognition Models.* Bristol, Pa.: Open University Press, 2001. Used with permission. We are indebted to Alexander Rothman and Stephen Sutton for their assistance in clarifying the characteristics and testing of stage theories and to Cara Cuite, May Lou Klotz, Judith Lyon, Paul Miller, and Nancy Roberts for their contributions to our radon research. We gratefully acknowledge the funding for the radon research from the New Jersey Department of Environmental Protection, the New Jersey Agricultural Experiment Station, and the National Cancer Institute.

AIDS is a fatal, progressive disease. Few have any idea how to answer most of your questions. Still, their behaviors differ. Some have many sexual partners; some have one regular partner; some are abstinent. Some use condoms, and some do not. Nevertheless, neither their current behaviors nor the likelihood that they will change these behaviors can be explained or predicted by their beliefs about HIV. As yet, they have few such beliefs.

As this example shows, theories that seek to explain health behaviors in terms of beliefs about the pros and cons of action could not explain risky sexual behavior in 1987. These theories apply only to a particular phase of precaution adoption—a period when people have already been engaged by the threat and have formed beliefs about possible responses. The idea that there are different phases to precaution taking—and that we need to develop different explanations for what goes on in these different phases—is the fundamental assumption of stage theories of health behavior. But this has not been the way that most theories have explained health actions.

How Traditional Theories Approach the Issue of Explaining and Changing Health Behavior

Because significant changes in behavior seem to require conscious decision making, the theories used most frequently to explain individual preventive health behavior (Theory of Reasoned Action—Ajzen & Fishbein, 1980, Fishbein & Ajzen, 1975, and Fishbein & Middlestadt, 1989; Theory of Planned Behavior—Ajzen, 1985, Ajzen & Madden, 1986; Health Belief Model—Janz & Becker, 1984, Kirscht, 1988, Rosenstock, 1974; Protection Motivation Theory—Rogers, 1983, Prentice-Dunn & Rogers, 1986; Subjective Expected Utility Theory—Edwards, 1954, Ronis, 1992, Sutton, 1982) view action as the outcome of a cognitive process in which expected benefits are weighed against expected costs. The first goal of these theories is to identify the variables—including beliefs, experiences, social pressures, and past behaviors—that have the greatest impact on such decisions.

The second goal of these theories is to predict behavior. The theories combine the variables they have identified in an equation that is either prescribed by the theory or derived empirically from collected data (for examples, see Weinstein, 1993). Each theory has a single prediction equation. Substituting the variables into this equation leads to a single numerical value for each individual, and this value is interpreted as the relative probability that this person will act. Thus, the prediction rule places each person along a continuum of action likelihood, and such theories might be labeled continuum theories.

The goal of interventions, according to this perspective, is to move people along the continuum toward a position of higher probability, although action can occur from any point along the continuum. If different interventions increase the value of the prediction equation by the same amount, they are all expected to produce the same change in behavior regardless of the fact that they may focus on quite different variables.

How Stage Theories Approach the Issue of Explaining and Changing Behavior

In the health arena, advocates of stage theories question whether change in health-relevant behaviors can be described by a single prediction equation. In effect, they suggest that we must try to understand a whole series of changes, identifying for each stage transition the relevant variables and the way in which they combine. This is a much more complicated goal than finding a single prediction rule, but it offers the possibility of greater intervention efficiency and effectiveness. An example may help make this claim clearer.

Consider pregnancy prevention. A great many variables—social norms, knowledge, efficacy beliefs, risk perceptions—are likely to influence whether a person engages in behavior that could lead to an unwanted pregnancy. However, given a list of such variables, how do we design a program to encourage safe behavior? Should every intervention address all these variables? Do certain topics (such as general knowledge and personal vulnerability) need to be addressed before others (such as practicing how to discuss one's preferences with a potential sexual partner)?

Identify the dominant stage or stages, and focus available resources on those factors that are most important in moving people to the next stage.

A stage theory of pregnancy prevention would specify an ordered set of categories into which people can be classified and identify the factors that could induce movement from one category to the next. Given such a theory, a health educator approaching a new population (or individual) could identify the dominant stage or stages and focus available resources on those factors that are most important in moving people to the next stage. The greatest attraction of stage theories, thus, is the potential they offer for tailoring messages to audiences.

Continuum theories acknowledge quantitative differences among people in their likelihood of action and in their standing on various influential variables. Such theories do not, however, acknowledge changes in the barriers that people must overcome to progress toward action. For everyone, the goal of interventions is to maximize the variables that increase the value of the prediction equation.

The notion of matching interventions to people is either incidental or completely missing in continuum theories.

Essential Elements of Stage Theories

Stage theories of health behavior have four principal elements (Weinstein, Rothman, & Sutton, 1998):

1. *A category system to define the stages.* Stages are theoretical constructs. A prototype can be defined for each stage, but few people will match this ideal perfectly, and the actual boundaries between stages may not be as clear as the theories or measurements suggest.

2. *An ordering of the stages.* Stage theories assume that people generally pass through all the stages to reach the end point of action or maintenance. However, progression is neither inevitable nor irreversible (Bandura, 1995). There is no minimum length of time people must spend in a particular stage. Sometimes they may progress so rapidly (for example, when a doctor recommends an action that someone had never thought about before) that, for practical purposes, people can be said to skip stages. Also, some stages may lie on side paths that are not on the route to action, and people taking precautions do not need to pass through them.

3. *Common barriers to change facing people in the same stage.* Stage ideas will be helpful in designing programs that encourage people to move toward action if people at one stage have to address similar types of issues before they can progress to the next stage.

4. *Different barriers to change facing people in different stages.* If the factors producing movement toward action were the same regardless of a person's stage, the same intervention could be used for all, and the concept of stages would be superfluous.

Thus, a completely specified theory would describe both the criteria that define the stages and the issues that represent barriers between stages. Most stage theories, regardless of what particular stages they claim exist, assume that this set of stages applies to many or all health behaviors. For example, the stage when people have decided to act but have not yet acted may be identified by a theory and be considered relevant to a wide range of preventive actions. Although the stages may transcend particular behaviors, many of the barriers to progress between stages may be action specific. Thus, the particular factors that help people make a decision to lose weight, for example, may be quite different from the factors that help people make a decision to use condoms, even though the process of reaching a decision is common to both actions. A model that proposes a particular sequence of stages in the change process can be correct about these stages even if it has not identified all the barriers at each stage. The stages should be seen as a framework that needs to be filled in with details about the barriers relevant to the adoption of a specific behavior.

How Stage Theories Can Be Tested

A variety of approaches have been used to determine whether a particular behavior change passes through the sequence of stages proposed by a stage theory (Weinstein, Rothman, et al., 1998). The most common approach is to use cross-sectional data from surveys or questionnaires to look for differences among people thought to be in different stages. Simply finding differences among stages tells us little, however, since nonstage processes will also produce such differences. Finding specific hypothesized characteristics of people in various stages is more convincing. Another test sometimes used to verify a stage theory is to compare the success of an intervention that is tailored to a person's stage with a standardized intervention. This is also a poor test. Tailoring usually involves considerable personalization and extra attention, and the latter ingredients, rather than the tailoring, could easily account for greater success in the tailored condition.

Much more definitive are experimental studies using matched and mismatched interventions. If it is true that different variables influence movement at different stages, treatments designed to influence these variables should be most effective when applied to people in the appropriate stage. Thus, individuals in a given stage should respond better to an intervention that is matched to their stage than to one that is mismatched (that is, matched to a different stage).

Only stage models predict that the sequencing of treatments is important. For maximum effectiveness, the order of interventions should follow the hypothesized order of stages. Consequently, sequence effects provide further evidence of a stage process. Unfortunately, because testing for sequence effects requires sequential interventions, such tests are quite difficult to carry out.

An elegant data analysis method for testing whether different variables are significant at different stages has been developed by Hedeker, Mermelstein, and Weeks (1999). It can be used with experimental, prospective, and cross-sectional research designs.

The Precaution Adoption Process Model

The adoption of a new precaution or the abandonment of a risky behavior requires deliberate action. Such actions, rather than the gradual development of habitual patterns of behavior, such as exercise or diet, constitute the domain in which the Precaution Adoption Process Model (PAPM) is applicable. It can also be used to explain why and how people make deliberate changes in their habitual patterns.

The goal of the PAPM is to explain how a person comes to the decision to take this action and manages to translate that decision into action. For this reason, the PAPM focuses on psychological processes within the individual. As a consequence, its stages are defined in terms of the mental states that appear to be important rather than in terms of factors external to the person, such as current behavior, past behavior, or some combination of these with the person's mental state. Stages should not be defined in terms of criteria that are salient only to health professionals, such as the percentage of fat in a person's diet, since they are unlikely to explain a layperson's behavior.

Although several aspects of the model were discussed in 1988 (Weinstein, 1988), the formulation now used was published in 1992 (Weinstein & Sandman, 1992). The PAPM identifies seven stages along the full path from ignorance to action. At some initial point in time, people are unaware of the health issue (Stage 1). When they first learn something about the issue, they are no longer unaware, but they are not necessarily engaged by it either (Stage 2). People who reach the decision-making stage (Stage 3) have become engaged by the issue and are considering their response. This decision-making process can result in one of two outcomes. If the decision is to take no action, the precaution adoption process ends (Stage 4), at least for the time being. But if people decide to adopt the precaution (Stage 5), the next step is to initiate the behavior (Stage 6). A seventh stage, if appropriate, indicates that the behavior has been maintained over time (Stage 7).

Although the stages have been labeled with numbers, there is certainly no implication that these numbers have any more than ordinal value. They should never be used to calculate correlation coefficients, nor should one ever calculate the mean stage for a sample. Both calculations assume that the stage represents not only a single underlying dimension but also equal intervals along this dimension. Both of these assumptions contravene the basic idea of a stage model.

The PAPM is relatively new and has been applied to a limited number of health behaviors: osteoporosis prevention, mammography, hepatitis B vaccination, and home testing to detect radioactive radon gas (Blalock et al., 1996; Clemow et al., 2000; Hammer, 1997; Weinstein & Sandman, 1992; Weinstein, Lyon, Sandman, & Cuite, 1998). Two specific examples, the stages relevant to radon testing and to taking calcium for osteoporosis prevention, are shown in Figure 2.1. (Although repeat radon testing is recommended by experts under some circumstances, radon testing is still largely a one-time process. Therefore, the maintenance phase for radon testing is not shown in the figure.)

FIGURE 2.1. STAGES OF THE PRECAUTION ADOPTION MODEL.

Precaution Adoption Process Model Stages	Precaution Adoption Process Model for Radon Testing	Precaution Adoption Process Model for Osteoporosis Prevention
Stage 1 Unaware of Issue	Never Heard of Radon	Never Heard of Taking Calcium to Prevent Osteoporosis
Stage 2 Unengaged by Issue	Never Thought About Testing	Never Thought About Taking Calcium
Stage 3 Deciding About Acting	Undecided About Testing	Undecided About Taking Calcium
Stage 4 Decided Not to Act	Decided Not to Test	Decided Not to Take Calcium
Stage 5 Decided to Act	Decided to Test	Decided to Take Calcium
Stage 6 Acting	Testing	Started Taking Calcium
Stage 7 Maintenance	N.A.	Takes Calcium Regularly

The PAPM asserts that people usually pass through the stages in sequence, without skipping any. Although not shown in Figure 2.1, movement backward toward an earlier stage can also occur, without necessarily going back through all the intermediate stages, though obviously it is not possible to go from later stages to Stages 1 or 2. The PAPM appears to resemble another stage theory, the Transtheoretical Model, developed by Prochaska and colleagues (Prochaska, Velicer, DiClemente, Guadagnoli, & Rossi, 1991; Prochaska & DiClemente, 1983). However, it is mainly the names that have been given to the stages that are similar. A closer examination shows that the number of stages is not the same in the two theories, and even the stages with similar names are actually defined quite differently.

Justification for the PAPM Stages

This section sets out the rationale behind the stages of the PAPM.

Stage 1 (Unaware). Much health research deals with well-known hazards, like smoking, AIDS, and high-fat diets. In such cases, asking someone about his or her beliefs and plans is quite reasonable, since most people have thought about the relevance of these threats to their own lives. But if people have never heard of a hazard, they certainly have no opinions about it. The reluctance of respondents to answer survey questions about less familiar issues suggests that investigators ought to allow people to say that they do not know or have no opinion rather than forcing them to state a position. Participants in health behavior research are seldom given this opportunity.

Stage 2 (Unengaged) Versus Stage 3 (Deciding About Acting). Once people have heard about a hazard and have begun to form opinions about it, they are no longer in Stage 1. However, so many issues compete for our limited time and attention that people can know a moderate amount about a hazard without ever having considered whether they need to do anything about it. We believe that this condition of awareness without personal engagement is quite common. In a 1986 survey of radon testing (Weinstein, Sandman, & Klotz, 1987), for example, 50 percent of respondents in a high-risk region said that they had never thought about testing their own homes; all had previously indicated that they knew what radon was, and most had correctly answered more than half the questions on a knowledge test.

The PAPM suggests further that it is important to distinguish between the people who have never thought about an action and those who have given the action some consideration but are undecided. There are several reasons for making this distinction. First, people who have thought about acting are likely to be more knowledgeable. Furthermore, attitudes based on experience with an issue are more predictive of future behavior than attitudes generated on the spot, without such experience (Fazio & Zanna, 1981). Thus, whether a person has or has not thought about taking action appears to be an important distinction.

Stage 3 (Deciding About Acting) Versus Stage 4 (Decided Not to Act) And Stage 5 (Decided to Act). Research reveals important differences between people who have not yet formed an opinion and those who have come to a decision. People who have come to a definite position on an issue—especially an issue regarding their own behavior—have different responses to information and are more resistant to persuasion than people who have never formed an opinion (Anderson, 1983; Brockner & Rubin, 1985; Cialdini, 1988; Jelalian & Miller, 1984; Nisbett & Ross, 1980). This tendency to adhere to one's own position has been termed *confirmation bias, perseverance of beliefs,* and *hypothesis preservation.* It manifests itself in a variety of ways. According to Klayman (1995), these include overconfidence in one's beliefs, searches for new evidence that are biased to favor one's beliefs, biased interpretations of new data, and insufficient adjustment of one's beliefs in the light of new evidence.

For these reasons, the PAPM holds that it is significant when people say that they have decided to act or have decided not to act, and that the implications of someone saying that he or she has decided to act are not the same as saying it is "very likely" he or she will act.

We believe that cost-benefit theories of health behavior, such as the Health Belief Model, the Theory of Reasoned Action, the Theory of Planned Behavior, Protection Motivation Theory, and Subjective Expected Utility Theory, are really dealing with the factors that govern how people get to Stage 3, where they decide what to do. The issues identified by these theories are important, but they relate mainly to this one portion of the precaution adoption process. One factor that frequently influences what people decide is perceived susceptibility (or, equivalently, perceived personal likelihood), which is included in most theories of health behavior (Connor & Norman, 1995). Because people are reluctant to acknowledge personal susceptibility to harm even when they acknowledge the risk that others face (Weinstein, 1987), it appears that overcoming this reluctance is one of the major barriers to getting people to decide to act.

Stage 5 (Decided to Act) Versus Stage 6 (Acting). The distinction between decision and action is not an original idea. Ajzen's Theory of Planned Behavior (Ajzen, 1985; Ajzen & Madden, 1986), for example, distinguishes between intentions and action. Similarly, Schwarzer's Health Action Process Approach (Schwarzer, 1992; Schwarzer & Fuchs, 1996) distinguishes between two phases. During the initial, motivation phase, people develop an intention to act, based on beliefs about risk, outcomes, and self-efficacy. After a goal has been established within this motivation phase, people enter the volition phase in which they plan the details of action, initiate action, and deal with the difficulties of carrying out that action successfully.

Protection Motivation Theory is not a stage theory, but its developers implicitly recognize the need for sequencing of interventions. According to Rogers and Prentice-Dunn (1997), Protection Motivation Theory experiments always present information in the same order of threatening information followed by coping information. These researchers also talk in terms of developing motivation first and then coping skills.

A growing body of research (Gollwitzer, 1999) suggests that there are important gaps between intending to act and carrying out this intention and that helping people develop specific implementation plans can reduce these barriers. The PAPM suggests that detailed implementation information that would be uninteresting to people in early stages, and even to those who try to decide what to do, will often be essential to help them make the transition from decision to action.

Stage 6 (Acting) Versus Stage 7 (Maintenance). The distinction between action and maintenance is widely recognized (Dishman, 1988; Marlatt & Gordon, 1985; Meichenbaum & Turk, 1987) and will not be discussed here.

Stages of Inaction. One value of the PAPM is its recognition of important differences among people who are not acting and not even thinking about acting. People in Stage 1 (unaware), Stage 2 (unengaged), and Stage 4 (decided not to act) all fit in this broad category. Those in Stage 1 obviously need basic information about the hazard and the recommended precaution. People in Stage 2 need something that makes the threat and action seem personally relevant. Personalized messages and contact with friends and neighbors who have considered action should help these individuals move to the next stage. People who have thought about and rejected action, Stage 4, are a particularly difficult group. Evidence shows that they can be quite well informed (Blalock et al., 1996; Weinstein & Sandman, 1992), and they will tend to dispute or ignore information that challenges their decision that action is unnecessary in their case.

Suggestions about other factors that may be important at different transitions are given in Weinstein (1988).

Application to Mammography Testing

One use of the PAPM is to help identify barriers that inhibit preventive action. Clemow and colleagues (2000) conducted telephone interviews with 2,382 women between the ages of fifty and eighty who had never had a mammogram or had not been getting mammograms at least every twenty-four months. Rather than treating this as a homogeneous group, they examined whether women in various preaction stages differed in ways that might suggest ways to encourage movement toward screening.

Respondents were first asked whether they were definitely planning on having a mammogram in the next year or two (Stage 5; 53.2 percent), were thinking of having a mammogram in the next year or two (Stage 3; 25.4 percent), or were not planning on having a mammogram at all in the next year or two. No one said they had never heard of a mammogram (Stage 1). The "not planning" group was subdivided according to whether they had never seriously considered getting a mammogram (Stage 2; 10.8 percent), had considered having a mammogram but had decided against it (Stage 4; 8.2 percent), or had thought about it but were still undecided (6.3 percent).

This last category is not a stage of the PAPM but could be seen as similar to the undecided people in Stage 3. Its presence should remind us that small changes in the wording of questions can affect responses. Women who said they were thinking about acting in the next year or two and those who were not planning to act but were undecided might have given the same answers if one response to the initial question had been "undecided about having a mammogram in the next year or two." Similarly, people may respond differently to the wording "planning to act" as compared to "decided to act." The PAPM is too new to have codified any particular wording, but the wording shown in Figure 2.1 is recommended.

Many differences between the people in the various stages were found, despite the fact that all might be classified together as noncompliant by some theories. Certain of the variables differentiated among all the main groups. For example, people who were planning to act saw more pros to getting a mammogram than people who were only thinking about it, and the latter group saw more pros than people who were planning not to act. The undecideds were also not planning to act. Other variables differentiated among only some of the groups. For example, people planning to act scored no higher in general knowledge about mammograms and did not see themselves as any more vulnerable to breast cancer than people who were only thinking about acting, but the latter were more knowledgeable and felt more vulnerable than people who were planning not to act. People who were planning not to act were more likely than any other group to say that they were frightened of getting a mammogram.

Once the attributes of people in particular stages were identified in this study by the researchers, they were used to help health care professionals, who easily and quickly identified a woman's stage, decide what topics to focus on during a brief clinical encounter.

As this research suggests, some variables may be important at all stages, and others may be important at particular stages. It is important to keep in mind, though, that these are basically correlational data, and one cannot tell whether differences between stages in such a survey represent causal factors. Once the attributes of people in particular stages were identified in this study by the researchers, they were used to help health care professionals, who easily and quickly identified a woman's stage, decide what topics to focus on during a brief clinical encounter.

PAPM Radon Testing Experiment

A field experiment focusing on radon testing (Weinstein, Lyon, et al., 1998) was designed to examine several aspects of the PAPM. The experiment is described here in some detail to show how experiments with stage theories can be constructed and analyzed and to explain what the results of the study tell us about the validity of the model.

Radon is an invisible, odorless, radioactive gas produced by the decay of small amounts of naturally occurring uranium in soil. It enters homes through foundation cracks and other openings. Radiation from the decay of radon can damage cells in the lungs, and radon is the second leading cause of lung cancer after smoking (National Academy of Sciences, 1988; U.S. Environmental Protection Agency, 1992). Radon tests can be carried out by homeowners with a modest degree of effort. A single do-it-yourself test typically costs between ten and fifty dollars. Testing is also provided by private companies.

The experiment focused on two stage transitions: from being undecided about testing one's home for radon (Stage 3) to deciding to test (Stage 5), and from deciding to test (Stage 5) to actually ordering a test (Stage 6). The study did not look at the transition from being unaware of the radon issue (Stage 1) to being aware but not engaged (Stage 2), or from being unengaged (Stage 2) to thinking about testing (Stage 3), because merely agreeing to participate in a radon study and answering questions about testing would probably be sufficient to produce these changes. People who had already decided not to test (Stage 4) were excluded because a brief intervention would probably be unable to reverse that decision.

To determine whether the two transitions studied involve different barriers, as the theory claims, two interventions were used, one matched to each transition. Previous surveys and experiments (Sandman & Weinstein, 1993; Weinstein, Sandman, & Roberts, 1990) gave insights into the potential barriers. They suggested that increasing homeowners' perceptions of their own risk—that is, increasing the perceived likelihood of having unhealthy radon levels in their homes—is important in getting undecided people to decide to test. This was chosen as the goal of one intervention.

Interventions focusing on risk had not been effective, however, in getting people to order tests (Weinstein, Sandman, & Roberts, 1990, 1991). Instead, several studies had found that test orders could be increased by increasing the ease of testing (Doyle, McClelland, & Schulze, 1991; Weinstein, Sandman, & Roberts, 1990, 1991). Thus, for people who had already decided to test, the second intervention was intended to lower barriers to action by providing information about do-it-yourself test kits and a test order form.

Study Design

The study took place in Columbus, Ohio, a city with high radon levels. Because the issue had received only scant attention for several years, we were concerned that homeowners' thoughts about testing might be weakly held and that any stage assessment would be unstable. Consequently, all participants viewed a general informational video before receiving any experimental treatment. Their stage of testing was assessed after this first video (preintervention measurement).

After the questionnaire had been returned and eligibility to continue had been ascertained, the experimental videos were delivered to participants. One intervention (High Likelihood) focused on increasing the perceived likelihood of having a home radon problem. The second (Low Effort) focused on decreasing the perceived and actual effort required to test. These two treatments were combined factorially to create four conditions: Control (no intervention), High Likelihood, Low Effort, and Combination (High Likelihood + Low Effort). Stage of testing was assessed immediately after the experimental treatment (postintervention measurement) and several months later.

Intervention Videos

Three videos were developed for the experiment. All participants viewed the six-minute preintervention tape, *Basic Facts About Radon,* which provided an overview of the topic but included only general information about radon risk and testing procedures.

The High-Likelihood treatment consisted of a five-minute video, *Radon Risk in Columbus Area Homes,* and an accompanying cover letter. The goal of the video was to convince people that they had a moderate to high chance of finding unhealthy radon levels in their own homes. Results of radon studies indicating high local levels, pictures of actual local homes with high levels, and testimony by a local homeowner and a city health official all presented evidence of the problem. Myths about radon levels that had been identified in past research were presented and refuted. The cover letter mentioned that test kits could be ordered from the American Lung Association (ALA) but did not include an order form.

Participants in the Low-Effort condition received a five-minute video, *How to Test Your Home for Radon,* an accompanying cover letter, and a form to order test kits through the ALA. The video described how to select a kit type (making an explicit recommendation in order to reduce uncertainty), locate and purchase a kit, and conduct a test. The process was represented as simple and inexpensive.

Participants in the Combination condition received a ten-minute video that was the combination of the two separate treatments. They received the same letter and order form as people in the Low-Effort condition. Participants in the Control condition received a letter stating that their assistance in viewing a second video was not needed (recall that they had already screened *Basic Facts About Radon*).

Procedure and Stage Assessment

Study participants were initially contacted by telephone. Homeowners who had at least heard of radon, who had not tested, and who agreed to take part ($n = 4,706$) were mailed *Basic Facts About Radon* and a questionnaire assessing their reactions. The particular question designed to assess stage of testing asked, "What are your thoughts about testing your home for radon?" The choices offered were, "I have already completed a test, have a test in progress, or have purchased a test" (Stage 6); "I have never thought about testing my home" (Stage 2); "I'm undecided about testing" (Stage 3); "I've decided I *don't* want to test" (Stage 4); and "I've decided I *do* want to test" (Stage 5)."

Those individuals who were either in the "undecided" stage or "decided to test" stage after watching *Basic Facts About Radon* were assigned at random to one of the four experimental conditions and were mailed the intervention materials appropriate for that condition and a feedback questionnaire. The response rate to the second video was 73.2 percent, with no significant differences among conditions.

Follow-up telephone interviews (completion rate was 94.5 percent) were carried out nine to ten weeks after respondents returned the second video questionnaire. These asked whether participants had purchased a radon test kit and, if not, determined their final stage.

Results

The final sample consisted of 1,897 homeowners. After watching *Basic Facts About Radon*, the division among stages of those retained in the study was 28.8 percent undecided and 71.2 percent decided to test.

Predicting Progress Toward Action. Table 2.1 shows the percentage of people from each preintervention stage who progressed one or more stages toward testing. This criterion (rather than progress of only a single stage toward testing) was chosen because although people stopped at one stage were hypothesized to lack the requirements to get to the next stage, there was no a priori reason to assume that they did not already possess the information or skills needed to overcome later barriers. The upper half of the table indicates the percentage of people at follow-up who had moved from the undecided stage to either the decided-to-test or the testing stage. The lower half of the table shows the percentage of decided-to-test people who had moved on to the testing stage.

Statistical analyses showed more people progressing from the undecided stage than from the decided-to-test stage, $F(1, 1886) = 61.6$, $p < .0001$, and more progress from those who received the High-Likelihood treatment than from those who did not, $F(1, 1886) = 31.5$, $p < .0001$. Most important, as expected from the use of matched and mismatched interventions, there was a significant stage by High-Likelihood Treatment interaction, $F(1, 1886) = 18.5$, $p < .0001$, indicating that the High-Likelihood treatment was much more effective for undecided participants than for decided-to-act participants.

There was also a large main effect of the Low-Effort treatment, $F(1, 1886) = 89.4$, $p < .0001$. The stage by Low-Effort treatment interaction, $F(1, 1886) = 5.9$, $p < .02$, indicated that, as hypothesized, the Low-Effort treatment in the Low-Effort and Combination conditions had a relatively bigger effect on people already planning to test than on people who were undecided. The High-Likelihood by Low-Effort interaction and the three-way interaction were not significant.

Predicting Test Orders. The follow-up interviews revealed that radon tests were ordered by 342 study participants, or 18.0 percent of the sample. The data concerning test orders are presented in Table 2.2. For people initially planning to test, "progress" and testing are the same according to the PAPM, so the data in the lower half of Table 2.2 are identical to those in the lower half of Table 2.1. As

TABLE 2.1. RESPONDENTS WHO PROGRESSED ONE OR MORE STAGES TOWARD PURCHASING A RADON TEST.

Preintervention Stage	Condition			
	Control	High Likelihood	Low Effort	Combination
Undecided	18.8% (138)	41.7% (144)	36.4% (130)	54.5% (139)
Decided to test	8.0% (339)	10.4% (338)	32.5% (329)	35.8% (345)

Note: The group size in each cell is shown in parentheses.

expected, there was more testing from the decided-to-test stage than from the undecided stage, $F(1, 1887) = 42.3, p < .0001$. In addition, there was much more testing from people exposed to a Low-Effort treatment than from those who did not receive this treatment, $F(1, 1887) = 87.9, p < .0001$. The High-Likelihood treatment effect and the Low-Effort by High-Likelihood interaction were not significant, p's > .1 Most important was the highly significant interaction between stage and Low-Effort treatment, $F(1, 1887) = 18.2, p < .0001$. The other interactions (stage by High-Likelihood and stage by Low-Effort by High-Likelihood) were not significant (p's > .1).

More specific tests concern predicted cell-by-cell contrasts. In subsequent paragraphs, the predictions are presented in brackets and experimental groups are labeled with letters that refer to the cells in Table 2.2.

Test order rates of both undecided and decided-to-test participants in the Control condition were expected to be quite low since both groups were viewed as lacking information needed to progress to action. The main problems facing people who had decided to test were hypothesized to be the difficulties in choosing, purchasing, and using radon test kits. Thus, the Low-Effort treatment was expected to be much more helpful than the high-risk treatment in getting people in this stage to order tests [g > f]. In fact, past research (Weinstein et al., 1990, 1991) suggested that the High-Likelihood treatment would be ineffective in eliciting testing from people planning to test and, more obviously, unable to elicit test orders from undecided people. Furthermore, because it was anticipated that people in the decided-to-test stage did not need more information about risk, we predicted that testing in the Combination condition would not be significantly greater than testing in the Low-Effort condition.

According to the PAPM, people who are undecided have to decide to test before acting, so a Low-Effort intervention alone was not expected to produce test orders from this group. However, undecided people in the Combination condition received both high-likelihood information (seen as important in deciding to test) and low-effort assistance (seen as important for carrying out action intentions).

TABLE 2.2. RADON TEST ORDERS.

Preintervention Stage	Condition			
	Control	High Likelihood	Low Effort	Combination
Undecided	(a) 5.1%	(b) 3.5%	(c) 10.1%	(d) 18.7%
Decided to test	(e) 8.0%	(f) 10.4%	(g) 32.5%	(h) 35.8%

Some of these people might be able to make two stage transitions [d > c], but not as many as decided-to-test people in the Combination condition who needed to advance only one stage [d < h].

T-tests comparing the means of the cells mentioned in the preceding eight hypotheses demonstrated that none of the pairs predicted to be approximately the same were significantly different (p's > .3), but all pairs predicted to be different were significantly different (all p's < .0001 except for the hypothesis that d > c, p = .03).

Implications for Theory and Practice

The radon study has obvious theoretical implications.

Implications for Theory

First, it provides support for our claim that never having thought about an action, being undecided, and having decided to act represent distinct stages, with different barriers between stages. Second, the data support the suggestion that information about risk is helpful in getting people to decide to act, even though this same information may have little value in producing action among individuals who have already decided to act. Third, information that increases the perceived and actual ease of action appears to aid people who have decided to act greatly, but it is less important among people who are still undecided. Obviously, more research is needed to determine whether these same factors are important at the same stages for other health behaviors.

Acceptance of the idea that stages exist also has implications for theory development. If the factors facilitating movement toward action vary from stage to stage, few, if any, factors will be important at all stages. Thus, the standard approach of comparing people who have acted with everyone who has not will be a poor strategy for discovering variables important for precaution adoption. A variable may be a powerful determinant of progress at an early stage, but it may look rather weak if all one does is to compare actors with a combined group of everyone else. In fact, when everyone who has not acted is lumped together, some stage may happen to be completely missing. In this case, it would be impossible to discover the role of a variable that is crucial to people reaching or leaving this stage but not relevant to other transitions. Stage theories suggest that we will be better able to identify important barriers if we compare people who are in adjacent stages.

Implications for Practice

The results of the radon testing experiment are strong enough to have practical implications. When viewed in terms of odds ratios—for example, the threefold difference in test orders between the undecided and decided-to-test stages in the Low-Effort condition or the tenfold difference between cells with the highest and lowest testing rates—the effects observed were quite large.

Stage-targeted communications have never been used in actual radon testing promotions and until recently have not been used for any health behaviors. The most widely disseminated radon communications, national television public service advertisements, have focused on persuading viewers that the radon hazard is substantial for people in general. To the extent that a target audience stage can be inferred, these public service advertisements appeared to be aimed primarily at viewers who are unaware of the radon problem (Stage 1) or had never thought about their own response (Stage 2). This was a defensible choice when the issue was new and the medium used (national television) was scattershot. But fifteen years after radon started to receive substantial public attention, most radon communication campaigns have retained the same focus, even though there is reason to think that much of the audience is beyond Stages 1 and 2.

Criteria for Applying Stage-Based Interventions

A variety of issues need to be considered to determine the practical utility of the PAPM or of any other stage theory.

Superiority over Unstaged Messages. The practical utility of a stage model obviously depends on the extent to which it leads to interventions that are more effective than generic messages. For the radon testing study described here, we needed to develop two different interventions. The interventions chosen were based on years of research on radon testing, plus a sizable pilot project in the target community.

As predicted, individual vulnerability turned out to be a particularly useful message for people in the Columbus area at the undecided stage of the radon testing decision. We suggest that vulnerability is usually a key issue for transitions from Stage 3 to Stage 5—as opposed to, say, information about illness severity—but this suggestion requires verification. Ease of testing turned out to be particularly useful to those Columbus residents who had already decided to test but had not yet done so. We suggest that detailed instructions for carrying out precautions is key to transitions from Stage 5 to Stage 6, but this idea also needs testing.

Since the combination treatment in our experiment produced the greatest progress among both undecided and decided-to-test participants, one might be tempted to conclude that the PAPM did not provide any new treatment ideas. "Just use the combination treatment," someone might say.

There are several flaws in this reasoning. First, it is important to recall that the combination treatment was approximately twice as long as each of its two components. Media time is expensive; speakers usually have a fixed length of time for their presentations; audiences have a limited attention span. Thus, attempting to replace the Low-Effort or High-Likelihood interventions with their combination would involve substantial costs. Second, although no evidence is available on this point, people seem likely to be more engaged by a treatment that matches their stage, and a mismatched treatment may deter them from attending to the properly matched treatment to come. For example, unlike people who have agreed to participate in a research study, members of the general public who are undecided about taking a precaution may not pay attention to the detailed procedural information they might need later to carry out that precaution. Worse, among people who had decided to act, risk information was superfluous and might deter attention to the more relevant information about how to test. Nevertheless, if only a single message can be given to a mixed-stage audience, the combination intervention would probably be the most appropriate.

Stage Assessment. A second relevant criterion is the ability to identify stages accurately and efficiently. The PAPM requires only a single question to assess a person's stage, so it can be used easily in individual or small-group settings. Even in a large audience, a show of hands might be used to determine quickly the distribution of stages present. However, if the audience is dispersed, the budget is small, or time is tight, efforts to measure stage may be impractical. Furthermore, a single assessment may not be enough. Progress toward action may need to be monitored over time so that the interventions or messages can change to match the current stages of the intended audience.

Also requiring consideration is the accuracy and reliability of stage assessments, since in all current stage theories, these are based on self-reports. Furthermore, accuracy and reliability are likely to depend on the frequency and recency with which audience members have considered the health topic. When people are asked about new hazards or new precautions or about old ones that they have not thought about for years, their responses may be unreliable and reveal little about their actions or concerns. Essentially nothing is known about factors determining the accuracy of stage assessments. One might expect that people will overstate their interest in actions that are socially desirable, possibly making a written assessment method superior to a verbal assessment.

Delivery of Targeted Messages. The feasibility of delivering stage-targeted messages in different situations varies greatly. If communication is one-on-one, as in a doctor's office or counseling session, delivering the message appropriate for the individual is quite easy. In group settings, such as public lectures, messages can be chosen to fit the overall audience, though not individual members. In mass communications, a stage approach is more often useful with print than with broadcast media. Within print channels, pamphlets and magazines offer more opportunities for stage targeting than newspapers; within broadcasting, cable offers more opportunities for stage targeting than networks.

A closely related question is the browsability or searchability of the medium. Although we tend to think of targeting as something the communicator does, audience members can also target the content they need. The more browsable and searchable a medium is, the easier it is for each audience member to seek out content appropriate to his or her stage. A lecture, videotape, or broadcast program is extremely low on this dimension. Whatever comes next comes next, and the audience's only choice is whether to continue listening. By contrast, print messages are much more browsable and searchable, and well-designed aids such as subheads and indexes take advantage of this capacity. The Internet and interactive computer programs, of course, are more browsable and searchable still. If each audience member could be relied on to find the most stage-relevant information, it would be possible to reap the advantages of stage targeting without actually having to target simply by facilitating audience self-targeting. Of course, this is not just a matter of choosing and using the medium wisely. Self-targeting takes motivation. Audiences to whom the issue is hot probably will seek out what they need to know (or at least what they think they need to know). Audiences for whom the issue is either unfamiliar or boringly familiar probably will not.

The ability to deliver targeted messages to members of a group also depends on the range of stages present in that group. The greater the range of stages present, the more difficult it is to choose a single message. For a mass audience, the most efficient way to encourage a new health-protective action may be with a comprehensive broadcast message that ignores stage or assumes everyone to be at a very early stage. As the issue matures, however, distinctive audiences, separable by stage, merit distinctive messages, and print or "narrowcasting" becomes the medium of choice for mass communications. Thus, stage-based messages are likely to be more important for relatively mature health issues than for emerging ones.

Difficulty of Behavior Change. A final criterion of importance concerns the difficulty of the action being advocated and the expected resistance of the audience to the behavior change recommendation. When a behavior is easy and resistance is low, stage may matter little. In such situations, the interventions or messages needed to help people progress from stage to stage can be brief, and several may be combined into a single comprehensive treatment. In contrast, when change is difficult and resistance is high, there is a greater need to have separate messages for each stage.

When a behavior is easy and resistance is low, stage may matter little. In such situations, the interventions or messages needed to help people progress from stage to stage can be brief, and several may be combined into a single comprehensive treatment. In contrast, when change is difficult and resistance is high, there is a greater need to have separate messages for each stage.

In our radon testing experiment, the general preintervention videotape moved many participants through two stages from "never thought about acting" to "decided to act." Similarly, the Low-Effort intervention persuaded many undecided people to progress two stages and order test kits. In this second case, we can imagine homeowners who had been reluctant to test telling themselves, "If it is really that simple and inexpensive, I might as well do it"—in effect skipping the decision-making process on the grounds that such a low-effort behavior would be easier to implement than to evaluate. It is easy to imagine people adopting many other simple precautions—changing to a fluoridated toothpaste, bypassing a brand of food reported to be contaminated, or avoiding a street on which a crime has occurred—on the strength of a single message that informs them about the risk, describes who is susceptible, and recommends a particular response.

Radon testing is so easy and radon test kits so accessible that it comes as a surprise to many professionals that there is any need for an effort-reducing intervention. Even apparently simple actions may raise questions that need to be answered before people feel confident they can carry out the behavior successfully. It seems much more difficult to the public than to the professional. Other lifestyle changes—exercise, smoking cessation, dietary change, cancer screening, and others—are obviously difficult or frightening, and it is hard to convince audiences that action is needed. In cases like these, matching interventions to stage would be expected to matter more. Furthermore, the targeted messages would need to be spaced so audiences have time to digest what they have learned and move on to the next stage before getting the message designed for that new stage.

Clearly, stage-based tailored interventions are more complex, and thus usually more expensive, than standardized, one-size-fits-all interventions. They may be more complex and expensive than targeted interventions based on psychological or demographic distinctions other than stages. Thus, it seems certain that there will be situations in which the improvement produced by a stage-based intervention is not large enough to justify its use. Nevertheless, there are numerous health behaviors that have proved resistant to standard health promotion approaches. Examples include automobile seat belt use, weight loss, smoking prevention, adherence to medication programs, and condom use. In such situations, the need to try new approaches seems undeniable. Furthermore, in many one-on-one interactions (such as doctor-patient and health educator–client), a stage-based approach would cost no more than a standardized approach and might receive a much better welcome.

References

Ajzen, I. (1985). From intentions to actions: A theory of planned behavior. In J. Kuhl & J. Beckmann (Eds.), *Action control: From cognition to behavior* (pp. 11–40). New York: Springer-Verlag.

Ajzen, I., & Fishbein, M. (1980). *Understanding attitudes and predicting behavior.* Upper Saddle River, NJ: Prentice Hall.

Ajzen, I., & Madden, T. J. (1986). Prediction of goal-directed behavior: Attitudes, intentions, and perceived behavioral control. *Journal of Experimental Social Psychology, 22,* 453–474.

Anderson, C. A. (1983). Abstract and concrete data in the perseverance of social theories: When weak data lead to unshakable beliefs. *Journal of Experimental Social Psychology, 19,* 93–108.

Bandura, A. (1995, March). *Moving into forward gear in health promotion and disease prevention.* Address presented at the annual meeting of the Society of Behavioral Medicine, San Diego, CA.

Blalock, S. J., DeVellis, R. F., Giorgino, K. B., DeVellis, B. M., Gold, D., Dooley, M. A., Anderson, J. B., & Smith, S. L. (1996). Osteoporosis prevention in premenopausal women: Using a stage model approach to examine the predictors of behavior. *Health Psychology, 15,* 84–93.

Brockner, J., & Rubin, J. Z. (1985). *Entrapment in escalating conflicts: A social psychological analysis.* New York: Springer-Verlag.

Cialdini, R. B. (1988). *Influence: Theory and practice.* Glenview, IL: Scott, Foresman.

Clemow, L., Stoddard, A. M., Costanza, M. E., Haddad, W. P., Luckmann, R., White, M. J., & Klaus, D. (2000). Underutilizers of mammography screening today: Characteristics of women planning, undecided about, and not planning a mammogram. *Annals of Behavioral Medicine, 22,* 80–88.

Connor, M., & Norman, P. (1995). *Predicting health behavior.* Bristol, PA: Open University Press.

Dishman, R. K. (1988). *Exercise adherence: Its impact on public health.* Champaign, IL: Human Kinetics.

Doyle, J. K., McClelland, G. H., & Schulze, W. D. (1991). Protective responses to household risk: A case study of radon mitigation. *Risk Analysis, 11,* 121–134.

Edwards, W. (1954). The theory of decision making. *Psychological Bulletin, 51,* 380–417.

Fazio, R. H., & Zanna, M. P. (1981). Direct experience and attitude-behavior consistency. In L. Berkowitz (Ed.), *Advances in experimental social psychology* (Vol. 14, pp. 161–202). Orlando, FL: Academic Press.

Fishbein, M., & Ajzen, I. (1975). *Belief, attitude, intention and behavior: An introduction to theory and research.* Reading, MA: Addison-Wesley.

Fishbein, M., & Middlestadt, S. E. (1989). Using the theory of reasoned action as a framework for understanding and changing AIDS-related behaviors. In V. M. Mays, G. W. Albee, & S. F. Schneider (Eds.), *Primary prevention of AIDS: Psychological approaches* (pp. 93–110). Thousand Oaks, CA: Sage.

Gollwitzer, P. (1999). Implementation intentions: Strong effects of simple plans. *American Psychologist, 54,* 493–503.

Hammer, G. P. (1997). *Hepatitis B vaccine acceptance among nursing home workers.* Unpublished doctoral dissertation, Johns Hopkins University.

Hedeker, D., Mermelstein, R. J., & Weeks, K. A. (1999). The thresholds of change model: An approach to analyzing stages of change data. *Annals of Behavioral Medicine, 21,* 61–70.

Janz, N. K., & Becker, M. H. (1984). The health belief model: A decade later. *Health Education Quarterly, 11,* 1–47.

Jelalian, E., & Miller, A. G. (1984). The perseverance of beliefs: Conceptual perspectives and research developments. *Journal of Social and Clinical Psychology, 2,* 25–56.

Kirscht, J. P. (1988). The health belief model and predictions of health actions. In D. Gochman (Ed.), *Health behavior* (pp. 27–41). New York: Plenum.

Klayman, J. (1995). Varieties of confirmation bias. In K. W. Spence & J. T. Spence (Eds.), *The psychology of learning and motivation* (Vol. 32, pp. 385–418). Orlando, FL: Academic Press.

Marlatt, G. A., & Gordon, J. R. (1985). *Relapse prevention: Maintenance strategies in the treatment of addictive behaviors.* New York: Guilford Press.

Meichenbaum, D., & Turk, D. C. (1987). *Facilitating treatment adherence: A practitioner's handbook.* New York: Plenum.

National Academy of Sciences. (1988). *Health effects of radon and other internally deposited alpha-emitters: BEIR IV.* Washington, DC: National Academy Press.

Nisbett, R., & Ross, L. (1980). *Human inference: Strategies and shortcomings of social judgment.* Upper Saddle River, NJ: Prentice Hall.

Prentice-Dunn, S., & Rogers, R. W. (1986). Protection motivation theory and preventive health: Beyond the Health Belief Model. *Health Education Research, 1,* 153–161.

Prochaska, J. O., & DiClemente, C. C. (1983). Stages and processes of self-change in smoking: Toward an integrative model of change. *Journal of Consulting and Clinical Psychology, 51,* 390–395.

Prochaska, J. O., Velicer, W. F., DiClemente, C. C., Guadagnoli, E., & Rossi, J. S. (1991). Patterns of change: Dynamic typology applied to smoking cessation. *Multivariate Behavioral Research, 26,* 83–107.

Rogers, R. W. (1983). Cognitive and physiological processes in fear appeals and attitude change. In J. T. Cacioppo & R. E. Petty (Eds.), *Social psychophysiology* (pp. 153–176). New York: Guilford Press.

Rogers, R. W., & Prentice-Dunn, S. (1997). Protection motivation theory. In D. Gochman (Ed.), *Handbook of health behavior research: Vol. 1. Determinants of health behavior: Personal and social* (pp. 113–132). New York: Plenum.

Ronis, D. L. (1992). Conditional health threats: Health beliefs, decisions, and behaviors among adults. *Health Psychology, 11,* 127–134.

Rosenstock, I. M. (1974). The Health Belief Model: Origins and correlates. *Health Education Monographs, 2,* 36–353.

Sandman, P. M., & Weinstein, N. D. (1993). Predictors of home radon testing and implications for testing promotion programs. *Health Education Quarterly, 20,* 1–17.

Schwarzer, R. (1992). Self-efficacy in the adoption and maintenance of health behaviors: Theoretical approaches and a new model. In R. Schwarzer (Ed.), *Self-efficacy: Thought control of action* (pp. 217–242). Washington, DC: Hemisphere.

Schwarzer, R., & Fuchs, R. (1996). Self-efficacy and health behaviors. In M. Conner & P. Norman (Eds.), *Predicting health behavior: Research and practice with social cognition models* (pp. 163–196). Bristol, PA: Open University Press.

Sutton, S. R. (1982). Fear arousing communications: A critical examination of theory and research. In J. R. Eiser (Ed.), *Social psychology and behavioral medicine* (pp. 303–338). New York: Wiley.

U.S. Environmental Protection Agency, Office of Radiation Programs, and U.S. Department of Health and Human Services Centers for Disease Control. (1992). *A citizen's guide to radon* (2nd ed.). Washington, DC: Author.

Weinstein, N. D. (1987). Unrealistic optimism about susceptibility to health problems: Conclusions from a community wide sample. *Journal of Behavioral Medicine, 10,* 481–500.

Weinstein, N. D. (1988). The precaution adoption process. *Health Psychology, 7,* 355–386.

Weinstein. N. D. (1993). Testing four competing theories of health-protective behavior. *Health Psychology, 12,* 324–333.

Weinstein, N. D., Lyon, J. E., Sandman, P. M., & Cuite, C. L. (1998). Experimental evidence for stages of precaution adoption. *Health Psychology, 17,* 445–453.

Weinstein, N. D., Rothman A., & Sutton, S. (1998). Stage theories of health behavior. *Health Psychology, 17,* 290–299.

Weinstein, N. D., & Sandman, P. M. (1992). A model of the precaution adoption process: Evidence from home radon testing. *Health Psychology, 11,* 170–180.

Weinstein, N. D., Sandman, P. M., & Klotz, M. L. (1987). *Public response to the risk from radon, 1986.* New Brunswick, NJ: Environmental Communications Research Program, Rutgers University.

Weinstein, N. D., Sandman, P. M., & Roberts, N. E. (1990). Determinants of self-protective behavior: Home radon testing. *Journal of Applied Social Psychology, 20,* 783–801.

Weinstein, N. D., Sandman, P. M., & Roberts, N. E. (1991). Perceived susceptibility and self-protective behavior: A field experiment to encourage home radon testing. *Health Psychology, 10,* 25–33.

CHAPTER THREE

THE INFORMATION-MOTIVATION-BEHAVIORAL SKILLS MODEL

Jeffrey D. Fisher
William A. Fisher

The Information-Motivation-Behavioral Skills (IMB) model has been used as a basis for understanding human immunodeficiency virus (HIV) risk and prevention across populations and behaviors of interest and for the focused conceptual analyses of HIV risk behavior seen among adolescents (J. Fisher, Fisher, Misovich, Kimble, & Malloy, 1996; Fisher, Fisher, Bryan, & Misovich, in press), individuals in close relationships (Misovich, Fisher, & Fisher, 1997), those who are severely mentally ill (Carey, Carey, & Kalichman, 1997; Carey, Carey, & Weinhardt, 1997), homosexual men (DeVroome, deWit, Sandfort, & Strobe, 1996), people who are infected with HIV (J. Fisher Kimble, Misovich, & Weinstein, 1998), and injection drug users (Bryan, Fisher, Fisher, & Murray, 2000), among others. The model has also been used as a basis for understanding and promoting adolescent contraception (Byrne, Kelley, & Fisher, 1993), sexually transmitted disease (STD) risk reduction (W. Fisher, 1997), and reproductive health promotion education (Connecticut Department of Public Health, 1997; Health Canada, 1994; W. Fisher & Fisher, 1999). More recently, the IMB model has been articulated as a general model of health behavior change (W. Fisher & Fisher, in press) and has received support in that context (Misovich, Martinez, Fisher, Bryan, & Catapano, in press; Murray, 2000). Standardized measures of the IMB model's constructs

We acknowledge National Institute of Mental Health grant RO1 MH59473, which supported work on this manuscript.

have been developed and validated for use within a number of populations and for a number of health behaviors of interest (J. Fisher & Fisher, 1996; J. Fisher, Fisher, Williams, & Malloy, 1994; W. Fisher & Fisher, 1993; Misovich, Fisher, & Fisher, 1996; Misovich, Fisher, & Fisher, 1998; Murray, 2000; Williams et al., 1998). Although the model has broad application potential in health promotion practice, it was originally developed in response to the HIV epidemic. Consequently, we systematically examine the utility of the IMB model with special reference to that context.

Epidemiology of HIV

The HIV epidemic has had catastrophic effects in the United States and worldwide. In the United States, 753,103 people have been infected with HIV and 438,795 have died from HIV-related causes (Centers for Disease Control, 2000). These effects have been felt disproportionately among certain groups: minorities, injection drug users, and men who have sex with men (Centers for Disease Control, 2000). Worldwide, the consequences have been nothing less than catastrophic. Projections indicate that 36.1 million have been infected with HIV, and 21.8 million have died of HIV-related illnesses (UNAIDS, 2000). Worldwide, estimates of the numbers of adults and children newly infected with HIV during the year 2000 approximate 5.3 million, with 15,000 new infections occurring each day in developing countries (UNAIDS, 2000). Especially hard hit during 2000 were sub-Saharan Africa, South and Southeast Asia, and Latin America (UNAIDS, 2000).

Limitations of HIV Prevention Approaches

Over the course of the HIV epidemic, large numbers of HIV prevention interventions have been implemented in a broad array of settings. Unfortunately, there has typically been an enormous gap between what is known about effective HIV prevention interventions at a conceptual level and HIV prevention practice as typically implemented (J. Fisher & Fisher, 2000; Gluck & Rosenthal, 1995). To date, as with other public health interventions, the vast majority of those targeting groups that practice HIV risk behavior are implemented directly by state or local health departments, or funded by them and administered by community-based organizations. All too often, neither behavioral scientist input nor well-tested theories of behavior change are incorporated into the intervention design process (J. Fisher & Fisher, 2000; Holtgrave, Qualls, Curran, Valdiserri, Guinan, & Parra, 1995; Kelly, Murphy, Sikkema, & Kalichman, 1993). In addition, rigorous evaluations of the efficacy of these programs are all too rare. A large number of HIV prevention interventions have also been undertaken by public schools (Kirby & DiClemente, 1994), and in many jurisdictions there are laws mandating that HIV education be provided, but without stipulations concerning how this should be done. Primary and secondary educational institutions have generally fielded extremely weak, atheoretical interventions, with content that is highly unlikely to change HIV risk behavior. Until relatively recently, of the entire portfolio of HIV prevention interventions that have been implemented, most have focused primarily—and in many cases solely—on providing information about HIV. Such information has consistently been shown to be unrelated to HIV risk behavior change (Brunswick & Banaszak-Hol, 1996; Exner, Seal, & Ehrhardt, 1997; J. Fisher & Fisher, 1992, 2000; Helweg-Larsen & Collins, 1997).

In the past few years, a greater level of sophistication has begun to emerge in public health sector HIV prevention programs, especially since the U.S. Centers for Disease Control mandated that behavioral scientists become involved in intervention design, implementation, and evaluation (Holtgrave et al., 1995; U.S. Department of Health and Human Services, 1993). Recently, greater sophistication has been found in some school-based programs (J. Fisher, Fisher, Bryan, & Misovich, 2002). Nevertheless, over the course of the HIV epidemic, the primary domain in which cutting-edge research has consistently been done involves interventions designed, implemented, and evaluated by behavioral scientists—generally based at academic institutions—with funding from government agencies. This work has been much more theoretically elegant, and much more likely to have been rigorously evaluated and proven to be effective, than other interventions. Unfortunately, such interventions comprise only a very small percentage of those that have been undertaken and only a small proportion of the total HIV prevention intervention funds spent. Furthermore, very few, if any, of these interventions have been broadly disseminated or disseminated at all.

When one reviews the entire body of HIV prevention intervention work conducted to date, a number of limitations that curtail intervention impact become clear (Coates, 1990; J. Fisher & Fisher, 1992, 2000; Gluck & Rosenthal, 1995; Kelly et al., 1993). First, although relevant conceptual frameworks for HIV risk behavior change have been proposed (for example, the Health Belief Model, Rosenstock, Stretcher, & Becker, 1994; the AIDS Risk Reduction Model, Catania, Gibson, Chitwood, & Coates, 1990; the Theory of Reasoned Action, Fishbein, Middlestadt, & Hitchcock, 1994; Social Cognitive Theory, Bandura, 1994; the Information-Motivation-Behavioral Skills Model of HIV Risk Behavior Change, J. Fisher & Fisher, 1992, 2000; the Transtheoretical Model, Prochaska, Redding, Harlow, Rossi, & Velicer, 1994), most interventions have been intuitively and not conceptually based and have failed to benefit from the substantial theoretical literature that is available to provide guidance for them (see Coates, 1990; deWit, 1996; J. Fisher & Fisher, 1992, 2000; W. Fisher & Fisher, 1993; Gluck & Rosenthal, 1995; Holtgrave et al., 1995, and Wingood & DiClemente, 1996, for discussion of this issue).

Second, relatively few interventions have systematically assessed target group members' preintervention HIV prevention information base, their HIV risk reduction motivation, and their behavioral skills with respect to HIV prevention in order to tailor interventions to target group needs. Consequently, most interventions have involved empirically untargeted "shooting in the dark" (see J. Fisher & Fisher, 1992, 2000, and W. Fisher & Fisher, 1993, 2000, for discussion of this issue).

Third, interventions often focus on efforts to change general patterns of behavior (for example, encouraging people to practice "safer sex") as opposed to focusing on increasing individuals' inclination and ability to practice specific risk-reduction acts, even though a great deal of social psychological research suggests that it is more effective to focus on specific acts than on general patterns of behavior (see Ajzen & Fishbein, 1980; Fishbein & Ajzen, 1975; and Fishbein et al., 1994, for discussion of this issue).

Fourth, as already noted, most existing interventions focus solely on providing information about HIV. Even within this narrow focus, the information that they provide is often not directly relevant to preventive behavior (for example, information about modes of infection is not *directly* relevant to enacting specific behaviors that are instrumental to HIV prevention), difficult to comprehend, unnecessarily frightening, sexist, or overtly risk provoking (see W. Fisher & Fisher, 1993, for discussion of this issue).

Fifth, interventions often fail to motivate individuals to change their risky behavior or to provide training to help them acquire, rehearse, and refine the requisite behavioral skills for HIV risk behavior change (Bandura, 1994; J. Fisher & Fisher, 1992, 2000; W. Fisher & Fisher, 1993; Kelly, 1995).

Sixth, the vast majority of HIV prevention interventions have focused on low-risk individuals who are not likely to be HIV infected. Although this is an important aspect of HIV prevention, we have often neglected the need for similar behavior change interventions tailored for people living with HIV. It is critical to recognize the importance of HIV risk-reduction interventions for HIV-infected people because they can transmit the virus. In addition to behavior change, medical adherence interventions for HIV-infected individuals (for example, to increase adherence to combination therapies) are also critical to avoid the development and transmission of treatment-resistant strains of HIV (J. Fisher, Fisher, Amico, & Harmon, 2001; J. Fisher, 2000, 2001; Popp & Fisher, 2002). Finally, existing interventions have often not been evaluated with sufficient rigor to determine whether intended changes in mediating factors, such as knowledge, motivation, and behavioral skills, and in HIV preventive behavior have actually occurred in the short or long term and in relation to both direct and indirect and nonreactive indicators of intervention outcome (see Exner et al., 1997; Gluck & Rosenthal, 1995; Johnson, Ostrow, & Joseph, 1990; Kelly et al., 1993; Leviton & Valdiserri, 1990; Oakley, Fullerton, & Holland, 1995; and Wingood & DiClemente, 1996, for discussion of this issue).

Origins and Roots of the IMB Model

The IMB model was created, in part, in an attempt to apply social-psychological conceptualizations, methodologies, and measurement techniques to address the problems with extant work cited above. The model is rooted in an analysis and integration of theory and research in the HIV prevention and social-psychological literatures (J. Fisher & Fisher, 1992, 2000; W. Fisher & Fisher, 1993, in press). It was also influenced by earlier work by J. Fisher (1988) and J. Fisher and Misovich (1990) on the effects of social influence on HIV preventive behavior and on the conditions under which behavior change is likely and unlikely (J. Fisher et al., 1989). Furthermore, it was influenced by earlier conceptual and empirical work by W. Fisher on affective determinants of sexual and reproductive health behavior (Fisher, Fisher, & Byrne, 1977; Fisher, Byrne, Kelly, & White, 1988; Fisher & Fisher, 1999), on the Sexual Behavior Sequence theory of the determinants of sexual behavior (Byrne, Jazwinski, DeNinno, & Fisher, 1977; Fisher, 1986) and work on changing risky sexual behavior (Fisher, Byrne, & White, 1983). Since its initial publication in *Psychological Bulletin* in 1992, the IMB model has been widely cited and tested in the context of HIV prevention with diverse populations and has received support in both correlational work and in experimental intervention research in the context of HIV prevention and other health behaviors (J. Fisher & Fisher, 1992, 2000; W. Fisher & Fisher, in press).

The IMB model has been widely cited and tested in the context of HIV prevention and has received support in correlational and experimental intervention research in HIV prevention and other health behaviors.

The IMB Model of HIV Preventive Behavior

The IMB model conceptualizes the psychological determinants of HIV preventive behavior and provides a general framework for understanding and promoting prevention across populations and preventive behaviors of interest (J. Fisher &

Fisher, 1992, 2000; W. Fisher & Fisher, 1993, in press). The model focuses comprehensively on the set of informational (U.S. Department of Health and Human Services, 1988), motivational (Fishbein & Middlestadt, 1989), and behavioral skills (Kelly & St. Lawrence, 1988) factors that are conceptually and empirically associated with HIV prevention but which are often dealt with in isolation (J. Fisher & Fisher, 1992, 2000). It specifies a set of causal relationships among these constructs and a set of operations to be used in translating this approach into conceptually based and empirically targeted HIV prevention interventions (J. Fisher & Fisher, 1992, 2000; W. Fisher & Fisher, 1993, 1999).

Fundamental Assumptions

The IMB model asserts that HIV prevention information, HIV prevention motivation, and HIV prevention behavioral skills are the fundamental determinants of HIV preventive behavior (J. Fisher & Fisher, 1992, 2000; J. Fisher et al., 1996; W. Fisher & Fisher, 1993). To the extent that individuals are well informed, motivated to act, and possess the behavioral skills required to act effectively, they will be likely to initiate and maintain patterns of HIV preventive behavior.

The IMB model asserts that HIV prevention information, HIV prevention motivation, and HIV prevention behavioral skills are the fundamental determinants of HIV preventive behavior.

According to the IMB model, HIV prevention information that is directly relevant to preventive behavior and can be enacted easily in the social ecology of the individual is a prerequisite of HIV preventive behavior (J. Fisher & Fisher, 1992, 2000; Kelly & St. Lawrence, 1988). HIV prevention information that is closely related to preventive behavior enactment can include specific facts about HIV transmission (for example, "Oral sex is a safer alternative to vaginal intercourse"), as well as facts relevant to HIV prevention (for example, "Consistent condom use can prevent HIV"), that serve as guides for personal preventive actions.

In addition to easy-to-translate-into-behavior facts, the IMB model recognizes additional cognitive processes and content categories that significantly influence performance of preventive behavior. Individuals often rely heavily on HIV prevention heuristics—simple decision rules that permit automatic and cognitively effortless (but often incorrect) decisions about whether to engage in HIV preventive behavior, and endorsement of such heuristics appears to be strongly negatively related to HIV preventive practices (Hammer, Fisher, & Fitzgerald, 1996; Misovich et al., 1996; Offir, Fisher, & Williams, 1993). For example, reliance on HIV prevention heuristics that hold that "monogamous sex is safe sex" and "known partners are safe partners" is ubiquitous and substantially interferes with performance of truly effective preventive behaviors (Hammer et al., 1996; Misovich et al., 1996).

Individuals also operate on the basis of implicit theories of HIV risk that (again incorrectly) hold that it is possible to detect and avoid HIV risk on the basis of assessment of a partner's externally visible characteristics such as dress, demeanor, personality, or social associations. Based on estimates of HIV risk made by assessing a partner's overtly accessible profile of supposed risk cues, people often decide that the partner poses little risk and that preventive behaviors are not warranted (Hammer et al., 1996; Misovich et al., 1996, 1997; Offir et al., 1993; Williams et al., 1992).

Motivation to engage in HIV preventive acts is an additional determinant of preventive behavior and influences whether even well-informed individuals will be inclined to act on what they know about prevention. According to the IMB model (J. Fisher & Fisher, 1992, 2000; W. Fisher & Fisher, 1993, in press), HIV prevention motivation includes personal motivation to practice preventive behaviors, such as attitudes toward practicing specific preventive acts; social motivation to engage in prevention, such as perceptions of social support for performing such acts (Fishbein & Ajzen, 1975); and perceptions of personal vulnerability to HIV infection (Rosenstock, 1996).

Behavioral skills for performing HIV preventive acts are an additional prerequisite of HIV preventive behavior and determine whether even well-informed and highly motivated individuals will be capable of practicing prevention effectively. The behavioral skills component of the IMB model is composed of an individual's objective ability and perceived self-efficacy concerning performance of the sequence of HIV-preventive behaviors involved in the practice of prevention (Bandura, 1989, 1994; J. Fisher & Fisher, 1992, 2000; W. Fisher, 1990; Kelly & St. Lawrence, 1988). Behavioral skills involved in HIV prevention can include objective and perceived abilities to purchase and to put on condoms, to negotiate consistent condom use before or during sexual contact, to negotiate HIV testing and monogamy, and the ability to reinforce the self and the partner for maintaining patterns of preventive behaviors across time, among many other such behaviors.

The IMB model (see Figure 3.1) specifies that HIV prevention information and HIV prevention motivation work primarily through HIV prevention behavioral skills to influence HIV preventive behavior. In essence, effects of prevention information and prevention motivation are expressed mainly as a result of the development and deployment of prevention behavioral skills that are directly applied to the initiation and maintenance of preventive behavior. The IMB model also specifies that prevention information and prevention motivation may have direct effects on preventive behavior in cases in which complicated or novel behavioral skills are not necessary to effect prevention. For example, HIV prevention information may have a direct effect on preventive behavior when a pregnant woman learns of the benefits of prenatal HIV antibody testing and simply agrees with her physician's suggestion that she undergo such testing. Motivation may have a direct effect on behavior when a motivated adolescent maintains a sexually absti-nent pattern of behavior as opposed to using condoms consistently, which might require relatively complicated or novel behavioral skills, including those involved in condom acquisition, discussion, negotiation, and consistent use. Finally, from the perspective of the IMB model, information and motivation are regarded as generally independent constructs in that well-informed individuals are not neces-sarily well motivated to practice prevention, and well-motivated individuals are not always well informed about prevention (J. Fisher & Fisher, 1992, 2000; J. Fisher et al., 1994). The model's basic constructs and the relationships among them are depicted in Figure 3.1.

The IMB model's information, motivation, and behavioral skills constructs are regarded as highly generalizable determinants of HIV preventive behavior across populations and preventive behaviors of interest (J. Fisher & Fisher, 1992, 1996, 2000; W. Fisher & Fisher, 1993). At the same time, however, it is asserted that these constructs should have specific content that is most relevant to the pre-vention needs of particular populations and particular preventive practices. Thus, within the IMB model, it is presumed that specific HIV prevention information, motivation, and behavioral skills can be especially relevant to understanding and promoting prevention among specific target populations. Similarly, specific HIV prevention information, motivation, and behavioral skills content will be especially

FIGURE 3.1. THE IMB MODEL OF HIV PREVENTION HEALTH BEHAVIOR.

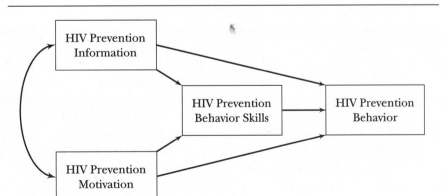

Source: J. Fisher and Fisher (1992) and W. Fisher and Fisher (1993), *Psychological Bulletin, 111,* 455–474. Copyright by APA. Reprinted with permission.

relevant to specific HIV preventive practices, such as abstinence, male and female condom use, and HIV antibody testing, within specific populations of interest. Also following this logic, the IMB model proposes that particular constructs of the model and particular causal pathways among them will emerge as more or less powerful determinants of HIV preventive practices for specific populations and specific preventive behaviors (J. Fisher & Fisher, 1992, 1996, 2000; W. Fisher & Fisher, 1993).

The IMB approach specifies measurement and statistical procedures for eliciting information, motivation, and behavioral skills content that is relevant to HIV prevention for particular populations and behaviors of interest. These procedures may then be used for the purpose of identifying specific causal elements and paths in the model that are especially influential in determining a given population's practice of a particular preventive behavior (J. Fisher & Fisher, 1992, 2000; Fisher et al., 1996; W. Fisher & Fisher, 1993). According to the IMB model, specification of the information, motivation, and behavioral skills content most relevant to a population's practice of a particular preventive behavior and identification of IMB model constructs that most powerfully influence the population's practice of the preventive behavior are crucial to the design of effective conceptually based and empirically targeted prevention interventions for specific target populations and preventive behaviors (J. Fisher & Fisher, 1992, 2000; Fisher et al., 1996; W. Fisher & Fisher, 1993).

The IMB approach to understanding and promoting HIV preventive behavior specifies a set of generalizable operations for constructing, implementing, and evaluating HIV prevention interventions for particular target populations and behaviors (J. Fisher & Fisher, 1992, 1996, 2000; W. Fisher & Fisher, 1993). See Figure 3.2.

On the basis of the model, the first step in the process of changing HIV preventive behavior involves elicitation research conducted with a subsample of a population of interest, to identify empirically population-specific deficits and assets in HIV prevention information, motivation, behavioral skills, and HIV risk and preventive behavior. The use of open-ended data collection techniques such as focus groups and open-ended questionnaires to avoid providing occasions for prompted responses is advocated, in addition to the use of close-ended techniques that lend themselves to quantitative analyses (W. Fisher & Fisher, 1993). The second step in this process of changing HIV risk behavior involves the design and implementation of conceptually based, empirically targeted, population-specific interventions, constructed on the basis of elicitation research findings. These targeted interventions address identified deficits in HIV prevention information, motivation, behavioral skills, and behavior and capitalize on assets in these factors that may characterize a population. The third step in the process of HIV risk behavior

FIGURE 3.2. THE IMB MODEL APPROACH TO THE PROMOTION OF HEALTH BEHAVIOR.

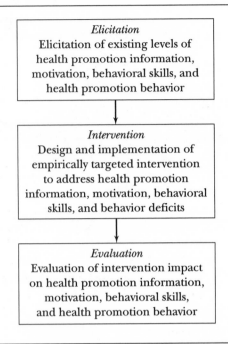

Source: J. Fisher and Fisher (1992) and W. Fisher and Fisher (1993), *Psychological Bulletin, 111,* 455–474. Copyright by APA. Reprinted with permission.

change involves methodologically rigorous evaluation research conducted to determine whether an intervention has had significant and sustained effects on the information, motivation, and behavioral skills determinants of HIV preventive behavior and on HIV preventive behavior itself. The IMB approach advocates evaluation research that relies on convergent sources of data, at least some of which are collected in a context and manner that appears to participants to be unrelated to the intervention itself (J. Fisher & Fisher, 1992, 1996, 2000; W. Fisher & Fisher, 1993).

Empirical Support for the IMB Model

Considerable empirical support for the fundamental assumptions of the IMB model has been provided in multivariate correlational research concerning informational, motivational, and behavioral skills determinants of HIV preventive behavior across populations and preventive behaviors of interest (for example, DeVroome et al., 1996; J. Fisher et al., 1994; W. Fisher, Williams, Fisher, & Malloy, 1999). Confirmatory evidence concerning the IMB model's risk-reduction behavior change implications has also been accumulated in model-based experimental intervention research, which has resulted in significant and sustained increases in HIV risk-reduction information, motivation, behavioral skills, and preventive behavior over time and across diverse populations at risk for HIV (for example, Fisher et al., 1996; Fisher et al., 2002).

Multivariate correlational evidence consistently supports the IMB model's assumptions concerning the determinants of HIV preventive behavior. In an initial study in this research line, J. Fisher et al. (1994) used a structural equation modeling approach to test empirically the IMB model's assumptions concerning the determinants of HIV preventive behavior within a primarily heterosexual university student sample. In this sample, HIV prevention information and motivation were statistically independent factors; each was related to HIV prevention behavioral skills, and HIV prevention behavioral skills were related to HIV preventive behavior. Each of these relationships was precisely as predicted by the IMB model. In an additional study in this series, J. Fisher et al. (1994) examined HIV preventive behavior from the perspective of the IMB model within a community sample of adult homosexual men. Once again, it was found that information and motivation were independent constructs, that each had a direct link to behavioral skills, and that behavioral skills were associated with preventive behavior, as predicted by the model. A direct link between HIV prevention motivation and HIV preventive behavior was observed as well, also in accord with the model's assumptions. Subsequent research has substantially confirmed the IMB model's propositions concerning the determinants of HIV preventive behavior in populations of sexually active minority high school students (W. Fisher et al., 1999), among African American and white very low-income women (Anderson, Winett, Wagstaff, Sikkema, & Heckman, 1997), in a cohort of gay men in the Netherlands (DeVroome et al., 1996), in a sample of heroin users on methadone (Bryan et al., 2000), and among Indian truck drivers (Bryan, Fisher, & Benziger, 2001).

The relationships observed across multiple empirical tests of the IMB model's relationships are summarized in Table 3.1. It is clear that the central propositions of the IMB model are consistently supported and that the data are in accord with the assertion that HIV prevention information and motivation stimulate the application of HIV prevention behavioral skills to effect HIV preventive behavior. It is also clear that there is often a direct link between HIV prevention motivation and HIV preventive behavior, in accord with the model's supposition that motivation may directly influence the practice of preventive behaviors that are not complicated or novel. In addition, it is evident that the IMB model's constructs generally account for a substantial proportion of the variance in HIV preventive behavior.

With respect to HIV risk-reduction behavior change, IMB model-based experimental intervention research has demonstrated the utility of this approach and has produced sustained and significant changes in HIV prevention information, motivation, behavioral skills, and behavior. In research reported by J. Fisher et al. (1996), samples of primarily heterosexual university students participated in elicitation studies to identify deficits in their HIV prevention information, motivation, and behavioral skills and to determine their most significant HIV risk behaviors. Based on elicitation findings, an IMB model-based, empirically targeted HIV risk-reduction intervention was designed to address HIV prevention information gaps, motivational obstacles, and behavioral skills deficits related to this population's primary HIV risk behaviors. The intervention was a field experiment in which paired male and female dormitory floors received an IMB model-based intervention—consisting of information, motivation, and behavioral skills—focused slide shows, videos, group discussions, and role plays, delivered by a health educator and peer educators—or they were assigned to a control condition. Evaluation research showed that the intervention had significant effects on multiple measures of HIV prevention information, motivation, and behavioral skills at four weeks postintervention and significant effects on discussing condom use with sexual partners, keeping condoms accessible, and using condoms during sexual intercourse at this interval. Results of a follow-up assessment indicated that the intervention had significant and sustained effects on condom accessibility and condom use and on HIV antibody testing two to four months postintervention.

With respect to HIV risk-reduction behavior change, IMB model-based experimental intervention research has produced sustained and significant changes in HIV prevention information, motivation, behavioral skills, and behavior.

In a related experimental intervention, Carey, Maisto, Kalichman, Forsyth, Wright, and Johnson (1997) used the IMB model to guide HIV risk-reduction elicitation, intervention, and evaluation research in a sample of primarily African American, economically disadvantaged, urban women. The model-based intervention focused on information concerning HIV transmission and prevention, increasing motivation to practice HIV preventive behavior, and the development of HIV prevention behavioral skills, and it was delivered in the context of four ninety-minute intervention sessions. Evaluation research indicated that the intervention had a significant impact on HIV risk-reduction information, motivation, and behavioral skills and on HIV risk behavior, such that participants were significantly less likely than controls to engage in unprotected vaginal intercourse at a three-week follow-up. The mean effect size for the behavioral outcome measures

Table 3.1. TESTS OF THE IMB MODEL: SUMMARY OF REPORTED ASSOCIATIONS.

Sample	Information-Motivation	Information-Behavioral Skills	Motivation-Behavioral Skills	Behavioral Skills-Behavior	Information-Behavior	Motivation-Behavior	Percentage Variance
Heterosexual university males and females (Fisher et al., 1994)		✓	✓	✓		✓	10
Homosexual adult males (Fisher et al., 1994)		✓	✓	✓		✓	35
Urban minority high school males (Fisher et al., 1999)			✓	✓		✓	75
Urban minority high school females (Fisher et al., 1999)		✓	✓	✓			46
Netherlands adult homosexual males (deVroom et al., 1996)	✓	✓	✓	✓	✓	✓	26
Low-income African American females (Anderson et al., 1997)	✓	✓	✓	✓	✓	✓	36
Low-income white females (Anderson et al., 1997)	✓		✓	✓		✓	57
Indian truck drivers (Bryan et al.,2001)				✓	✓	✓	40–51%

Source: From Fisher, J. D., & Fisher, W. A. (2000). Theoretical approaches to individual-level change. In Peterson, J. and DiClemente, R. (Eds.), *HIV Prevention Handbook* (pp. 3–55). New York: Kluwer Academic/Plenum Press (permission granted).

at this time was reported to be a robust .94, and most effects of the intervention persisted at a twelve-week follow-up assessment.

In other research, St. Lawrence, Brasfield, and Jefferson (1995) found strong experimental support for the intervention efficacy of the IMB model in an HIV prevention intervention with minority adolescents. In a further application of the model, Weinhardt, Carey, and Carey (1997) conducted an uncontrolled pilot investigation of an IMB model–based intervention for seriously mentally ill men and women. Results of this pilot study indicated that an IMB approach to HIV risk reduction among chronically mentally ill individuals resulted in pre- to postintervention increases in HIV prevention information and trends toward enhanced prevention behavioral skills and preventive behavior. These findings are consistent with the IMB model, and the investigators suggest that IMB model–based risk-reduction research, with larger controlled samples, has promise for the amelioration of the high levels of HIV risk behavior seen among chronically mentally ill individuals. More recently, Kalichman, Cherry, and Browne-Sperling (1999) report that an IMB model–based intervention led to lower rates of unprotected vaginal intercourse and to higher condom use among minority men recruited from a public clinic, and Kalichman et al. (1999) observed that an intervention with information, motivation, and skills elements led to greater use of female condoms in women. Additional research by Kalichman et al. (2001) reported that an intervention containing IMB elements was effective at reducing HIV transmission risk behavior in HIV-infected people. Finally, meta-analytic work has strongly demonstrated the efficacy of including information, motivation, and behavioral skills elements in HIV risk behavior change interventions (Albarracin, Johnson, Fishbein, & Muellerleile, 2001; Johnson, Marsh, & Carey, 2001).

Case Application of the IMB Model

Just completed work by Fisher et al. (2002) will be used to provide a more extensive case example of the use of the IMB model in HIV prevention intervention research. These researchers used the IMB model to promote change in HIV risk behavior among inner-city minority adolescent high school students at substantial risk for HIV. Half of all new U.S. HIV infections are among young people between the ages of thirteen and twenty-four, and among newly infected teens, 49 percent are African American and 20 percent are Hispanic. Overall, young Americans between the ages of thirteen and twenty-four are contracting HIV at a rate of two per hour (Thurman, 2000). It has been emphasized that school-based HIV prevention interventions may represent the most efficient and universal delivery channel available for targeting adolescents at risk of HIV infection (Basen-Engquist et al., 1997; U.S. Office of National AIDS Policy, 2000).

Reviews of school-based HIV prevention interventions (Coyle et al., 1999; Kirby, 1999; Kirby & DiClemente, 1994) indicate that with very few exceptions (Coyle et al., 1999; Kirby & DiClemente, 1994; Walter & Vaughn, 1993; J. Fisher et al., 2002), school-based interventions have not been based on well-articulated and well-tested behavior change theory (J. Fisher et al., 2002; J. Fisher & Fisher, 2000) and have not demonstrated a significant impact on students' HIV risk behavior. The research at focus applied the IMB model to design, implement, and evaluate an HIV prevention intervention procedure in inner-city minority high school settings. The standard-of-care control condition did not receive any of the experimental interventions. They were, however, exposed to their school's standard HIV/AIDS curriculum, known as AIDS Week. During this week, health classes focused on HIV/AIDS, and the curriculum consisted largely of HIV prevention information.

Participants were students in inner-city high schools in Connecticut. The sample was predominantly female, reflecting the gender breakdown in the schools at focus. Participants ranged in age from thirteen to nineteen, the mean age was about fifteen years, and the great majority were in the ninth grade. More than half were African American, about a third were Hispanic American, and about 10 percent classified their race as Caucasian, "mixed," or "other."

The study employed a quasi-experimental nonequivalent control group design. One high school participated in the classroom intervention; another quite similar high school served as a standard-of-care comparison group. Equating nonequivalent groups at pretest as much as possible is strongly recommended in this type of design (West, Biesanz, & Pitts, 2000). The HIV prevention intervention examined in this research was empirically targeted to address deficits in inner-city high school students' HIV prevention information, motivation, and behavioral skills identified in population-specific elicitation research.

The intervention was delivered by high school teachers during five successive class sessions between Monday and Friday of a given week for a class that met daily. In each school, all students present, including special education students who were mainstreamed, were included in the intervention sessions. During the first intervention class, activities focused on providing factual information about HIV transmission and prevention and on correcting widespread misperceptions, including HIV prevention heuristics and implicit theories about HIV. Classroom activities to address such information deficits included viewing *Knowing the Facts* (1997), a video created specifically to address HIV prevention information deficits identified in elicitation research in this population. Students also used flashcards in an exercise designed to reinforce the information in this video.

The second classroom intervention session was designed to increase HIV prevention motivation by influencing students' attitudes and social norms concerning HIV risk and prevention. Attitudinal and normative change were addressed by showing *Just Like Me* (1997), a video created specifically for this research, which consisted of interviews with an ethnically diverse group of HIV-infected young people, selected on the basis of their social comparability (that is, similarity) to intervention participants. The video was designed to demonstrate to students that adolescents who look and act as they do are at considerable risk of HIV infection. This video had a visible impact on adolescent viewers. The young people in the video directly implored students to alter their attitudes and norms about HIV risk and prevention, lest students in the audience experience the catastrophe that has befallen them. After viewing *Just Like Me,* teachers prompted students to consider and discuss how unfavorable attitudes and norms about HIV prevention led to the infection of the young people in the video (and the death of two of them) and how the same attitudes and norms are common—and in need of change—among high school students such as themselves.

The third classroom intervention session continued to focus on enhancing HIV prevention motivation. An additional video, *Stakes Are High (Part 1)* (1997), conveyed strong attitudinal and normative support for HIV prevention, and supportive attitudes and norms were reinforced in associated teacher-led group activities following the video. *Stakes Are High (Part 1)* featured attractive ethnically diverse social comparison urban high school students encountering and overcoming typical HIV prevention obstacles, such as discussing abstinence or condom use with a resistant partner, assertively negotiating abstinence or safer sex, and physically leaving risky situations. The benefits of abstaining from sex or using condoms were discussed, ways of reducing the social costs of these practices were illustrated, and the youths in the video supported and encouraged one another's HIV prevention efforts. Associated classroom activities demonstrated to students that there is support for HIV prevention among classmates and a degree of rejection of HIV risk behaviors, and they provided an opportunity for students to consider the benefits of HIV prevention and to problem-solve with their classmates to overcome perceived obstacles to prevention.

The fourth class focused on developing HIV prevention behavioral skills for abstinence and condom acquisition and use. Students viewed a fourth specially produced video, *Stakes Are High (Part 2)* (1997), which featured ethnically diverse social comparison inner-city high school students skillfully enacting behaviors to protect themselves from HIV (for example, assertively maintaining abstinence from intercourse; purchasing, carrying, discussing, and using condoms) and included a demonstration of condom use. After the video, the teacher repeated the condom demonstration for the class, and students practiced unrolling a condom over their fingers. Next, students discussed how to apply the abstinence and safer-sex skills depicted in the video in their own social environment. To learn the safer-sex script, each student was given a large card depicting a step in the safer-sex process (for example, deciding whether to have intercourse and communicating this decision to a partner, discussing safer sex, putting on a condom, and removing a condom). Students arranged the cards in sequence by placing themselves appropriately into a line with the initial behavior (deciding whether to have intercourse) first and succeeding behaviors (acquiring condoms, taking condom out of package) later.

During the final classroom session, students augmented their skills by reviewing and discussing rules for effective safer-sex communication. Next, they formed small groups and generated effective verbal responses to a series of common HIV risk scenarios—for example, a partner refuses to use condoms during sexual intercourse or insists on engaging in sexual intercourse when the other person wants to abstain. Responses were critiqued and modified according to rules for effective communication that had been discussed, and students were then given the opportunity to role-play and rehearse modified and improved safer-sex statements. Finally, the teacher answered any remaining student questions related to the intervention.

To evaluate intervention efficacy, one-year postintervention, participants who indicated that they had been sexually active reported how often they had used condoms during sexual intercourse in the preceding twelve months. Examination of path coefficients indicated that the classroom-based intervention resulted in increased condom use for the year following completion of the intervention, in comparison to the control group ($B = .19$, $p < 01$). At one year postintervention, the classroom intervention–induced changes resulted in shifts of fully one unit on a five-unit scale measuring condom use, a statistically significant shift that has clinically meaningful public and personal health implications (see Fisher et al., 2002, for a detailed discussion of the procedures used, additional intervention conditions, and additional results of this research).

This research study demonstrates that an IMB model–based, empirically targeted HIV prevention intervention, delivered in inner-city high school classrooms to generally high-risk minority students by their own teachers, had significant effects on a critical HIV preventive behavior—condom use during sexual intercourse—one year postintervention. These findings represent one of the only reports of a rigorously evaluated controlled trial, conducted within existing, intact high school settings, that has demonstrated success at increasing long-term HIV preventive behavior among inner-city youth at high risk of infection (Fisher et al., 2002).

The classroom-based intervention we have described can be broadly deployed in urban high schools. It was designed to be cheaply, easily, and widely applied within actual inner-city high school settings and included the existing teaching staff and entire intact classrooms rather than the use of specially selected teachers, charismatic intervenors, select student volunteers, or expensive intervention materials. The intervention procedures require only the availability of currently employed teaching staff and a modest investment in intervention training and deployment. All intervention materials (including manuals, videos, and flashcards) are ready to implement and are available from the senior author or on-line (www.films.com/Dynamic/Item/Item8801.asp). On a per-student basis, calculations indicate that the cost of the classroom-based intervention, using existing teaching personnel, amounted to only $2.22 per student.

Future Directions: The IMB Model as a General Health Behavior Change Conceptualization

Beyond its established strength in predicting, understanding, and intervening to change HIV risk behavior, the IMB model is viewed as a generalizable approach to understanding and promoting heath behavior more broadly defined (W. Fisher & Fisher, 1999, in press). As a preliminary step in establishing the generality of the model, we conducted a review of the correlational research literature concerning psychological factors linked to performance of diverse health behaviors. We found that in correlational research, information, motivation, and behavioral skills elements are consistently related to health behavior performance across diverse areas such as exercise behavior, smoking cessation, and breast and cardiovascular health. In effect, correlational evidence supports the IMB model's assertion that the three factors in the model are critical determinants of health behavior outside the domain of HIV prevention (for further details, see W. Fisher & Fisher, in press).

We next reviewed experimental intervention research across the same health domains. In this review, we observed that interventions that contain information, motivation, and behavioral skills elements were more effective in promoting health behavior change than interventions that lacked one or more of these elements. Furthermore, we compared the strength of the information, motivation, and behavioral skills content of interventions that had strong health behavior change effects, versus those

Overall, the findings provide support for IMB model elements as determinants of intervention efficacy across diverse domains of health behaviors.

with weak effects, and found that the former had greater information, motivation, and behavioral skills–related content than the latter (for further details, see W. Fisher & Fisher, in press). Overall, the findings provide support for IMB model elements as determinants of intervention efficacy across diverse domains of health behaviors.

We then applied the IMB model directly in an effort to account for health behavior in two diverse areas, breast self-examination (BSE), a detection and screening behavior, and motorcycle safety gear use, an injury prevention behavior, both of which are quite different from HIV preventive behavior, which is a disease prevention behavior.

Breast Self-Examination

BSE is a critical health behavior, both because it is regarded as effective in the early detection and subsequent cure of breast cancer (American Cancer Society, 1998) and because relatively few women practice it (W. Fisher, Dervatis, Bryan, Silocx, & Kohn, 2000; Misovich et al., in press). In research by Misovich et al. (in press), women who were recruited in workplace settings completed questionnaires measuring levels of BSE-relevant information, motivation, behavioral skills, and behavior. In addition to identifying critical deficits in BSE-relevant information, motivation, behavioral skills, and behavior (see Misovich et al., in press, for the specifics), we tested the hypothesized interrelations among the IMB model constructs (depicted in Figure 3.3 for the context of BSE) using structural equation modeling procedures. Results showed that each of the relationships specified by the model was confirmed and that it provided an acceptable fit to the data (CFI = .96, RMSEA = .07). As can be seen in Figure 3.3, BSE information and motivation are statistically independent constructs, each is significantly linked with BSE behavioral skills, and behavioral skills are significantly associated with performance of BSE-related behaviors, all as specified by the IMB model. In addition, and also predicted by the model, there is an independent link between BSE motivation and BSE-related behavioral performance. The three components of the IMB model account for 70 percent of the variance in BSE-related behaviors, which is regarded as a large effect size for a prediction model in the behavioral sciences (Cohen, 1988).

Motorcycle Safety

As an additional test of the IMB model as a generalizable account of the psychological determinants of health behavior performance, we report the findings of model-based research concerning determinants of motorcycle safety gear use (Murray, 2000). Motorcycle accidents and associated injury and death are very common occurrences (U.S. Department of Transportation, 1997). Although motorcycle safety gear use has been demonstrated to save hundreds of lives annu-

Figure 3.3. EMPIRICAL TEST OF THE IMB MODEL OF THE DETERMINANTS OF BREAST SELF-EXAMINATION BEHAVIOR.

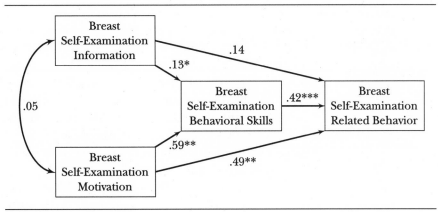

*p < .05
**p < .01
***p < .001

Source: Misovich et al. (in press).

ally (U.S. Department of Transportation, 1997), it is inconsistently practiced by those at risk.

First, Murray (2000) created elicitation research–based sets of information, motivation, behavioral skills, and behavior questionnaire items relating to motorcycle safety gear use. Data collection for the research to test the IMB model in the context of motorcycle safety then took place with samples of motorcycle riders recruited at a biker event, at motorcycle shops, and using flyers posted on a university campus (n = 180). A large additional Internet sample (n = 710) was recruited through motorcycle-related Web sites and Web-based mailing lists, and questionnaires completed on the Internet were returned by e-mail.

Findings from this cross-sectional study revealed that motorcycle riders had significant information, motivation, behavioral skills, and behavior deficits with respect to motorcycle safety gear use (for specific findings, see Murray, 2000). For example, motorcycle helmets, which are particularly critical for saving lives, were reportedly used only 80 percent of the time in states without helmet laws. Concerning the IMB model, results of structural equation modeling analyses again showed that the relationships specified by the IMB approach were confirmed and that the model provided an acceptable fit to the data (CFI = .97, RMSEA = .07). As can be seen in Figure 3.4 and as predicted by the IMB model, for complex tasks (wearing helmets, jackets, and pants can be challenging to put on since they involve multiple fasteners and, more important, can impair a rider's sense of control and mobility while riding), both information and motivation were linked to behavioral skills for motorcycle safety gear use. In addition, behavioral skills were significantly associated with reported complex motorcycle safety gear use behavior. Further, information and motivation concerning motorcycle safety gear use are statistically related constructs. Note that although the IMB model suggests that information and motivation are often independent constructs because well-informed persons are not necessarily well motivated to practice health behaviors, the model does not require the statistical independence of the information and motivation constructs.

Overall, these findings contribute to establishing the generalizability and strength of the IMB model across diverse domains of health behavior, including disease preventive behavior (for example, HIV prevention), disease screening and detection behavior (for example, BSE), and injury prevention behavior (for example, motorcycle safety gear use).

Other Applications

In addition to establishing the empirical generalizability of the IMB model, we wish to demonstrate its utility as a conceptual basis for analysis and insight into the determinants and dynamics of still other health-related behaviors. To illus-

FIGURE 3.4. EMPIRICAL TEST OF THE IMB MODEL OF THE DETERMINANTS OF COMPLEX MOTORCYCLE SAFETY GEAR USE.

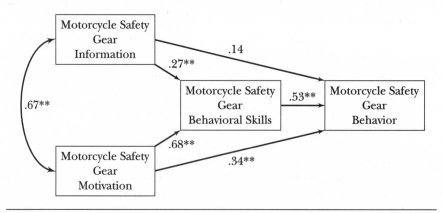

*p < .05.

**p < .01.

Source: Murray (2000).

trate, we present an IMB model–based conceptualization of factors implicated in adherence to active antiretroviral therapy (ART) among people living with HIV. Understanding and promoting ART adherence in HIV-positive individuals is of enormous individual and public health significance. On the one hand, ART has proven dramatically effective in reducing the viral load and associated morbidity of persons living with HIV and has contributed directly to dramatic declines in HIV-related mortality (Greenberg et al., 1999; Montaner et al., 1998). On the other hand, adherence to ART must be highly consistent, in the range of 90 percent, but in actuality it is generally much lower (W. Fisher et al., 2001). When ART adherence is suboptimal, treatment failure, viral mutation, and development of multidrug-resistant HIV can take place (Hogg, Yip, Chanm, O'Shaughnessy, & Montaner, 2000). HIV-positive individuals who inconsistently adhere to their medication are at significant personal health risk and may pose a substantial public health threat involving the potential development and transmission of multidrug-resistant HIV to others.

From the perspective of the IMB model, adherence to medical regimen shares much in common with other critical health behaviors (J. Fisher, Fisher, Amico, & Harman, 2001; W. Fisher & Fisher, in press). Therefore, ART adherence is conceptualized to occur as a function of the presence of a specific set of relevant information, motivation, and behavioral skills factors. All else being equal, to the extent that an HIV-positive individual is well informed about ART, motivated to act, and possesses the requisite behavioral skills to act effectively, he or she will be likely to adhere to ART regimens and reap substantial health benefits. To the extent that an HIV-positive individual is poorly informed, unmotivated to act, and lacks the requisite behavioral skills for effective adherence, the individual will be nonadherent to ART and will fail to realize its health benefits. An IMB model analysis of ART adherence is presented in Figure 3.5. It describes specific information, motivation, behavioral skills, and adherence behavior parameters and the relationships among them, as well as a set of moderating factors relevant in the context of ART adherence.

According to the IMB model, information that is directly relevant to antiretroviral medication use is an initial prerequisite for ART adherence. Motivation and behavioral skills are also critical for adherence (see Figure 3.5 for the specific types of information, motivation, and behavioral skills that may be most important). Consistent with other health behaviors, the IMB model of adherence specifies that adherence information and motivation are often statistically independent factors that work primarily through behavioral skills to affect adherence behavior (see Figure 3.5). Adherence information and motivation may also have direct effects on adherence behavior in situations in which novel or complicated behavioral skills may not be required for ART adherence. Currently, ART adherence

FIGURE 3.5. AN IMB MODEL ANALYSIS OF ADHERENCE TO ANTIRETROVIRAL MEDIATION.

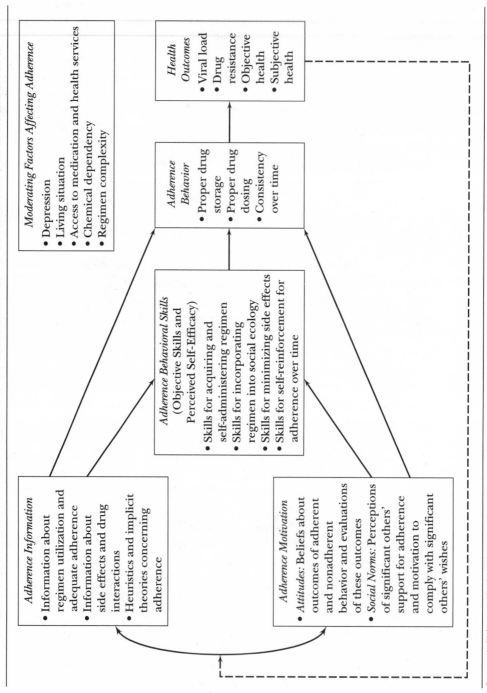

Source: J. Fisher et al. (2001).

clearly does require complex behavioral skills. If in the future antiretroviral regimens are developed that are delivered by daily or weekly dosages or transdermal patches and that have very low cost and few side effects, the IMB model would anticipate that adherence information or motivation, or both, could have direct effects on adherence behavior. The IMB approach described in Figure 3.5 includes some critical additional elements and feedback loops (see J. Fisher et al., 2001, and W. Fisher & Fisher, in press, for details), and is in the process of being tested in a large-scale field study in Puerto Rico.

Critique of the IMB Model

Overall, the IMB model provides a comprehensive conceptual approach to understanding the determinants of HIV prevention and other health behaviors and may constitute a generalizable methodology for intervening to promote such behavior. The model's assumptions concerning the determinants of HIV prevention and other health behaviors have been consistently confirmed in multivariate correlational research conducted across a diversity of populations and behaviors (J. Fisher et al., 1994; W. Fisher et al., 1999; W. Fisher & Fisher, in press), and its constructs account for a substantial proportion of the variance in HIV prevention and other health behaviors. The IMB model's approach to HIV risk and other health behaviors has been supported in elicitation, experimental intervention, and evaluation research conducted with diverse populations. Results of this research are consistent with the IMB model's focus on identifying and addressing deficits in HIV- and health-relevant information, motivation, and behavioral skills as an effective means for promoting health behavior change. Effects of IMB model–based interventions on health behavior change have been significant and sustained.

Empirical tests of the IMB model have also suggested criticisms of the IMB approach to understanding and promoting health behavior change that need to be addressed in future conceptual and empirical work. First, given the relatively recent genesis of the IMB model, first published in 1992, it is not surprising that some areas of IMB model–based research are somewhat sparse. Prospective studies of the determinants of health behavior (J. Fisher et al., 1998) are far fewer in number than cross-sectional studies (J. Fisher et al., 1994), and experimental intervention research, while consistently confirming the utility of the model with diverse populations, remains limited. Moreover, much IMB model–based research is still in the process of being submitted for publication or in press and is not yet widely available.

Second, on a conceptual level, this review raises questions about the role of the IMB model's information construct, which across studies appears to be a relatively inconsistent contributor to the prediction of preventive behavior. Although the model has specified situations in which information is expected to be a substantial contributor to health behavior (such as early in epidemics such as the HIV epidemic) and when it will not (later in epidemics; J. Fisher & Fisher, 1992, 2000), further empirical study of the model's conceptualization of the role of information is necessary. Our review also raises questions concerning the relationship of the information and motivation constructs, which are sometimes independent and sometimes not. The model's logic, which holds that well-informed people are not necessarily well motivated to practice prevention, and vice versa (J. Fisher & Fisher, 1992, 2000), would appear to permit at least the possibility of a relationship between informational and motivational factors. Other questions remaining for future conceptual and empirical consideration involve specification of when—in terms of populations at risk and preventive behaviors of interest—specific model constructs may prove to be most important.

References

Ajzen, I., & Fishbein, M. (1980). *Understanding attitudes and predicting social behavior.* Upper Saddle River, NJ: Prentice Hall.

Albarracin, D., Johnson, B. T., Fishbein, M., & Muellerleile, P. A. (2001). Theories of reasoned action and planned behavior as models of condom use: A meta-analysis. *Psychological Bulletin, 127,* 142–161.

American Cancer Society. (1998). What are the key statistics about breast cancer? Available: www.cancer.org/ben/info/brstats.html.

Anderson, E. S., Winett, E. A., Wagstaff, D. A., Sikkema, K. J., & Heckman, T. G., et al. (1997, April). *AIDS prevention among low-income, urban African-American and white women: Testing the Information-Motivation-Behavioral Skills (IMB) Model.* Poster presented at the 18th Annual Scientific Session of the Society of Behavioral Medicine, San Francisco.

Bandura, A. (1989). Perceived self-efficacy in the exercise of control over AIDS infection. In V. M. Mays, G. W. Albee, & S. M. Schneider (Eds.), *Primary prevention of AIDS* (pp. 128–141). Thousand Oaks, CA: Sage.

Bandura, A. (1994). Social cognitive theory and exercise control of HIV infection. In R. J. DiClemente & J. L. Peterson (Eds.), *Preventing AIDS: Theories and methods of behavioral interventions* (pp. 25–59). New York: Plenum.

Barrett, M., Fisher, W. A., & McKay, A. (Eds.). (1994). *Canadian guidelines for sexual health education.* Ottawa: Health Canada.

Basen-Engquist, K., Parcel, G. S., Harrist, R., Kirby, D., Coyle, K., Banspach, S., & Rugg, D. (1997). The safer choices project: Methodological issues in school-based health promotion intervention research. *Journal of School Health, 67,* 365–371.

Brunswick, A. F., & Banaszak-Hol, J. (1996). HIV risk behavior and the health belief model: An empirical test in an African American community sample. *Journal of Community Psychology, 24,* 44–65.

Bryan, A. D., Fisher, J. D., & Benziger, T. J. (2000, December). HIV prevention information, motivation, behavioral skills among Indian truck drivers in Chennai, India. *AIDS, 14,* 756–758.

Bryan, A. D., Fisher, J. D., & Benziger, T. J. (2001). Determinants of HIV risks among Indian truck drivers: An information, motivation, behavioral skills approach. *Social Science and Medicine, 53,* 1413–1426.

Bryan, A. D., Fisher, J. D., Fisher, W. A., & Murray, D. M. (2000). Understanding condom use among heroin addicts in methadone maintenance using the information, motivation, behavioral skills model. *Substance Use and Misuse, 35,* 451–471.

Byrne, D., Jazwinski, C., DeNinno, J. A., & Fisher, W. A. (1977). Negative sexual attitudes and contraception. In D. Bryne & L. A. Byrne (Eds.), *Exploring human sexuality.* New York: HarperCollins.

Byrne, D., Kelley, K., & Fisher, W. A. (1993). Unwanted teenage pregnancies: Incidence, interpretation, intervention. *Applied Prevention Psychology, 2,* 101–113.

Carey, M. P., Carey, K. B., & Kalichman, S. C. (1997). Risk for human immunodeficiency virus (HIV) infection among persons with severe mental illnesses. *Clinical Psychological Review, 17,* 271–291.

Carey, M. P., Carey, K. B., & Weinhardt, L. S. (1997). Behavioral risk for HIV infection among adults with a severe and persistent mental illness: Patterns and psychological antecedents. *Journal of Community Mental Health, 33,* 133–142.

Carey, M. P., Maisto, S. A., Kalichman, S. C., Forsyth, A. D., Wright, E. M., & Johnson, B. T. (1997). Enhancing motivation to reduce the risk of HIV infection for economically disadvantaged urban women. *Journal of Consulting Clinical Psychology, 65,* 531–541.

Catania, J. A., Gibson, D. R., Chitwood, D. D., & Coates, T. J. (1990). Methodological problems in AIDS behavioral research: Influences on measurement error and participation bias in studies of sexual behavior. *Psychological Bulletin, 108,* 339–362.

Centers for Disease Control and Prevention. (2000). *HIV/AIDS Surveillance Report. National Center for HIV, STD and TB Prevention.* Atlanta, GA: Centers for Disease Control and Prevention. Available: www.cdc.gov/hiv/stats/cumulati.html.

Coates, T. J. (1990). Strategies for modifying sexual behavior patterns for primary and secondary prevention of HIV disease. *Journal of Consulting and Clinical Psychology, 58,* 57–69.

Cohen, J. (1988). *Statistical power analysis for the behavioral sciences* (2nd ed.). Hillsdale, NJ: Erlbaum.

Connecticut Department of Public Health. (1997). *Program goals: AIDS prevention education services.* Hartford, CT: Connecticut Department of Public Health.

Coyle, D., Basen-Engquist, K., Kirby, D., Parcel, G., Banspach, S., Harrist, R., Baumier, E., & Well, M. (1999). Short-term impact of safer choices: A multi-component, school-based HIV, other STD, and pregnancy prevention program. *Journal of School Health, 69,* 181–188.

DeVroome, E. M., deWit, J. B., Sandfort, T. G., & Stroebe, W. (1996). Comparing the Information-Motivations Behavioral Skills Model and the Theory of Planned Behavior in explaining unsafe sex among gay men. Unpublished manuscript, Department of Gay and Lesbian Studies and Department of Social and Organizational Psychology, Utrecht University, The Netherlands.

deWit, J. B. (1996). The epidemic of HIV among young homosexual men. *AIDS, 10* (Suppl. 3), 21–25.

deWit, J.B.F., Stroebe, W., DeVroome, E.M.M., Sandfort, T.G.M., & VanGriensven, G.J.P. (2000). Comparing the Information-Motivation-Behavioral Skills Model and the theory of planned behavior in explaining unsafe sex among gay men. *Psychology & Health, 15*(3), 325–340.

Exner, T. M., Seal, D. W., & Ehrhardt, A. A. (1997). A review of HIV interventions for at-risk women. *AIDS and Behavior, 1,* 93–124.

Fishbein, M., & Ajzen, I. (1975). *Belief, attitude, intention and behavior: An introduction to theory and research.* Reading, MA: Addison-Wesley.

Fishbein, M., & Middlestadt, S. E. (1989). Using the theory of reasoned action as a framework for understanding and changing AIDS-related behaviors. In V. M. Mays, G. W. Albee, & S. M. Schneider (Eds.), *Primary prevention of psychopathology* (pp. 93–110). Thousand Oaks, CA: Sage.

Fishbein, M., Middlestadt, S. E., & Hitchcock, P. J. (1994). Using information to change sexually transmitted disease-related behaviors. In R. J. DiClemente & J. L. Peterson (Eds.), *Preventing AIDS: Theories and methods of behavioral interventions* (pp. 61–78). New York: Plenum.

Fisher, J. D. (1988). Possible effects of reference group-based social influence on AIDS-risk behavior and AIDS-prevention [Special issue]. *American Psychologist, 43,* 914–920.

Fisher, J. D. (2000, June). *The IMB model of adherence.* Invited presentation at the First International Workshop on the Information-Motivation-Behavioral Skills Model, Naples, Italy.

Fisher, J. D. (2001, August). *Physician-delivered interventions: The Options Project.* Paper presented at the HIV Prevention in Treatment Settings: U.S. and International Priorities conference, Washington, DC

Fisher, J. D., & Fisher, W. A. (1992). Changing AIDS risk behavior. *Psychological Bulletin, 111,* 455–474.

Fisher, J. D., & Fisher, W. A. (1996). The Information-Motivation-Behavioral Skills Model of AIDS risk behavior change: Empirical support and application. In S. Oskamp & S. Thompson (Eds.), *Understanding and preventing HIV risk behavior: Safer sex and drug use* (pp. 100–127). Thousand Oaks, CA: Sage.

Fisher, J. D., & Fisher, W. A. (2000). Theoretical approaches to individual-level change. In J. Peterson & R. DiClemente (Eds.), *HIV prevention handbook* (pp. 3–55). New York: Kluwer Academic/Plenum Press.

Fisher, J. D., Fisher, W. A., & Amico, R. (2001, July). An *Information-Motivation-Behavior Skills Model of adherence to highly active antiretroviral therapy.* Paper presented at AIDS Impact: Biopsychosocial Aspects of HIV Infection, Fifth International Conference, Brighton, UK.

Fisher, J. D., Fisher, W. A., Amico, K. R., & Harman, J. J. (2001). *An information-motivation-behavioral skills model of adherence to antiretroviral therapy.* Manuscript in preparation.

Fisher, J. D., Fisher, W. A., Bryan, A. D., Misovich, S. J. (2002). Information-Motivation-Behavioral Skills Model-Based HIV risk behavior change intervention for inner city high school youth. *Health Psychology, 21*(2), 177–186.

Fisher, J. D., Fisher, W. A., Misovich, S. J., Kimble, D. L., & Malloy, T. E. (1996). Changing AIDS risk behavior: Effects of an intervention emphasizing AIDS risk reduction information, motivation, and behavioral skills in a college student population. *Health Psychology, 15,* 114–123.

Fisher, J. D., Fisher, W. A., Williams, S. S., & Malloy, T. E. (1994). Empirical tests of an Information-Motivation-Behavioral Skills Model of AIDS preventive behavior in gay men and heterosexual university students. *Health Psychology, 13,* 238–250.

Fisher, J. D., Kimble, D. L., Misovich, S. J., & Weinstein, B. (1998). Dynamic of sexual risk behavior in HIV-infected men who have sex with men. *AIDS and Behavior, 2,* 101–113.

Fisher, J. D., & Misovich, S. (1990). Evolution of college students' AIDS-related behavioral responses, attitudes, knowledge, and fear. *AIDS Education and Prevention: An Interdisciplinary Journal, 2,* 322–337.

Fisher, J. D., Silver, R., Chinksy, J., Goff, B., Klar, Y., & Zagieboylo, C. (1989). Psychological effects of participation in a large group awareness training. *Journal of Consulting and Clinical Psychology, 57*, 747–755.

Fisher, W. A. (1986). A psychological approach to human sexuality: The sexual behavior sequence. In D. Byrne & K Kelley (Eds.), *Approaches to human sexuality*. Hillsdale, NJ: Erlbaum.

Fisher, W. A. (1990). Understanding and preventing adolescent pregnancy and sexually transmissible disease/AIDS. In J. Edwards, R. S. Tindale, L. Health, & E. J. Posavac (Eds.), *Social influence processes and prevention* (pp. 71–101). New York: Plenum Press.

Fisher, W. A. (1997). A theory-based framework for intervention and evaluation in STD/HIV prevention. *Canadian Journal of Human Sexuality, 6*, 105–111.

Fisher, W. A., & Fisher, J. D. (1993). A general social psychological model for changing AIDS risk behavior. In L. Pryor & G. Reeder (Eds.), *The social psychology of HIV infection* (pp. 127–153). Hillsdale, NJ: Erlbaum.

Fisher, W. A., & Fisher, J. D. (1999) Understanding and promoting sexual and reproductive health behavior: Theory and method. In R. C. Rosen, C. M. Davis, & H. J. Ruppel, Jr. (Eds.), *Annual review of sex research* (Vol. 9, pp. 39–76). Lake Mills, IA: Society for the Scientific Study of Sex.

Fisher, W. A., & Fisher, J. D. (2000). Understanding and promoting sexual and reproductive health behavior: Theory and method. In R. Rosen, C. Davis, & H. Ruppel (Eds.), *Annual review of sex research* (Vol. 9, pp. 39–76). Mason City, IA: Society for the Scientific Study of Sex.

Fisher, W. A., & Fisher, J. D. (in press). The Information-Motivation-Behavioral Skills Model as a general model of health behavior change: Theoretical approaches to individual-level change. In J. Suls & K. Wallston (Eds.), *Social psychological foundations of health*. Cambridge, MA: Blackwell.

Fisher, W. A., Fisher, J. D., & Byrne, D. (1977). Consumer reactions to contraception purchasing. *Personality and Social Psychology Bulletin, 3*, 293–296.

Fisher, W. A., Byrne, D., Kelley, K., & White, L. A. (1988). Erotophobia-erotophilia as a dimension of personality. *Journal of Sex Research, 25*, 123–151.

Fisher, W. A., Byrne, D., & White, L. A. (1983). Emotional barriers to contraception. In D. Byrne & W. A. Fisher (Eds.), *Adolescents, sex, and contraception*. Hillsdale, NJ: Erlbaum.

Fisher, W. W., Dervatis, K. A., Bryan, A. D., Silcox, J., & Kohn, H. (2000). Sexual health, reproductive health, sexual coercion, and partner abuse indicators in a Canadian obstetrics and gynaecology outpatient population. *Journal of the Society of Obstetricians and Gynaecologists of Canada, 22*, 714–724.

Fisher, W. A., Gilmore, J., Clark, F., Pook, T., Wilson, T., Wilbur, C., & Shuper, P. (2001). *Patterns and correlates of HIV transmission risk behavior among HIV+ patients in clinical care*. Manuscript in preparation.

Fisher, W. A., Williams, S. S., Fisher, J. D., & Malloy, T. E. (1999). Understanding AIDS risk behavior among sexually active urban adolescents. An empirical test of the Information-Motivation-Behavioral Skills Model. *AIDS and Behavior, 3*, 13–23.

Gluck, M., & Rosenthal, E. (1995). *OTA Report: The effectiveness of AIDS prevention efforts*. Washington, DC: American Psychological Association.

Greenberg, B., Berkman, A., Thomas, R., Hoos, D., Finkelstein, R., Astemborski, J., & Vlahov, D. (1999). Evaluating supervised ART in late-stage HIV among drug users: A preliminary report. *Journal of Urban Health, 76*, 468–480.

Hammer, J. C., Fisher, J. D., & Fitzgerald, P. (1996). When two heads aren't better than one: AIDS risk behavior in college-age couples. *Journal of Applied Social Psychology, 26,* 375–397.

Health Canada. (1994). *Canadian guidelines for sexual health education.* Ottawa: Ministry of National Health and Welfare.

Helweg-Larsen, M., & Collins, B. E. (1997). A social psychological perspective on the role of knowledge about AIDS in AIDS prevention. *Current Directions in Psychological Science, 6,* 23–53.

Hogg, R. S., Yip, B., Chanm, K., O'Shaughnessy, M. V., & Montaner, S. G. (2000, January–February). *Nonadherence to triple combination therapy is predictive of AIDS progression and death in HIV-positive men and women.* Program and abstracts of the Seventh Conference on Retroviruses and Opportunistic Infections, San Francisco.

Holtgrave, D. R., Qualls, N. L., Curran, J. W., Valdiserri, R. O., Guinan, M. E., Parra, W. C. (1995). An overview of the effectiveness and efficiency of HIV prevention programs. *Public Health Report, 110,* 134–146.

Johnson, B. T., Marsh, K. L., & Carey, M. P. (2001). *Factors underlying the success of behavioral interventions to reduce sexual HIV transmission.* Paper presented at the Fifth International Conference of AIDS Impact, Brighton, England.

Johnson, R. W., Ostrow, D. G., & Joseph, J. G. (1990). Educational strategies for prevention of sexual transmission of HIV. In D. G. Ostrow (Ed.), *Behavioral aspects of AIDS* (pp. 43–73). New York: Plenum.

Just Like Me. (1997). [Video]. (Available from Films for the Humanities & Sciences, P.O. Box 2053, Princeton, NJ 08543–2053)

Kalichman, S. C., Cherry, C., & Browne-Sperling, F. (1999). Effectiveness of a video-based motivational skills-building HIV risk-reduction intervention for inner-city African American men. *Journal of Consulting and Clinical Psychology, 67,* 959–966.

Kalichman, S. C., Rompa, D., Cage, M., DiFonzo, K., Simpson, D., Austin, J., Luke, W., Buckles, J., Kyomugisha, G., Benotsch, E., Pinkerton, S., Graham, J. (2001). Effectiveness of an intervention to reduce HIV transmission risks in HIV-positive people. *American Journal of Preventive Medicine, 21,* 84–92.

Kelly, J. A. (1995). *Changing HIV risk behavior: Practical strategies.* New York: Guilford Press.

Kelly, J. A., Murphy, D. A., Sikkema, K. L., & Kalichman, S. C. (1993). Psychological interventions to prevent HIV infection are urgently needed: New priorities for behavioral research in the second decade of AIDS. *American Psychologist, 48,* 1023–1034.

Kelly, J. A., & St. Lawrence, J. S. (1988). *The AIDS health crisis: Psychological and social interventions.* New York: Plenum Press.

Kirby, D. (1999). Reflections on two decades of research on teen sexual behavior and pregnancy. *Journal of School Health, 69,* 89–94.

Kirby, D., & DiClemente, R. J. (1994). School-based interventions to prevent unprotected sex and HIV among adolescents. In R. J. DiClemente & J. L. Peterson (Eds.), *Preventing AIDS: Theories and methods of behavioral interventions* (pp. 117–139). New York: Plenum Press.

Knowing the Facts. (1997). [Video]. (Available from Films for the Humanities & Sciences, P.O. Box 2053, Princeton, NJ 08543–2053)

Leviton, L. C., & Valdiserri, R. O. (1990). Evaluating AIDS prevention: Outcome, implementation, and mediating variables. *Evaluation and Program Planning, 13,* 55–66.

Misovich, S. J., Fisher, J. D., & Fisher, W. A. (1996). The perceived AIDS-preventive utility of knowing one's partner well: A public health dictum and individual's risky sexual behavior. *Canadian Journal of Human Sexuality, 5,* 83–90.

Misovich, S. J., Fisher, J. D., & Fisher, W. A. (1997). Close relationships and HIV risk behavior: Evidence and possible underlying psychological processes. *General Psychology Review, 1,* 72–107.

Misovich, S. J., Fisher, W. A., & Fisher, J. D. (1998). A measure of AIDS prevention information, motivation and behavioral skills. In C. M. Davis, R. Yarber, G. Bauserman, G. Schreer, & S. L. Davis (Eds.), *Sexuality related measures: A compendium.* Thousand Oaks, CA: Sage.

Misovich, S. J., Martinez, T., Fisher, J. D., Bryan, A. D., & Catapano, N. (in press). Breast self-examination: A test of the information, motivation, and behavioral skills model. *Journal of Applied Social Psychology.*

Montaner, J. D., Reiss, P., Cooper, D., Vella, S., Harris, M., Conway, B., Weinberg, M. A., Smith, D., Robinson, P., Hall, D., Myers, M., & Lange, J.M.A. (1998). A randomized, double-blind trial comparing combinations of nevirapine, didanosine, and zidovudine for HIV-infected patients. *Journal of the American Medical Association, 279,* 930–937.

Murray, D. M. (2000). *Exploring motorcycle safety gear use: A thoeretical approach.* Unpublished master's thesis, University of Connecticut, Storrs, Connecticut.

Oakley, A., Fullerton, D., & Holland, J. (1995). Behavioral interventions for HIV/AIDS prevention. *AIDS, 9,* 479–486.

Offir, J. T., Fisher, J. D., & Williams, S. S. (1993). Possible reasons for inconsistent AIDS prevention behaviors among gay men. *Journal of Sex Research, 30,* 62–69.

Popp, D., & Fisher, J. D. (2002). First, do no harm: A call for emphasizing adherence and HIV prevention interventions in ART programs in the developing world. *AIDS, 16*(4), 676–678.

Prochaska, J. O., Redding, C. A., Harlow, L. L., Rossi, J. S., & Velicer, W. F. (1994). The transtheoretical model of change and HIV prevention: A review. *Health Education Quarterly, 21,* 471–486.

Rosenstock, I. M. (1996). Why people use health services. *Milbank Memorial Fund Quarterly, 44,* 94–124.

Rosenstock, I. M., Stretcher, V. J., & Becker, M. H. (1994). The health belief model and HIV risk behavior change. In R. J. DiClemente & J. L. Peterson (Eds.), *Preventing AIDS: Theories and methods of behavioral interventions* (pp. 5–25). New York: Plenum.

St. Lawrence, J. S., Brasfield, T. L., & Jefferson, K. W. (1995). Cognitive-behavioral intervention to reduce African American adolescents' risk for HIV infection. *Journal of Consulting Clinical Psychology, 63,* 221–237.

Stakes Are High, Part 1. (1997). [Video]. (Available from Films for the Humanities & Sciences, P.O. Box 2053, Princeton, NJ 08543–2053)

Stakes Are High, Part 2. (1997). [Video]. (Available from Films for the Humanities & Sciences, P.O. Box 2053, Princeton, NJ 08543–2053)

Thurman, S. L. (2000, October). Youth and HIV/AIDS 2000: A new American agenda: A message from the director of National AIDS policy. Available: www.thebody.com/whitehouse/youthreport/director.html

UNAIDS. (2000, October). *Joint United Nations Programme on HIV/AIDS: Report on the global HIV AIDS epidemic.* New York: United Nations.

U.S. Department of Health and Human Services. (1988). *Understanding AIDS.* Rockville, MD: Centers for Disease Control.

U.S. Department of Health and Human Services (1993). *Planning and evaluating HIV/AIDS prevention programs in state and local health departments: A companion to program announcement 300.* Rockville, MD: Centers for Disease Control.

U.S. Department of Transportation, National Highway Traffic Safety Administration. (1997). *Traffic safety facts: Motorcycles.* Washington, DC: U.S. Government Printing Office.

U.S. Office of National AIDS Policy. (2000). *Youth and HIV/AIDS 2000: A New American Agenda.* Washington, DC: U.S. Government Printing Office.

Walter, H., & Vaughn, R. D. (1993). AIDS risk reduction among a multi-ethnic sample of urban high school students. *Journal of the American Medical Association, 270,* 725–730.

West, S. G., Biesanz, J. C., & Pitts, S. C. (2000). Causal inference and generalization in field settings: Experimental and quasi-experimental designs. In H. T. Reis & C. M. Judd (Eds.), *Handbook of research methods in social and personality psychology* (pp. 40–84). Cambridge: Cambridge University Press.

Weinhardt, L. S., Carey, M. P., & Carey, K. B. (1997). HIV risk reduction for the seriously mentally ill: Pilot investigation and call for research. *Journal of Behavior Therapy and Experimental Psychiatry, 28,* 1–8.

Williams, S. S., Doyle, T. M., Pittman, L. D., Weiss, L. H., Fisher, J. D., & Fisher, W. A. (1998). Roleplayed safer sex skills of heterosexual college students influenced by both personal and partner factors. *AIDS and Behavior, 2,* 177–187.

Williams, S. S., Kimble, D. L., Covell, N. H., Weiss, L. H., Newton, K. S., Fisher, J. D., & Fisher, W. A. (1992). College students use implicit personality theory instead of safer sex. *Journal of Applied Social Psychology, 22,* 921–933.

Wingood, G. M., & DiClemente, R. J. (1996). HIV sexual risk reduction interventions for women: A review. *American Journal of Preventive Medicine, 12,* 209–217.

CHAPTER FOUR

THE ELABORATION LIKELIHOOD
MODEL OF PERSUASION

Health Promotions That Yield
Sustained Behavioral Change

Richard E. Petty
Jamie Barden
S. Christian Wheeler

The typical goal of health promotion campaigns and research is to induce positive change in health-related behaviors. For example, a media campaign might attempt to convince people to use their seat belts or to stop smoking. However, studies of the effectiveness of media and direct interventions have provided inconsistent results. In particular, efforts in critical areas such as drug and alcohol abuse and prevention of acquired immunodeficiency syndrome (AIDS) have sometimes proved disappointing in terms of concrete successes. This challenge has led to a number of responses. For example, an entire issue of the journal *Health Psychology* was dedicated to the notion that a distinction has to be made between initiation of behavior change and sustained behavioral change (Rothman, 2000). Numerous investigators have pointed out that simply increasing knowledge about a topic is not sufficient to lead to behavioral change (Helweg-Larsen & Collins, 1997; Petty, Baker, & Gleicher, 1991). In order to understand why certain interventions with high face validity fail to provide sustained behavioral change, health promotion researchers and practitioners have sought insight from basic research on influence processes.

Experimental research has shown that attitudes represent one of the most important theoretical constructs that determine behavior (Eagly & Chaiken, 1993; Fishbein & Ajzen, 1975; Petty & Cacioppo, 1981). As commonly conceived, an attitude is a relatively stable global evaluation of a person, object, or issue. Taking exercise behavior as an example, critical attitudes might include: "Exercise is good; I feel favorable toward running on the weekends; I feel good enough about myself to believe I can start exercising." Thus, multiple attitudes held toward different objects at different levels of specificity (in the example, the general concept of exercise, a specific behavior such as running, one's own self-efficacy) can affect the likelihood that any behavior is adopted. Thus, one job of those interested in health promotion is to determine which attitudes are the most important for predicting a particular health behavior and which procedures are best used for changing those attitudes and obtaining sustained behavioral change.

Of course, a number of factors other than attitudes determine whether people engage in a certain behavior. These include social norms (Fishbein & Ajzen, 1975), the strength of the attitude (Petty & Krosnick, 1995), feelings of self-efficacy and competence (Bandura, 1986), and prior behaviors and habits (Triandis, 1977). Although this might suggest that we should try to change these factors instead, many of these behavioral determinants result from attitudes as well. For example, when the attitudes of many people change, social norms change as well. Positive attitudes toward the self can increase feelings of self-efficacy, making behavioral change more likely. Negative attitudes toward past behaviors and habits can drive behavioral change. Thus, to change behavior, it is useful to understand how attitudes are changed.

Attitudes are most frequently measured using some type of direct self-report procedure, such as asking a person how favorable or unfavorable and positive or negative he or she is toward wearing seat belts (see Eagly & Chaiken, 1993, for more detail about common attitude measurement procedures). When planning a health promotion program, it is important to select the attitude or attitudes that the promotion is intended to change and to measure each attitude separately to determine the success of the program. Depending on one's goals, it can be useful to measure attitudes toward a general idea (safer sex), a specific object (condom), or a behavior (using a condom). The success of a persuasive attempt is then measured by assessing change in the attitudes targeted. Change can be assessed in a pre-post design or by comparing the attitudes of individuals who have and have not received some persuasion treatment (Campbell & Stanley, 1964).

When planning a health promotion program, it is important to select the attitude or attitudes that the promotion is intended to change and to measure each attitude separately to determine the success of the program.

The Elaboration Likelihood Model of Persuasion

Contemporary scientific research on attitude change began in the 1940s as an extension of the U.S. military's effort during World War II to understand propaganda and persuasion (Hovland, Lumsdaine, & Sheffield, 1949). The learning theories developed at that time viewed persuasion as a function of attention, comprehension, acceptance, and retention of the persuasive communication (Hovland, Janis, & Kelley, 1953). This early research identified many of the variables investigators continue to examine as determinants of attitude change. Beginning with the Hovland group and continuing today, researchers focus on features of the source of the message (Is the source attractive? Expert? A member of an ingroup?), the message itself (Is the message complex? Composed of cogent arguments? Rational or emotional?), the recipient of the communication (Is the recipient in a good mood? Intelligent? Involved in the topic?), and the context in which the message is presented (Is the environment quiet or distracting? Is the message on the radio, television, or the Internet?).

As the number of persuasion studies began to grow, numerous inconsistencies in findings appeared. For example, increasing the same variable, such as number of arguments, source expertise, or use of fear appeals, would increase persuasion in one experiment, decrease it in another, and have no effect in a third. Furthermore, numerous attitude change theories were developed to describe a number of processes through which persuasion takes place, but each theory seemed to predict persuasion only under certain conditions. Theories were also in disagreement about the effects of any one variable (for example, how source expertise influences attitude change; see Petty, 1994).

The Elaboration Likelihood Model (ELM) was developed to explain past inconsistencies in attitudes research. Whereas past models tended to emphasize one effect of a given variable and one process by which that effect occurred, the ELM organized multiple persuasion processes into two routes to attitude change. The central route involves change that occurs when people are relatively thoughtful in their consideration of the issue-relevant information presented. In contrast, the peripheral route to persuasion involves processes requiring relatively little thought about issue-relevant information. Instead, attitudes are changed by simple association processes (for example, classical conditioning) or the use of various mental shortcuts and heuristics. By noting that variables influence attitudes by different means at different points along an elaboration continuum, the ELM is able to explain seemingly inconsistent findings in the persuasion literature. After describing key ideas from the ELM, we discuss the utility of the model for understanding health communication.

Central Route

The ELM organizes attitude change processes into two routes to persuasion: the central route and the peripheral route. The central route to persuasion involves careful consideration of information pertaining to the attitude object and its relationship to pertinent knowledge stored in memory. Careful consideration of the issue-relevant information presented involves generating positive or negative thoughts (or both) toward the advocated position, such as seat belt usage). Under the central route, the valence of those thoughts (whether positive or negative) is related to the direction of persuasion, and the extent to which the thoughts are new and more positive or negative than they were previously determines the extent of attitude change. The thoughts about the message make up the key component that links internal knowledge to the information presented in the message. Also, the more confidence people have in the thoughts that they generate under the central route, the more these thoughts determine a person's attitude (Petty, Tormala, Briñol, & Jarvis, 2001). The focus of the thinking under the central route is often on the perceived desirability of the consequences in the communication and the perceived likelihood that they will occur (Petty & Wegener, 1991; Ajzen & Fishbein, 2000).

Two conditions are necessary for effortful processing to occur: the recipient of the message must be motivated and able to process it thoroughly. A person's motivation to consider message arguments can be influenced by a number of variables, including the perceived personal relevance of the message (Petty & Cacioppo, 1979b) and whether the person enjoys thinking in general (Cacioppo, Petty, & Morris, 1983). A person's ability to think can also be influenced by a number of variables, including the amount of distraction present in the persuasion context (Petty, Wells, & Brock, 1976) and the number of times the message is repeated (Cacioppo & Petty, 1979). If a person is both motivated and able to think about the issue-relevant information presented, the result of this careful processing is an attitude that is well articulated, readily accessible, and integrated into the person's overall belief structure (Petty & Cacioppo, 1986).

If a person is both motivated and able to think about the issue-relevant information presented, the result of this careful processing is an attitude that is well articulated, readily accessible, and integrated into the person's overall belief structure.

Peripheral Route

In our daily lives, we often lack either the motivation or the ability to thoughtfully consider every potential persuasive communication in the way characterized by the central route. Attitude change can occur nonetheless because many persuasion processes require little to no consideration of substantive information. In the ELM, such processes are organized into the peripheral route, and they include reliance on simple cues available in the persuasion context as well as mental shortcuts called heuristics. The persuasion context may elicit an affective state (like happiness) that becomes associated with the advocated position through classical conditioning (Staats & Staats, 1958), or a mental shortcut might be used so that a message from an expert is judged based on the heuristic that "experts are generally correct" rather than careful consideration of the substantive arguments (Chaiken, 1987). Another common method used when either motivation or ability is lacking is simply to count the number of arguments made rather than evaluating them based on their content (Petty & Cacioppo, 1984). Although the peripheral route to persuasion does not involve thoughtful consideration of message content, it can be effective in leading to persuasion, at least in the short term.

Elaboration Likelihood Continuum

To this point, it has been convenient to break processes of persuasion into two distinct routes for explanatory purposes. However, the ELM holds that persuasion occurs along an elaboration likelihood continuum. The continuum stretches from processes requiring no thinking, like classical conditioning that occurs outside awareness, to processes requiring some effort, like counting arguments or making inferences based on one's experienced affect, to processes requiring careful consideration, like listing the pros and cons to make an important life decision. Along much of the continuum, both peripheral and central processes take place and can influence attitudes simultaneously (Petty, 1994). But as the elaboration likelihood increases, central route processes, that is, careful evaluation of issue-relevant information, tend to dominate in their impact on attitudes over more peripheral processes, such as reliance on simple heuristics.

It is important to emphasize that the distinction between central and peripheral routes is made based on the extent of issue-relevant scrutiny and on how the information is processed rather than on the type of information itself (Petty, Wheeler, & Bizer, 1999). As an example, information about the source of a message can have an impact on attitudes under either the central or the peripheral routes depending on whether the recipient has the motivation and ability to evaluate it carefully. If Magic Johnson is the source of a message about human immunodeficiency (HIV) and we use the heuristic "famous is good," then persuasion will follow the peripheral route. However, if we are more persuaded because he has contracted HIV and knows what he is talking about, then we are examining the central merits of Magic Johnson as a source, as is likely to occur under the central route. Note that under the peripheral route, the use of Magic Johnson could be effective regardless of the message topic because if all one considers is his fame, this is constant across attitude objects. On the other hand, if one processes the information carefully for relevance, Magic Johnson should be more effective in an HIV message than in a message for swimming pools. We will discuss in more depth how the same variable can influence attitudes in multiple ways in different situations.

Support for the Central and Peripheral Routes

There is extensive empirical support for the utility of the central and peripheral distinction (see Petty & Cacioppo, 1986; Petty & Wegener, 1998a, for reviews). In one early and representative study, the presence or absence of a potential peripheral cue and the quality of the arguments, strong versus weak (as determined in pilot testing), were manipulated (Petty, Cacioppo, & Goldman, 1981).

In this study, college students were given one of four persuasive messages: (1) strong and compelling arguments attributed to an expert source, (2) weak and specious arguments presented by an expert source, (3) strong and compelling arguments attributed to a nonexpert source, or (4) weak arguments attributed to a nonexpert source. No distractions were present during the procedure and the message was easily comprehended, so all participants had the ability to process the message. However, motivation to process the message was manipulated by informing some of the students that the proposal (supporting a change in campus policy) would take effect in a year (high-relevance condition), whereas others were informed that the proposal would go into effect in ten years (low-relevance condition). The high-relevance condition should motivate effortful processing of the message (Petty & Cacioppo, 1979b). The low-relevance condition offers little motivation to process the message, so low-effort attitude change processes should have a greater impact on attitude change. This was in fact the observed pattern: those in the high-motivation condition processed the message arguments, so their level of persuasion was greatly influenced by the manipulation of argument strength. They responded based on whether the arguments offered good support for the advocated position. Those in the low-personal-relevance condition lacked the motivation to process the message thoroughly, and so their level of persuasion was a function of the expertise of the source rather than strength of the message. That is, they supported the policy change as long as the source was an expert, regardless of the quality of the arguments offered to support the policy.

Variables Influencing the Elaboration Likelihood

Taken as a whole, the evidence supporting the ELM shows that a number of variables exist that can have an impact on persuasion by influencing a message recipient's motivation or ability to think about the communication. In this way, these variables determine whether high or low effort processes are more likely to influence attitudes. For example, if a woman has a family history of breast cancer, then she might be motivated to think about a persuasive message about breast self-exams based on perceived self-relevance (Rothman & Schwarz, 1998). However, if the perceived self-relevance is so intense as to induce fear, defensive avoidance might occur (Janis & Feshbach, 1953). In addition to motivational variables, ability variables also influence processing. For example, if the message is delivered in the hall of a busy hospital, the ability to think will be lowered. Variables that influence motivation and ability to think can be part of the situation (context) or internal to the person (recipient).

The breast exam example mentioned variables that influence the extent of thinking (whether many or few thoughts are generated). Other variables influence the direction of thinking (whether favorable or unfavorable to the message). For example, telling an audience that they are about to receive an attempt to persuade them on an important issue can bias responses to the message because the audience becomes motivated to actively resist a change in their current opinion (Petty & Cacioppo, 1979a). Conversely, if a person is put in a good mood when exposed to a message on an important topic, the good mood increases the likelihood of generating positive thoughts to the communication (Petty, Schumann, Richman, & Strathman, 1993). Thus, responses to a persuasive message are determined by both situational and personal factors that influence motivation or ability to think in ways that change the extent or direction of thinking.

Consequences of the Route to Persuasion

The route used to produce attitude change is critical, because central route attitude changes tend to have different consequences and properties from peripheral route attitude changes (see Petty, Haugtvedt, & Smith, 1995, for a review). Overall, attitudes that result from central route processes tend to be stronger than those from peripheral route processes. As compared to weak attitudes, strong attitudes are more durable because they persist over time and resist change when challenged by contrary information. In addition, strong attitudes guide thinking, and, perhaps most important, strong attitudes guide behavior (Krosnick & Petty, 1995). As an example, consider an individual who engaged in thoughtful processing of a message on exercise that resulted in a strong positive attitude toward this behavior. Strong attitudes are more predictive of behavior, so thoughtful attitude change makes the initiation of exercise behavior more likely. In addition, because strong attitudes persist in memory, they will continue to influence behavior over time. Furthermore, when a friend suggests forgoing exercise to watch television, the strong attitude will be resistant to change. It will also bias thinking in favor of the attitude, so the friend's statement may be reinterpreted as, "Stay in and be a slob," increasing the likelihood of behavior maintenance. Thus, stronger attitudes produced through central route processes have a number of features that increase the chance of eliciting sustained behavioral change.

Stronger attitudes produced through central route processes have a number of features that increase the chance of eliciting sustained behavioral change.

A number of studies provide evidence that attitudes resulting from more effortful thinking better predict behavioral intentions and guide actions than do attitudes resulting from little thinking. As one example, Brown (1974) assessed the attitudes of high school students toward various health-related behaviors such as using drugs and obeying traffic safety laws. Students who reported giving the issues greater thought exhibited greater attitude-behavior consistency than those who reported giving the issues little thought.

Research on the need for cognition, a measure of the extent to which people engage in and enjoy thinking (Cacioppo & Petty, 1982), has also supported this proposition. For example, Cacioppo, Petty, Kao, and Rodriguez (1986) found that the attitudes toward presidential candidates of individuals who enjoy thinking were more predictive of their votes than the attitudes of individuals who did not enjoy thinking (see Cacioppo, Petty, Feinstein, & Jarvis, 1996, for a thorough review of work on need for cognition).

In these studies, existing attitudes based on high or low amounts of thought were examined. Other studies have created new attitudes and assessed how well the attitudes predict behavior. In one study, for example (Sivacek & Crano, 1982, experiment 2), undergraduate students were informed that their university was exploring the possibility of implementing senior comprehensive exams (an issue new to them), and they then read a message describing these exams. Then students reported their attitudes toward the proposal and were given the opportunity to sign petitions opposing the exams and to volunteer their services to a group that opposed the exams. The sample was divided into high- and low-relevance groups on the basis of the students' self-reports of whether the issue was high or low in perceived personal relevance (that is, whether it would affect them or not). The high-relevance group exhibited larger correlations between their attitudes toward senior comprehensive exams and their relevant behaviors (petition signing and volunteering). That is, students for whom the message was more personally relevant demonstrated higher attitude-behavior consistency than students who considered the message less relevant. Based on the assumption that students in the high-relevance group engaged in greater issue-relevant thought when forming their attitudes than students in the low-relevance group (as would be expected based on numerous experiments; Petty & Cacioppo, 1990), this study supports the notion that thoughtful attitudes are more predictive of behavior than unthoughtful attitudes. Other studies that have changed attitudes to a similar degree under conditions of high or low elaboration have also shown that thoughtful attitude changes are more predictive of behavioral intentions and actions than unthoughtful attitude changes (Leippe & Elkin, 1987; Petty, Cacioppo, & Schumann, 1983). Thus, attitudes formed by the central route exhibit greater attitude-behavior consistency.

Research evidence suggests that attitudes formed by the central route are more persistent over time and more resistant to counterpersuasive attempts than attitudes formed by the peripheral route. For example, in two studies (Haugtvedt & Petty, 1992), similar attitude changes were produced in individuals who differed in their need for cognition. In each study, college students were presented with a message containing strong arguments from a credible source, so there were two possible factors on which persuasion could be based. Both high- and low-need-for-cognition individuals became more favorable toward the position taken in the message, but what is critical is that they did so through different processes. Students who generally enjoy thinking changed based on a careful consideration of the high-quality arguments. Low-need-for-cognition students, who avoid thought, changed to the same extent but because of the positive source cue. When attitudes toward the issue were examined just two days after the persuasive message, recipients low in need for cognition had returned to their initial positions, but high-need-for-cognition students persisted in their new attitudes. In a second study, the students' new attitudes were challenged just a few minutes after they were created. High-need-for-cognition students resisted the message attacking their attitude to a greater extent than low-need-for-cognition individuals.

Taken together, these results suggest that attitude change might have less impact if it comes about through low rather than high amounts of issue-relevant thinking. Thus, although central route attitude changes are typically more difficult to produce than peripheral route changes, the benefits are considerable. A key contribution of the ELM is the finding that it is insufficient to know simply what a person's attitude is or how much change in attitude was produced. It is also important to know how the person's attitude was changed. Attitudes that are identical in valence can be quite different in terms of their underlying psychological antecedents (how they were formed or changed) and consequences (for example, whether they predict behavior; see Petty & Krosnick, 1995, for a review of attitude strength research).

The difficulties of creating central route attitude change are familiar to health promotion researchers. For example, there are great challenges in engaging young adults in health-related topics like safer-sex practices and substance abuse simply because they often do not see them as personally relevant or important to their lives (Scott, 1996; Scott & Ambroson, 1994). Due to these challenges, it is tempting to suggest that the use of peripheral cues and heuristics is the best way to create attitude change. However, attitude change produced through peripheral route processes can represent an empty victory, since weak attitudes produce little in the way of tangible results. Instead, more needs to be done to understand what variables successfully engage the thoughtful processing of such messages in each population. One possible hybrid strategy is to use the peripheral route in combination with the central route. That is, one might make a health position, such as using condoms, more acceptable to an unmotivated audience by the use of cues, and then when it is temporarily more desirable, more active processing techniques can be employed, such as getting people to justify their new attitudes in a role-playing exercise (Janis & King, 1954).

Multiple Roles of Variables in the ELM

One critical component of the ELM is that it allows for any one variable, such as the credibility of the message source or the mood a person is in, to influence persuasion through different processes in different situations. The capacity of one variable to affect judgments through different processes explains how such simple variables as the credibility of the source or one's mood can produce complex outcomes. It also makes it essential to identify the conditions under which a variable influences attitudes by one process rather than another. We have hinted at the limited number of ways that variables can affect attitudes according to the ELM: by serving as a simple cue, by serving as an argument, or by affecting one's thoughts (amount of thoughts, valence of thoughts, or confidence in thoughts).

Situations of low elaboration likelihood occur when people are unmotivated or unable to scrutinize the issue-relevant information presented. Under low elaboration conditions, then, persuasion-relevant variables such as a person's mood or the expertise of the source, to the extent that they have any impact at all, influence attitudes primarily through peripheral route processes. This is because people are either not motivated or not able to effortfully evaluate the merits of the information presented. Thus, if any evaluation is formed, it is likely to be the result of a relatively simple association or inference process that can occur without much cognitive effort (for example, "Experts are correct"). For example, under low-elaboration conditions, one's mood could serve as a simple cue either because the mood becomes associated with the advocated position through classical conditioning or because people infer their attitude from their mood ("I feel good, so I must like it"). Both of these peripheral processes assume that mood can influence attitudes without much issue-relevant thinking.

The ELM holds that under high elaboration conditions, however, people want to evaluate on the merits of the arguments presented, and they are able to do so.

In these high-elaboration situations, persuasion-relevant variables have relatively little impact by serving as simple cues. Instead, the variable is scrutinized, like a message argument, and can result in attitude change if the variable provides information relevant to the merits of the attitude object (for example, an emotional factor such as how much you "love" someone is central to the merits of selecting a spouse and can serve as an argument in favor of marriage). Even variables not central to the merits of the object can influence attitudes under high processing conditions by biasing the direction of thought taking place. For example, people might be motivated to generate mostly favorable thoughts about the message if the source is credible (Chaiken & Maheswaran, 1994), or they might overestimate the likelihood that some good consequence mentioned in the message will happen if they are in a good mood (Wegener, Petty, & Klein, 1994). Finally, if thoughts are generated when people are in a good mood or the source is expert, people might have more confidence in their thoughts than if the thoughts are generated when they are feeling bad or are in response to an unknowledgeable source (Petty, Briñol, & Tormala, in press). The more confidence one has in one's thoughts, the more they will impact attitudes.

The final role a variable can have is influencing the amount of thinking that takes place. For example, we previously noted that people are generally motivated to think more about messages of high rather than low personal relevance (Petty & Cacioppo, 1979b) and are generally unable to think carefully about messages when distraction is high (Petty et al., 1976). But many other variables can influence the extent of thinking when the elaboration is not already constrained to be high or low. For example, the variables of source expertise and a person's mood can influence the extent of thinking when other variables have not already constrained thinking to be very high or low. In such circumstances, people may be more motivated to pay attention to and think about what an expert rather than a nonknowledgeable source advocates (Heesacker, Petty, & Cacioppo, 1983). Or when in a happy mood, people will be more likely to think about a message that promises to be uplifting and less likely than individuals in a sad mood to think about a message that promises to be depressing (Wegener, Petty, & Smith, 1995). This suggests that positive mood influences message processing, at least in part, due to mood management concerns (Isen & Simmonds, 1978; Wegener & Petty, 1996). That is, people in a positive mood tend to avoid message processing when they think it might attenuate their good feelings such as when the message is expected to be unpleasant or counter to one's own attitude, but engage in message processing when it will maintain or enhance their mood, such as when it is pleasant or supports their own attitude (see Wegener & Petty, 1996; Petty, Febrigar, & Wegener, 2001, for reviews of research on mood and persuasion).

Summary of the Elaboration Likelihood Model

Figure 4.1 presents a schematic depiction of the ELM and highlights the major features of the model. In the simplest sense, the ELM does three things. First, it points to two routes to persuasion: a thoughtful and cognitively effortful route that occurs when the person is both motivated and able to think about the merits of the issue under consideration, and a less thoughtful route that occurs when motivation or ability is low. Second, the model points to consequences of these two routes. Thoughtful attitude changes are postulated to be more accessible to memory, persistent over time, resistant to counterpersuasive attempts, and predictive of behavior. Third, the model specifies how variables have an impact on persuasion. That is, the model specifies certain roles that variables can play in the persuasion process. Variables can influence a person's motivation to think or ability to think. They can influence the valence of one's thoughts or the confidence in the thoughts generated. Finally, they can serve as simple cues and change attitudes by one of several peripheral processes (for example, identification with the source, invocation of simple decision heuristics). With these features of the ELM in mind, we turn to the potential relevance of this model for health promotion.

Using the ELM to Understand Health Communication Efficacy

Over the past decade, researchers in the area of health promotion have made use of the ELM to develop health promotion campaigns and interventions including AIDS and condom use (Bakker, 1999; Dinoff & Kowalski, 1999; Helweg-Larsen & Collins, 1997; MacNair, Elliott, & Yoder, 1991; Mulvihill, 1996), exercise (Brock, Brannon, & Bridgwater, 1990; Rosen, 2000), diet counseling (Kerssens & van Yperen, 1996), substance abuse interventions (Scott, 1996; Scott & Ambroson, 1994), smoking cessation (Quinlan & McCaul, 2000), compliance in breast cancer screening (Drossaert, Boer, & Seydel, 1996), maternal attitudes toward baby bottle tooth decay (Kanellis, Logan, & Jakobson, 1997), compliance with hospital infection control procedures (Bartzokas & Slade, 1991), prenatal care for low-income Mexican women (Alcalay, Ghee, & Scrimshaw, 1993), and organ donor program participation (Skumanich & Kintsfather, 1996). Dissertations in the health domain have also made use of the ELM in research related to phenomena such as the fear associated with heart disease and ulcers (Rosenthal, 1997), adolescent AIDS interventions (Weiskotten, 1993), attitudes toward health maintenance organizations (Chan, 1999), and responses to unfavorable medical diagnosis (Lockhart, 1999).

FIGURE 4.1. THE ELABORATION LIKELIHOOD MODEL OF PERSUASION.

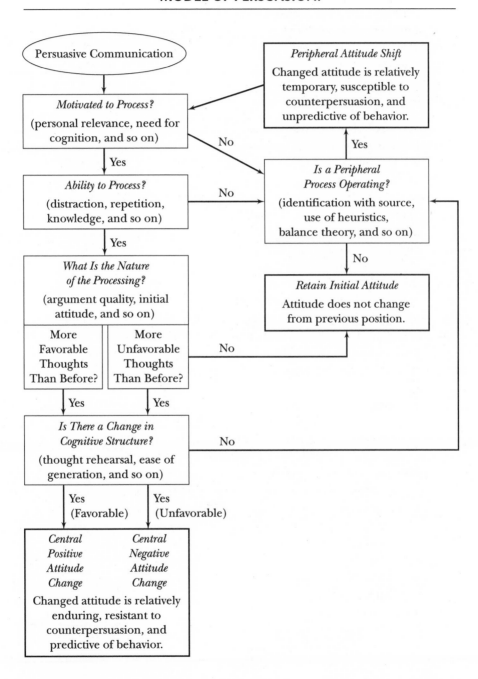

As a general theory of information processing, the ELM has considerable utility for understanding the outcomes of different persuasive attempts on resulting attitudes and behaviors. Because attitudes are a primary determinant of behavior, attitude change can be a central focus of any health promotion program.

Because attitudes are a primary determinant of behavior, attitude change can be a central focus of any health promotion program.

ELM Analysis of Message Tailoring

One area of health research in which the ELM has been fruitfully applied is in the domain of message tailoring. Although there are occasionally contradictory results (Quinlan & McCaul, 2000), the bulk of research has indicated that matching health messages to different aspects of an individual's personal characteristics can increase the effectiveness of the messages in changing attitudes and behavior (Kreuter, Bull, Clark, & Oswald, 1999; see Kreuter, Farrell, Olevitch, & Brennan, 2000, for a review). Although tailoring strategies have generally been successful, little is known about why tailoring is an effective strategy. Moreover, little is known about what differentiates the situations in which tailoring will or will not be effective in generating short-term or long-term behavioral change.

In this final section, we use the ELM to examine some mechanisms by which message tailoring could work and provide illustrative examples. In addition, we speculate about conditions that are likely to maximize the effectiveness of message tailoring, as well as those in which tailoring may lead to null or even reversed effects.

Tailoring. Within the health domain, tailoring typically refers to those instances in which the arguments contained in health communications are altered to match the particular concerns of the message recipient. For example, a pretest of Susie's concerns about condom use might indicate that she believes that they are awkward and inhibit pleasure. Susie may be less concerned about the cost of condoms or about their efficacy in preventing pregnancy or disease. A message tailored to Susie, then, would address the social and physical issues associated with condom use while leaving out information about their efficacy or cost.

Tailoring procedures can be used to match not only the types of concerns an individual has about a particular health behavior, but also the individual's stage of behavioral change. Stages of change models hold that there are a number of qualitatively distinct stages through which an individual must pass when adopting a health behavior (Prochaska, DiClemente, & Norcross, 1992; Weinstein, 1988; Weinstein & Sandman, 1992; also see Weinstein & Sandman, Chapter Two, this volume). For example, the Transtheoretical Model (Prochaska et al., 1992) suggests that individuals pass through five distinct stages (precontemplation, contemplation, preparation, action, and maintenance) on the path to behavioral change and that messages that match the individual's stage of change should be more effective in changing behavior. With some exceptions, the available literature generally indicates that this is the case.[1]

Matching Effects. The finding that tailoring arguments to personal health concerns can increase persuasion bears more than superficial similarity to findings in other persuasion domains showing that matching a persuasive message to various facets of the person or his or her attitude can increase persuasion. For example, matching a message to the functions of an individual's attitude can increase persuasion (for example, providing image-related arguments to a person concerned about social image; see Shavitt, 1989; Snyder & DeBono, 1985). Making an emotional appeal to a person whose attitude is based on emotion can be more effective than making a more rational or cognitive appeal (see Edwards, 1990; Fabrigar & Petty, 1999). Finally, matching a message to one's group identity can be effective (for example, framing the message as "for men" or "for women" for individuals highly identified with their gender; see Fleming & Petty, 2000; Mackie, Worth, & Asuncion, 1990).

Although some researchers (for example, Kreuter et al., 1999) draw a distinction between personalization (putting a person's name on the communication) and tailoring, we believe that these types of matching share important underlying conceptual similarities. Petty, Wheeler, and Bizer (2000) reviewed matching effects in a variety of social-psychological research traditions, including attitude function matching, self-schema matching, group identity matching, and affect-cognition matching. Noting the remarkable similarity in induction procedures and persuasion outcomes, they suggested that these matching effects might stem from the same underlying factor: establishing a link to the self.

Matching Under Low Elaboration Conditions. In line with the multiple roles postulate of the ELM, linking a message to some aspect of the self ("me-ness" matching) could influence persuasion in a number of different ways. Under low-elaboration conditions, the match could act as a simple cue, for example, "If it's for me [or "relates to me," or is "similar to me"], I like it." This notion derives support from the numerous findings indicating that objects or ideas that are associated with the self are preferred to those that are not. Thus, individuals prefer products that they own to those that they do not, whether the products were chosen by the individual (Brehm, 1956) or received as an unselected gift (Kahneman, Knetsch, & Thaler, 1991). Individuals prefer arguments that they have generated to those that others have generated (Greenwald & Albert, 1968) and even prefer the first

letters in their own names to other letters of the alphabet (Nuttin, 1985). Given
the typically high self-esteem that most individuals possess (Taylor & Brown, 1988),
it is not surprising that the self serves as a positive cue so frequently (an "own-ness"
bias; Perloff & Brock, 1980).

Thus, under low-elaboration conditions, matching a message to some aspect
of the individual's self, such as one's concerns, values, goals, groups, or posses-
sions, could act as a positive cue in the absence of much issue-relevant thinking.
Although this cue strategy could be fruitful in the short run, durable attitude
change is more likely when a message is processed under high-elaboration conditions. By engaging in active elaboration on the message topic, the individual forges
more linkages between the new information and knowledge already stored in memory. Greater elaboration is therefore likely to render the resulting attitude more persistent, more resistant, and more likely to influence thought and behavior.

Matching Under Moderate Elaboration Conditions. When baseline elaboration
likelihood conditions are moderate (that is, motivation and ability factors are not
constrained to be high or low), a persuasion variable can act to increase the
amount of elaboration that takes place. For example, we already noted that a variable that increases the perceived personal relevance of a message can increase the
extent to which an individual thinks carefully about all of the issue-relevant information presented (Petty & Cacioppo, 1979b). In line with this prediction, a
number of studies in the literature have provided evidence consistent with the idea
that tailoring a message to the recipient can increase elaboration (see Petty &
Wegener, 1998b). For example, Brug, Steenhaus, Van Assema, and deVries (1996)
found that tailored messages were perceived by recipients as more personally
relevant and as written especially for them. Perhaps because of this increased perception of relevance, tailored messages are more likely to be read by the recipients and result in greater recall for the message content (Brug et al., 1996;
Campbell et al., 1994; Skinner, Strecher, & Hospers, 1994).

Matching Under High-Elaboration Conditions. Under high-elaboration conditions, tailoring or matching a message to an individual could lead to biased message processing. For example, arguments that are tailored to address individual
concerns, such as those about cost, could be perceived to be stronger than those
that are not so tailored, such as messages about social benefits, even though there
are no differences (or even a reverse difference) in actual argument quality. For example, people may be more likely to fill in positive interpretations for matched
than mismatched arguments. Alternately, tailored arguments could address health
concerns about which the individual has a biased store of issue-relevant knowledge. This could lead to an ability bias even when the individual has an accu-

racy motivation. That is, the person's biased store of knowledge might enable the person to see the merits in some types of arguments more easily than other types. Finally, people might have more confidence in the thoughts that they generate to tailored rather than nontailored messages, leading thoughts in response to tailored messages to have a greater impact on attitudes.

Illustrative Research on Tailoring

In a prototypical tailoring experiment, Kreuter et al. (1999) collected an initial set of data on participants' beliefs, motives, perceived barriers, and so forth concerning weight loss. Participants were then sent one of three messages. Tailored messages included participants' names and fourteen arguments tailored toward their particular concerns. Another group received messages from the American Heart Association that were not tailored but contained general information and tips concerning weight loss. In a third condition, people received a message that contained the exact same information as the nontailored message group, but the message was formatted to resemble the tailored pamphlets in appearance. Results indicated that participants who received the tailored materials generated more positive personal connections (that is, links between the materials and their lifestyle, attitudes, social norms, or behavior) and more positive thoughts than those who received materials that were not tailored. In addition, participants indicated that the tailored messages elicited more attention. Although results on the attitude measures were somewhat equivocal, the experiment generally supported the conclusion that tailored messages can be effective in increasing message processing.

Although many studies within the health literature have tailored arguments to match the specific dimensions of concern the individual had expressed in that particular health domain, messages have also been matched on the basis of more general characteristics. For example, Brock et al. (1990) conducted a study in which they tailored persuasive messages to match the self-schemas of the message recipients. To create the tailored messages, they first contacted a pool of over seven thousand former customers of a weight-loss company with a letter from the (fictitious) Center for Personality Research. Using a card-sorting procedure and adjective-rating task, participants indicated their overall personality types. Brock et al. (1990) used these data to classify participants into one of four schema sets (one was "warm-communicative-compassionate"). These same individuals were later sent a packet of materials from the weight loss company. The materials included an insert that was tailored to either match or mismatch the schema set of the recipient and a business reply card that could be used to reactivate membership with the company. Control group participants received an insert designed to be neutral with regard to schema set. Results indicated that individuals who received an insert stringently matched to their schema set were over 12 percent more likely to return the business reply card than were individuals who received a mismatched insert. These results lend support to the hypothesis that tailoring messages to individuals' self-schemas can be another effective means of tailoring.

In addition, some work has shown that simply tailoring the message format to match some aspect of the recipient can increase persuasion. For example, Bakker (1999) reasoned that individuals who are high or low in the need for cognition (Cacioppo & Petty, 1982) would respond differently to messages presented in a way that made them appear easy or more difficult to process. Need for cognition is an individual difference variable that corresponds to a person's propensity to engage in and enjoy effortful cognitive activities (Cacioppo & Petty, 1982).

In this experiment, high school students were exposed to one of two messages about AIDS and STDs. Although the messages contained essentially the same information, one message was presented in a concise, written format, whereas the other message was presented in a cartoon format. Bakker (1999) reasoned that low-need-for-cognition individuals should be particularly motivated to think about the cartoon message because it would appear easier and more enjoyable to process. High-need-for-cognition individuals, on the other hand, could be more motivated to process the written message because it would appear to be more interesting and important. He reasoned that the cartoon message could actually inhibit persuasion among high-need-for-cognition participants by creating additional distraction or by leading to negative cognitive responses, such as responses about the potentially "childish" or simplistic nature of the message format.

Results indicated that participants in both the cartoon and written message conditions had significantly more knowledge about AIDS after reading the message than did participants in a no-message control group. However, analyses on attitudes toward condom use indicated a main effect of message type as well as a significant need for cognition by message type interaction. The main effect was such that individuals in both the cartoon and written message conditions showed more positive attitudes toward condom use than did participants in the no-message control group. The interaction, however, indicated that low-need-for-cognition individuals expressed more positive attitudes toward condom use after reading the cartoon message than the written message, and high-need-for-cognition individuals indicated more positive attitudes toward condom use after reading the written message than the cartoon message. Thus, message format appears to be an

Message format appears to be an additional type of tailoring or matching variable that can have a significant impact on health attitudes and behaviors.

additional type of tailoring or matching variable that can have a significant impact on health attitudes and behaviors.

Interpreting Tailoring Research

The three research examples of tailoring described demonstrate self-matching effects with three different types of manipulations. Kreuter et al. (1999) tailored their arguments to match the specific concerns of the message recipients (the most typical tailoring procedure), Brock et al. (1990) matched the arguments to aspects of the individuals' personality schemas, and Bakker (1999) matched the format of the message to the individuals' cognitive processing style. Although it is certainly possible to obtain similar findings for different reasons, it is possible that each of these results shares an important underlying similarity. That is, each of the studies reviewed matched an aspect of the persuasive message to a corresponding aspect of the message participant and may have therefore influenced persuasion as a result of the self-match.

Although each of the studies found increased persuasion under matched rather than mismatched conditions, the precise mechanism responsible for each finding is not entirely clear. Recall that according to the ELM, a given variable like a message match can serve in multiple roles depending on the overall level of elaboration present in the persuasion context. Consequently, additional manipulations and measures are necessary to draw strong inferences about the processes operating in each experiment. The authors of the experiments just reviewed all favored the explanation that matching increased elaboration. If one assumes that the arguments presented were strong and that elaboration was not constrained at high or low levels by other variables, this explanation would be quite plausible and consistent with the ELM. However, other researchers have provided support for the idea that self-matching can have other effects besides increasing elaboration, such as biasing elaboration in a favorable direction (Cacioppo, Petty, & Sidera, 1982; Lavine & Snyder, 1996) or serving as a peripheral cue (DeBono, 1987), and so, in the absence of empirical process indicators, multiple accounts for the data reviewed above are possible. For example, in the Bakker (1999) study, was a cartoon more effective than a written message for individuals low in need for cognition because the cartoon served as a simple cue or because it increased processing of the strong message arguments? Given that the individuals were low in need for cognition, it seems unlikely that the cartoon served in one of the roles reserved for high-elaboration conditions, such as biasing processing. In any case, the multiple roles reviewed earlier provide examples of how the same effects could be obtained using different processes under different elaboration conditions. The

ELM holds that it is important to understanding the underlying processes of change because of the strength properties that follow from the different processes.

Of our example studies, the one that provided the most extensive process evidence was that of Kreuter et al. (1999), who included measures of self-reported attention and cognitive responses. These researchers found that participants found the tailored messages to be more attention getting and that participants generated more positive cognitive responses in response to tailored messages. Although not significant, results further indicated that the total number of thoughts generated in response to the message was highest among individuals who read the tailored messages. Thus, it seems plausible that in the Kreuter et al. experiment, tailoring increased message elaboration.

From the standpoint of understanding the processes responsible for self-matching effects, it would be very useful to include a manipulation of argument quality in future research designs.[2] Argument quality manipulations can provide an additional source of information about the role of the variable by indicating the extent of elaboration (Petty & Cacioppo, 1986). That is, if a variable (like tailoring) increases persuasion equally when both strong and weak arguments are presented and argument quality makes little difference, then tailoring is likely to be operating as a peripheral cue. If, on the other hand, tailoring increases sensitivity to differences in argument quality, then it may be increasing objective message elaboration. If that were the case, tailoring would increase persuasion when the message arguments were strong but decrease persuasion when the message arguments were weak. When an argument quality main effect is found in conjunction with a main effect of the experimental variable, the variable may be biasing the already high levels of elaboration. Of course, to examine the multiple roles for message tailoring fully, it would be necessary to include a manipulation of tailoring and argument quality along with a manipulation of the extent of thinking.

It is also useful to assess ancillary measures such as the number and valence of cognitive responses generated and the confidence in one's thoughts and attitudes to determine the underlying processes of persuasion more thoroughly. That is, the positivity of cognitive responses can also be indicative of the direction and extent of message processing. For example, cognitive responses should be more likely to mediate the impact of argument quality on attitudes under high-elaboration conditions. Thought positivity can be computed as the ratio of positive minus negative thoughts to the total number of thoughts generated (see Cacioppo, Harkins, & Petty, 1981, for more on thought-listing techniques). Finally, additional measures of cognitive processing such as message recall, reading times, or self-reported effort can provide further information about the extent of elaboration, although they are imperfect when used in isolation.

Of course, the use of multiple manipulations and measurements can be difficult to achieve in practice. Field settings can often provide pragmatic limitations on the types of manipulations and measures that one is able to implement. More important, there could be serious ethical concerns associated with providing weak arguments for engaging in positive health behaviors. No doubt, this is likely one of the reasons for the limited use of argument-quality manipulations in health communication research to date. However, argument-quality manipulations have been used in some experiments (Rosen, 2000), and when combined with a thorough debriefing, including distribution of appropriate materials, argument-quality effects can provide important insight into the functioning of variables like tailoring. More likely, treatments can be pilot-tested in a controlled laboratory context in which strong and weak arguments are used to understand the mechanisms behind an effect (such as whether the variable is operating as a cue or increasing thinking). Once the desired outcome is obtained, the treatment can be taken to the field where only strong arguments would be used.

Implications for Practitioners

Research shows that the ELM can be used to derive more effective health communications and persuasion interventions.

To effect durable and influential attitude change, practitioners should attempt to increase the elaboration of the message recipients, that is, the extent to which people relate the ideas in the message to their prior knowledge and beliefs (see Petty & Krosnick, 1995; Petty & Cacioppo, 1986). A common problem noted by researchers is that recipients of health communications are often unmotivated to process carefully the materials they receive (Scott, 1996; Scott & Ambroson, 1994). This might lead some to suggest that developers of health messages should put their energies toward injecting peripheral cues into their communications. Although this could have a positive short-term impact, long-lasting attitude changes are unlikely to result from this strategy. Instead, procedures that increase the formation of highly elaborated, accessible, and well-integrated attitudes will be most likely to result in actual and sustained behavioral change.

One means of inducing elaboration is by increasing the perceived personal relevance of the communication (Johnson & Eagly, 1989; Petty & Cacioppo, 1979b). Different kinds of message matching or tailoring could be effective in this regard (Kreuter et al., 1999; Petty et al., 2000), even for those who are dispositionally prone to engaging in low-effort cognitive strategies (Bakker, 1999). Making individuals feel personally responsible or accountable for their own health outcomes could also increase attention to health-related communications (see Petty, Harkins, & Williams, 1980; Tetlock, 1983). In addition, if individuals believe that their current health beliefs or practices place them in the minority, they may elaborate more on the message to resolve the surprise that can result from being discrepant from others (Baker & Petty, 1994). Other variables with an impact on message elaboration have been reviewed extensively elsewhere (Petty & Wegener, 1998a; Petty, Wheeler, & Tormala, in press) and could prove useful in health communication campaigns.

In addition to these motivational variables, ability variables can have an effect on message elaboration. Elaboration of health communications should be higher when the communications are presented in a medium that permits self-pacing, for example, by using a written medium rather than audio or video media (Chaiken & Eagly, 1976) in an environment without distractions (Petty et al., 1976) and in language that recipients easily understand (Hafer, Reynolds, & Obertynski, 1996). Because the language used to describe health conditions and treatments is often quite technical, this latter prescription may require pretesting of the recipient population to ensure that the language is not perceived to be too technical. Perceptions that the message is too technical can decrease elaboration by its impact on perceived ability, even though actual ability may be adequate for elaborative processing (see Yalch & Elmore-Yalch, 1984). Alternatively, the educational background of the targets of many health communications could inhibit their ability to process verbal information, and such limitations should be taken into account.

High levels of elaboration will increase the impact of argument quality. Thus, the use of strong arguments is another important aspect of any health intervention. Argument strength can be determined by pretesting arguments on subsets of the target population. Particularly effective messages can be developed when the concerns of the target population are measured and arguments are developed to address each concern. More finely grained procedures may isolate subpopulations of the larger population that share similar concerns. For example, single individuals with multiple partners may be more interested in the efficacy of condoms for preventing sexually transmitted diseases, whereas married individuals with a single partner may be more interested in the efficacy of condoms for preventing conception. Once developed, the tailored arguments can be pretested not only to ensure that they are perceived as cogent by the target segments, but that they also elicit favorable thoughts rather than counterarguments. Adjustments can be made on the basis of such pretests before a broader distribution of the materials. Argument tailoring can thus serve as one means of ensuring that each population receives arguments that are perceived to be relevant and are compelling (Kreuter et al., 2000). Recent technological advances have made tailoring procedures increasingly efficient and affordable (Kreuter et al., 2000). Of course, tailoring the message arguments is only one type of self-matching strategy that might be used effectively to increase message elaboration.

Finally, assessment of the intervention's efficacy should be made, and adjustments should be made on the basis of the assessment. An important element in such an assessment is a measure of the recipients' attitudes. Message learning can occur in the absence of attitude change (Helweg-Larsen & Collins, 1997; MacNair et al., 1991); and differing levels of attitude change can occur with equal increases in knowledge (Bakker, 1999). Also, since all attitude change is not the same, indicators of the strength of the changed attitude, such as the accessibility of the attitude or the confidence in the attitude, should also be taken (Petty & Krosnick, 1995).

Conclusion

The ELM, a useful framework for interpreting and predicting the impact that health communications have on subsequent attitudes and behavior, proposes that attitudes can be formed as the result of different types of processes. Peripheral route processes are those that involve minimal cognitive effort and instead rely on superficial cues or heuristics as the primary bases for attitude change. Central route processes are those that involve effortful cognitive elaboration and rely on careful scrutiny of issue-relevant information and one's own cognitive responses as the primary bases for attitude change. Although each process can sometimes result in attitudes with similar valence, the two processes typically lead to attitudes with different consequences. High-effort central route processes are more likely to lead to attitudes that are persistent over time, resistant to counterattack, and influential in guiding thought and behavior than are peripheral route processes (Krosnick & Petty, 1995). Because enduring attitude and behavioral change are likely to be key goals of any health communication campaign, promoting attitude formation by central route processes is important. Consequently, using techniques that increase the perceived relevance of the communication and the quality of the arguments will promote achievement of the communicators' goals. A thorough understanding of these principles should result in more effective health communication campaigns that efficiently promote the adoption of health-protective behaviors.

Notes

1. Our aim here is not to assess the validity of stage models. As Weinstein, Rothman, and Sutton (1998) noted, the fact that personalization or tailoring can alter persuasion outcomes does not bear on the validity of stage models.

2. It might be argued that tailoring itself constitutes a manipulation of argument quality. However, the goal of most tailoring research is to uncover the dimensions of an object or issue that are important for a person, such as price or social consequences. The information that is presented on these dimensions, however, can constitute strong (for example, "less expensive than all leading brands") or weak ("costs just slightly more than the leading brands") evidence in favor of the position advocated (see Petty & Wegener, 1998b).

References

Ajzen, I., & Fishbein, M. (2000). Attitudes and the attitude-behavior relation: Reasoned and automatic processes. In W. Stroebe & M. Hewstone (Eds.), *European review of social psychology* (Vol. 11, pp. 1–33). New York: Wiley.

Alcalay, R., Ghee, A., & Scrimshaw, S. (1993). Designing prenatal care messages for low-income Mexican women. *Public Health Reports, 108,* 354–362.

Baker, S. M., & Petty, R. E. (1994). Majority and minority influence: Source position imbalance as a determinant of message scrutiny. *Journal of Personality and Social Psychology, 67,* 5–19.

Bakker, A. B. (1999). Persuasive communication about AIDS prevention: Need for cognition determines the impact of message format. *AIDS Education and Prevention, 11,* 150–162.

Bandura, A. (1986). *Social foundations of thought and action.* Upper Saddle River, NJ: Prentice Hall.

Bartzokas, C., & Slade, P. (1991). Motivation to comply with infection control procedures. *Journal of Hospital Infection, 18* (Suppl. A), 508–514.

Brehm, J. W. (1956). Post-decision changes in the desirability of alternatives. *Journal of Abnormal and Social Psychology, 52,* 384–389.

Brock, T. C., Brannon, L. A., & Bridgwater, C. (1990). Message effectiveness can be increased by matching appeals to recipients' self-schemas: Laboratory demonstrations and a national field experiment. In S. J. Agres & J. A. Edell (Eds.), *Emotion in advertising: Theoretical and practical explorations* (pp. 285–315). Westport, CT: Quorum Books.

Brown, D. W. (1974). Adolescent attitudes and lawful behavior. *Public Opinion Quarterly, 38,* 98–106.

Brug, J., Steenhaus, I., Van Assema, P., & de Vries, H. (1996). The impact of computer-tailored nutrition intervention. *Preventive Medicine, 25,* 236–242.

Cacioppo, J. T., Harkins, S. G., & Petty, R. E. (1981). The nature of attitudes and cognitive responses and their relationship to behavior. In R. E. Petty, T. M. Ostrom, & T. C. Brock (Eds.), *Cognitive responses in persuasion* (pp. 31–54). Hillsdale, NJ: Erlbaum.

Cacioppo, J. T., & Petty, R. E. (1979). Effects of message repetition and position on cognitive response, recall, and persuasion. *Journal of Personality and Social Psychology, 37,* 97–109.

Cacioppo, J. T., & Petty, R. E. (1982). The need for cognition. *Journal of Personality and Social Psychology, 42,* 116–131.

Cacioppo, J. T., Petty, R. E., Feinstein, J. A., & Jarvis, W.B.G. (1996). Dispositional differences in cognitive motivation: The life and times of individuals varying in need for cognition. *Psychological Bulletin, 119,* 197–253.

Cacioppo, J. T., Petty, R. E., Kao, C. F., & Rodriguez, R. (1986). Central and peripheral routes to persuasion: An individual difference perspective. *Journal of Personality and Social Psychology, 51,* 1032–1043.

Cacioppo, J. T., Petty, R. E., & Morris, K. J. (1983). Effects of need for cognition on message evaluation, recall, and persuasion. *Journal of Personality and Social Psychology, 45,* 805–818.

Cacioppo, J. T., Petty, R. E., & Sidera, J. (1982). The effects of salient self-schema on the evaluation of proattitudinal editorials: Top-down versus bottom-up message processing. *Journal of Experimental Social Psychology, 18,* 324–338.

Campbell, D. T., & Stanley, J. C. (1964). *Experimental and quasi-experimental designs for research.* Skokie, IL: Rand McNally.

Campbell, M. K, DeVellis, B. M., Strecher, V. J., Ammerman, A. S., DeVillis, R. F., & Sandler, R. S. (1994). Improving dietary behavior: The effectiveness of tailored messages in primary care. *American Journal of Public Health, 84,* 783–787.

Chaiken, S. (1987). The heuristic model of persuasion. In M. P. Zanna & J. M. Olson (Eds.), *Social influence: The Ontario symposium* (Vol. 5, pp. 3–39). Hillsdale, NJ: Erlbaum.

Chaiken, S., & Eagly, A. H. (1976). Communication modality as a determinant of message persuasiveness and message comprehensibility. *Journal of Personality and Social Psychology, 34,* 605–614.

Chaiken, S., & Maheswaran, D. (1994). Heuristic processing can bias systematic processing: Effects of source credibility, argument ambiguity, and task importance on attitude judgment. *Journal of Personality and Social Psychology, 66,* 460–473.

Chan, S.S.W. (1999). Media use of expert sources and its effects on public opinion. *Dissertation Abstracts International Section A: Humanities and Social Sciences, 60,* 0577.

DeBono, K. G. (1987). Investigating the social-adjustive and value-expressive functions of attitudes: Implications for persuasion processes. *Journal of Personality and Social Psychology, 52,* 279–287.

Dinoff, B. L., & Kowalski, R. M. (1999). Reducing AIDS risk behavior: The combined efficacy of protection motivation theory and the Elaboration Likelihood Model. *Journal of Social and Clinical Psychology, 18,* 223–239.

Drossaert, C.H.C., Boer, H., & Seydel, E. R. (1996). Health education to improve repeat participation in the Dutch breast cancer screening program: Evaluation of a leaflet tailored to previous participants. *Patient Education and Counseling, 28,* 121–131.

Eagly, A. H., & Chaiken, S. (1993). *The psychology of attitudes.* Fort Worth, TX: Harcourt Brace.

Edwards, K. (1990). The interplay of affect and cognition in attitude formation and change. *Journal of Personality and Social Psychology, 59,* 202–216.

Fabrigar, L. R., & Petty, R. E. (1999). The role of the affective and cognitive bases of attitudes in susceptibility to affectively and cognitively based persuasion. *Personality and Social Psychology Bulletin, 25,* 363–381.

Fishbein, M., & Ajzen, I. (1975). *Belief, attitude, intention, and behavior: An introduction to theory and research.* Reading, MA: Addison-Wesley.

Fleming, M. A., & Petty, R. E. (2000). Identity and persuasion: An elaboration likelihood approach. In M. A. Hogg & D. J. Terry (Eds.), *Attitudes, behavior, and social context: The role of norms and group membership* (pp. 171–199). Hillsdale, NJ: Erlbaum.

Greenwald, A. G., & Albert, R. D. (1968). Acceptance and recall of improvised arguments. *Journal of Personality and Social Psychology, 8,* 31–34.

Hafer, C. L., Reynolds, K. L., & Obertynski, M. A. (1996). Message comprehensibility and persuasion: Effects of complex language in counterattitudinal appeals to laypeople. *Social Cognition, 14,* 317–337.

Haugtvedt, C. P., & Petty, R. E. (1992). Personality and persuasion: Need for cognition moderates the persistence and resistance of attitude changes. *Journal of Personality and Social Psychology, 63,* 308–319.

Heesacker, M., Petty, R. E., & Cacioppo, J. T. (1983). Field dependence and attitude change: Source credibility can alter persuasion by affecting message-relevant thinking. *Journal of Personality, 51,* 653–666.

Helweg-Larsen, M., & Collins, B. E. (1997). A social psychological perspective on the role of knowledge about AIDS in AIDS prevention. *Current Directions in Psychological Science, 6,* 23–26.

Hovland, C. I., Janis, I. L., & Kelley, H. H. (1953). *Communication and persuasion.* New Haven, CT: Yale University Press.

Hovland, C. I., Lumsdaine, A. A., & Sheffield, F. D. (1949). *Experiments on mass communication.* Princeton, NJ: Princeton University Press.

Isen, A. M., & Simmonds, S. F. (1978). The effect of feeling good on a helping task that is incompatible with good mood. *Social Psychology, 41,* 346–349.

Janis, I. L., & Feshback, S. (1953). Effects of fear arousing communications. *Journal of Abnormal and Social Psychology, 48,* 78–92.

Janis, I. L., & King, B. T. (1954). The influence of role-playing on opinion change. *Journal of Abnormal and Social Psychology, 49,* 211–218.

Johnson, B. T., & Eagly, A. H. (1989). Effects of involvement on persuasion: A meta-analysis. *Psychological Bulletin, 106,* 290–314.

Kahneman, D., Knetsch, J., & Thaler, R. (1991). The endowment effect, loss aversion, and status quo bias. *Journal of Economic Perspectives, 5,* 328–338.

Kanellis, M. J., Logan, L. L., & Jakobson, J. (1997). Changes in maternal attitudes toward baby bottle tooth decay. *Pediatric Dentistry, 19,* 57–60.

Kerssens, J. J., & van Yperen, E. M. (1996). Patient's evaluation of dietetic care: Testing a cognitive-attitude approach. *Patient Education and Counseling, 27,* 217–226.

Kreuter, M. W., Bull, F. C., Clark, E. M., & Oswald, D. L. (1999). Understanding how people process health information: A comparison of tailored and nontailored weight-loss materials. *Health Psychology, 18,* 487–494.

Kreuter, M. W., Farrell, D., Olevitch, L., & Brennan, L. (2000). *Tailoring health messages: Customizing communication with computer technology.* Hillsdale, NJ: Erlbaum.

Krosnick, J. A., & Petty, R. E. (1995). Attitude strength: An overview. In R. E. Petty & J. A. Krosnick (Eds.), *Attitude strength: Antecedents and consequences* (pp. 1–24). Hillsdale, NJ: Erlbaum .

Lavine, H., & Snyder, M. (1996). Cognitive processing and the functional matching effect in persuasion: The mediating role of subjective perceptions of message quality. *Journal of Experimental Social Psychology, 32,* 580–604.

Leippe, M. R., & Elkin, R. A. (1987). When motives clash: Issue involvement and response involvement as determinants of persuasion. *Journal of Personality and Social Psychology, 52,* 269–278.

Lockhart, L. K. (1999). Reactions to favorable and unfavorable medical diagnoses: Do individual difference factors make a difference? *Dissertation Abstracts International: Section B: The Sciences and Engineering, 60,* 0411.

Mackie, D. M., Worth, L. T., & Asuncion, A. G. (1990). Processing of persuasive in-group messages. *Journal of Personality and Social Psychology, 58,* 812–822.

MacNair, R. R., Elliott, T. R., & Yoder, B. (1991). AIDS prevention groups as persuasive appeals: Effects on attitudes about precautionary behaviors among persons in substance abuse treatment. *Small Group Research, 22,* 301–319.

Mulvihill, C. (1996). AIDS education for college students: Review and proposal for a research-based curriculum. *AIDS Education and Prevention, 8,* 11–25.

Nuttin, J. M. (1985). Narcissism beyond Gestalt and awareness: The name letter effect. *European Journal of Social Psychology, 15,* 353–361.

Perloff, R. M., & Brock, T. C. (1980). And thinking makes it so: Cognitive responses to persuasion. In M. Roloff & G. Miller (Eds.), *Persuasion: New directions in theory and research* (pp. 67–100). Thousand Oaks, CA: Sage.

Petty, R. E. (1994). Two routes to persuasion: State of the art. In G. d'Ydewalle & P. Eelen (Eds.), *International perspectives on psychological science, Vol. 2: The state of the art* (pp. 229–247). Hillsdale, NJ: Erlbaum.

Petty, R. E., Baker, S., & Gleicher, F. (1991). Attitudes and drug abuse prevention: Implications of the Elaboration Likelihood Model of persuasion. In L. Donohew, H. E. Sypher, & W. J. Bukoski (Eds.), *Persuasive communication and drug abuse prevention* (pp. 71–90). Hillsdale, NJ: Erlbaum.

Petty, R. S., Briñol, P., & Tormala, Z. L. (in press). Thought confidence as a determinant of persuasion: The self-validation hypothesis. *Journal of Personality and Social Psychology.*

Petty, R. E., & Cacioppo, J. T. (1979a). Effects of forewarning of persuasive intent and involvement on cognitive responses and persuasion. *Personality and Social Psychology Bulletin, 5,* 173–176.

Petty, R. E., & Cacioppo, J. T. (1979b). Issue involvement can increase or decrease persuasion by enhancing message-relevant cognitive responses. *Journal of Personality and Social Psychology, 37,* 1915–1926.

Petty, R. E., & Cacioppo, J. T. (1981). *Attitudes and persuasion: Classic and contemporary approaches.* Dubuque, IA: Brown.

Petty, R. E., & Cacioppo, J. T. (1984). The effects of involvement on responses to argument quantity and quality: Central and peripheral routes to persuasion. *Journal of Personality & Social Psychology, 46,* 69–81.

Petty, R. E., & Cacioppo, J. T. (1986). The Elaboration Likelihood Model of persuasion. In L. Berkowitz (Ed.), *Advances in experimental social psychology* (Vol. 19, pp. 123–205). Orlando, FL: Academic Press.

Petty, R. E., & Cacioppo, J. T. (1990). Involvement and persuasion: Tradition versus integration. *Psychological Bulletin, 107,* 367–374.

Petty, R. E., Cacioppo, J. T., & Goldman, R. (1981). Personal involvement as a determinant of argument-based persuasion. *Journal of Personality and Social Psychology, 41,* 847–855.

Petty, R. E., Cacioppo, J. T., & Schumann, D. (1983). Central and peripheral routes to advertising effectiveness: The moderating role of involvement. *Journal of Consumer Research, 10,* 135–146.

Petty, R. E., Fabrigar, L. R., & Wegener, D. T., (2001). Emotional impact on attitudes and attitude change. In R. J. Davidson, H. H. Goldsmith, & K. R. Scherer (Eds.), *Handbook of affective sciences.* Cambridge: Cambridge University Press.

Petty, R. E., Harkins, S. G., & Williams, K. D. (1980). The effects of group diffusion of cognitive effort on attitudes: An information-processing view. *Journal of Personality and Social Psychology, 38,* 81–92.

Petty, R. E., Haugtvedt, C. P., & Smith, S. M. (1995). Elaboration as a determinant of attitude strength: Creating attitudes that are persistent, resistant, and predictive of behavior. In R. E. Petty & J. A. Krosnick (Eds.), *Attitude strength: Antecedents and consequences* (pp. 93–130). Mahwah, NJ: Erlbaum.

Petty, R. E., & Krosnick, J. A. (Eds.). (1995). *Attitude strength: Antecedents and consequences.* Mahwah, NJ: Erlbaum.

Petty, R. E., Schumann, D. W., Richman, S. A., & Strathman, A. J. (1993). Positive mood and persuasion: Different roles for affect under high- and low-elaboration conditions. *Journal of Personality and Social Psychology, 64,* 5–20.

Petty, R. E., Tormala, Z. L., Briñol, P., & Jarvis, W.B.G. (2001). Meta-cognitive factors in persuasion. In S. E. Heckler, & S. Shapiro (Eds.), *Proceedings of the Society for Consumer Psychology Winter Conference* (pp. 170–173). Tempe, AZ: Society for Consumer Psychology.

Petty, R. E., & Wegener, D. T. (1991). Thought systems, argument quality, and persuasion. In R.S.J. Wyer & T. K. Srull (Eds.), *The content, structure, and operation of thought systems.* (pp. 147–161). Hillsdale, NJ: Erlbaum.

Petty, R. E., & Wegener, D. T. (1998a). Attitude change: Multiple roles for persuasion variables. In D. T. Gilbert & S. T. Fiske (Eds.), *The handbook of social psychology* (4th ed., Vol. 1, pp. 323–390). New York: McGraw-Hill.

Petty, R. E., & Wegener, D. T. (1998b). Matching verus mismatching attitude functions: Implications for scrutiny of persuasive messages. *Personality and Social Psychology Bulletin, 24,* 227–240.

Petty, R. E., Wells, G. L., & Brock, T. C. (1976). Distraction can enhance or reduce yielding to propaganda: Thought disruption versus effort justification. *Journal of Personality & Social Psychology, 34,* 874–884.

Petty, R. E., Wheeler, S. C., & Bizer, G. Y. (1999). Is there one persuasion process or more? Lumping versus splitting in attitude change theories. *Psychological Inquiry, 10,* 156–163.

Petty, R. E., Wheeler, S. C., & Bizer, G. Y. (2000). Attitude functions and persuasion: An elaboration likelihood approach to matched versus mismatched messages. In G. R. Maio & J. M. Olson (Eds.), *Why we evaluate: Functions of attitudes* (pp. 133–162). Hillside, NJ: Erlbaum.

Petty, R. E., Wheeler, S. C., & Tormala, Z. (in press). Persuasion and attitude change. In T. Millon & M. J. Lerner (Eds.), *Comprehensive handbook of psychology.* New York: Wiley.

Prochaska, J. O., DiClemente, C. C., & Norcross, J. C. (1992). In search of how people change: Applications to addictive behaviors. *American Psychologist, 47,* 1102–1114.

Quinlan, K. B., & McCaul, K. D. (2000). Matched and mismatched interventions with young adult smokers: Testing a stage theory. *Health Psychology, 19,* 165–171.

Rosen, C. S. (2000). Integrating stage and continuum models to explain processing of exercise messages and exercise initiation among sedentary college students. *Health Psychology, 19,* 172–180.

Rosenthal, L. H. (1997). A new perspective on the relation between fear and persuasion: The application of dual-process models. *Dissertation Abstracts International: Section B: The Sciences and Engineering, 58*(6-B), 3371.

Rothman, A. J. (2000). Toward a theory-based analysis of behavioral maintenance. *Health Psychology, 19* (Suppl. 1), 64–69.

Rothman, A. J., & Schwarz, N. (1998). Constructing perceptions of vulnerability: Personal relevance and the use of experiential information in health judgments. *Personality and Social Psychology Bulletin, 24,* 1053–1064

Scott, C. G. (1996). Understanding attitude change in developing effective substance abuse prevention programs for adolescents. *School Counselor, 43,* 187–195.

Scott, C. G., & Ambroson, D. L. (1994). The rocky road to change: Implications for substance abuse programs on college campuses. *Journal of American College Health, 42,* 291–296.

Shavitt, S. (1989). Operationalizing functional theories of attitude. In A. R. Pratkanis, S. J. Breckler, & A. G. Greenwald (Eds.), *Attitude structure and function* (pp. 311–338). Hillsdale, NJ: Erlbaum.

Sivacek, J., & Crano, W. D. (1982). Vested interest as a moderator of attitude-behavior consistency. *Journal of Personality and Social Psychology, 43,* 210–221.

Skinner, C. S., Strecher, V. J., & Hospers, H. J. (1994). Physician recommendations for mammography: Do tailored messages make a difference? *American Journal of Public Health, 84,* 43–49.

Skumanich, S., & Kintsfather, D. (1996). Promoting the organ donor card: A causal model of persuasion effects. *Social Science and Medicine, 43,* 401–408.

Snyder, M., & DeBono, K. G. (1985). Appeals to image and claims about quality: Understanding the psychology of advertising. *Journal of Personality and Social Psychology, 49,* 586–597.

Staats, A. W., & Staats, C. (1958). Attitudes established by classical conditioning. *Journal of Abnormal and Social Psychology, 67,* 159–167.

Taylor, S. E., & Brown, J. D. (1988). Illusion and well-being: A social psychological perspective on mental health. *Psychological Bulletin, 103,* 193–210.

Tetlock, P. E. (1983). Accountability and the complexity of thought. *Journal of Personality and Social Psychology, 45,* 74–83.

Triandis, H. C. (1977). *Interpersonal behavior.* Monterey, CA: Brooks/Cole.

Triandis, H. C. (1979). Values, attitudes, and interpersonal behavior. *Nebraska Symposium on Motivation* (Vol. 27, pp. 195–259). Lincoln: University of Nebraska Press.

Wegener, D. T., & Petty, R. E. (1996). Effects of mood on persuasion processes: Enhancing, reducing, and biasing scrutiny of attitude-relevant information. In L. L. Martin & A. Tesser (Eds.), *Striving and feeling: Interactions among goals, affect, and self-regulation* (pp. 329–362). Hillside, NJ: Erlbaum.

Wegener, D. T., Petty, R. E., & Klein, D. J. (1994). Effects of mood on high elaboration attitude change: The mediating role of likelihood judgments. *European Journal of Social Psychology, 24,* 25–43.

Wegener, D. T., Petty, R. E., & Smith, S. M. (1995). Positive mood can increase or decrease message scrutiny: The hedonic contingency view of mood and message processing. *Journal of Personality and Social Psychology, 69,* 5–15.

Weinstein, N. D. (1988). The precaution adoption process. *Health Psychology, 7,* 355–386.

Weinstein, N. D., Rothman, A. J., & Sutton, S. R. (1998). Stage theories of health behavior: Conceptual and methodological issues. *Health Psychology, 17,* 290–299.

Weinstein, N. D., & Sandman, P. M. (1992). A model of the precaution adoption process: Evidence from home radon testing. *Health Psychology, 11,* 170–180.

Weiskotten, D. R. (1993). The Elaboration Likelihood Model: Effects of a brief psycho-educational intervention on early adolescents' attitudes toward AIDS. *Dissertation Abstracts International, 54*(6-B), 3393.

Yalch, R. F., & Elmore-Yalch, R. (1984). The effect of numbers on the route to persuasion. *Journal of Consumer Research, 11,* 522–527.

CHAPTER FIVE

APPLICATION OF THE AUTHORITATIVE PARENTING MODEL TO ADOLESCENT HEALTH BEHAVIOR

Bruce Simons-Morton
Jessica Hartos

Sammy: Can I take the car?

  Mom: Where do you want to go?

Sammy: To Rick's.

  Mom: What are you two going to do?

Sammy: We are going to hang out there and maybe go to a movie later.

  Mom: What time are you going to be home?

Sammy: Midnight.

  Mom: You know you can't drive past 10 P.M.

Sammy: Okay, 10 P.M.

  Mom: All right, you can take the car. Remember what we talked about: drive carefully, just you and Rick, and no highway driving.

Sammy: I know, I know, and come home by 10 P.M. or I won't get to use the car next week, and call if we go to the movies or anywhere else.

  Mom: Okay. Tell Rick good job on his last English test and I will see you later.

Sammy: Thanks! Bye!

Sixteen year-old Sammy just got his driver's license and is eager to drive. We know that motor vehicle crashes are the leading cause of injury and death for adolescents sixteen through nineteen years of age. What can we learn about how parenting affects child and adolescent adjustment, development, and behavior that can be applied to the prevention of motor vehicle crashes among young drivers? Which aspects of parenting make a difference, and how can protective parenting behaviors be fostered in families with adolescent children?

Parenting is a complex and multifaceted activity for socializing children. There are parenting goals, for example, that aim to instill certain attitudes, behaviors, and qualities in children. There are overall qualities of the parent-child relationship, such as warmth and support, that provide context for parent-child interactions. In addition, there are many parenting practices, ranging from spanking to encouragement, that are specific to parent-child interactions. Over the years, different theories and theorists have focused on different facets of parenting as "good," "important," and "beneficial."

The parenting style approach attributed to Baumrind (1978) has gained rapid acceptance and growth in the past several decades as a robust and useful construct for expressing relations among parenting behavior and child and adolescent growth and development. Within this approach, what is of overall importance is the extent to which parents are responsive to their children's needs and demanding of their children's behaviors.

Authoritative parenting is related to multiple positive child and adolescent outcomes, ranging from higher academic achievement to a reduced amount of deviant behaviors.

Parents who are both highly demanding and highly responsive are considered authoritative. Substantial research indicates that authoritative parenting is related to multiple positive child and adolescent outcomes, ranging from higher academic achievement to a reduced amount of deviant behaviors.

The constellation of parenting behaviors related to the authoritative parenting construct, including parenting goals for children's behaviors, the emotional climate for parent-child interactions, and responsive and demanding parenting practices, can assist in the design of prevention programs to affect positively child outcomes of interest, including adolescent driving behaviors.

The Authoritative Parenting Style

Parents are responsible for socializing their children: teaching appropriate behaviors and values for social situations. They "have the complex task of adjusting their demands and disciplinary methods flexibly to the developing capacities of the child so as to encourage social responsibility without discouraging independence and individuality" (Baumrind, 1978, p. 249). This task will vary depending on the developmental period of the child. In infancy, primary socialization tasks are to meet children's physical needs and sustain their natural exploratory activity. For children, parents assume a much more directive role as they deal with important socialization processes such as parental control, maturity demands, and use of reasoning. During adolescence, teens' dependency on parental control diminishes as new reference groups, values, and behaviors emerge; thus, parental control decreases and independence granting increases. "At each stage, then, the duties and rights of parents and children differ, finally approximating the balance which characterizes adult relations" (Baumrind, 1978, p. 268).

Prior to Baumrind's work, theories and theorists basically agreed that parent socialization practices incorporated aspects of warmth and control and that a combination of high warmth and control related to positive child and adolescent adjustment. However, aspects of parenting were conceptualized in various ways. These included parental attitudes and beliefs toward child rearing, specific parenting practices and behaviors, and the emotional relationship between the parent and child. Baumrind's work revolutionized thinking by incorporating all three aspects into the conceptualization of parenting styles (for excellent reviews, see Darling & Steinberg, 1993; Maccoby & Martin, 1983).

In her early work (Baumrind, 1967, 1971), Baumrind was interested in which parenting practices related to children's adjustment. She collected data on the behaviors of preschool children (that is, self-control, approach-avoidance behavior, mood, self-reliance, and peer affiliation) and their parents (that is, control, maturity demands, communication, and nurturance) through interviews, home visits, and structured observations. She found that parents whose children were self-reliant, self-controlled, buoyant, and approach oriented were firm, loving, demanding, and understanding. In contrast, the parents of dependent, immature children lacked control and were reserved with their children, and parents of dysphoric and disaffiliative children were firm, punitive, and unaffectionate.

For Baumrind (1967), parental control, which she referred to as parents' attempts to integrate the child into the family and society by demanding behavioral compliance, was the defining feature of three qualitatively different parenting styles—authoritative, authoritarian, and permissive—each with its own characteristic parental attitudes, parenting practices, and parent-child interactions (Baumrind, 1978). Authoritative parents were rational and issue oriented, encouraged verbal give and take, reasoned with children, exerted control when children disobeyed, recognized children's developmental levels, and set standards for future conduct. In contrast, authoritarian parents valued children's obedience, restricted children's autonomy, favored forceful compliance measures, and were either very concerned and protective or neglectful. Permissive parents accepted child impulses and actions and considered themselves to be resources for the child rather than directive agents responsible for shaping child behavior and personality. Permissive parents could have been either very loving or self-involved.

Maccoby and Martin (1983) furthered this line of thinking by defining Baumrind's parenting styles along two dimensions: demandingness and responsiveness. Demandingness referred to the extent to which parents demand mature behavior, supervise activities, and discipline transgressions. Responsiveness referred to the extent to which parents are attuned to their children's physical, social, and emotional needs and support their growing autonomy. From these dimensions, four parenting styles emerge: authoritative, authoritarian, permissive-indulgent, and neglectful-indifferent. Authoritative and authoritarian parenting are very similar to Baumrind's initial conceptualization, but what she called permissive parenting was divided into two types: those that are responsive but not demanding (indulgent-permissive) and those that are neither responsive nor demanding (indifferent-neglectful). Features of each parenting style (Baumrind, 1991; Maccoby & Martin, 1983) are listed in Figure 5.1.

FIGURE 5.1. FEATURES OF PARENTING STYLES.

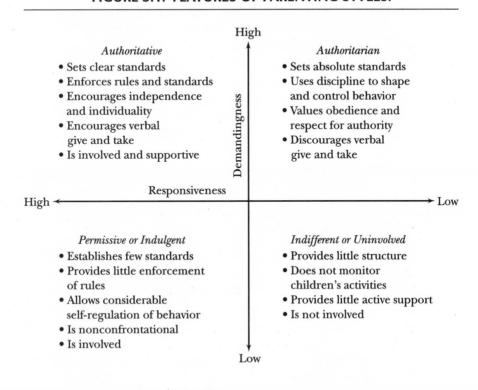

Whereas Baumrind (1971) defined parenting styles as qualitatively different, current thinking in parenting styles, attributable to Maccoby and Martin (1983), is based on the quantitative differences measured along the two dimensions of responsiveness and demandingness (Darling & Steinberg, 1993). Measures of parental responsiveness seek to quantify how frequently, consistently, and well parents attend to their children. Measures of demandingness seek to quantify how frequently, consistently, and clearly parents supervise and monitor their children, set standards for child behavior, and encourage specific, goal-directed behaviors. Research indicates that parental demandingness is positively related to behavioral adjustment and responsiveness is positively related to psychosocial development (Gray & Steinberg, 1999; Parish & McCluskey, 1994), suggesting that both contribute to positive psychosocial adjustment in children.

Thus, the fourfold classification of parenting styles describes how parents reconcile "joint needs of children for nurturance and limit-setting" (Baumrind, 1991, p. 62), and this union affects the development of instrumental competence, including social responsibility, independence, achievement orientation, and vigor (Baumrind, 1978). Despite some variation in the benefits of authoritative parenting across ethnicity, socioeconomic status, and family structure (Dornbusch, Ritter, Leiderman, Roberts, & Fraleigh, 1987; Jackson, Henriksen, & Foshee, 1998; Lamborn, Mounts, Steinberg, & Dornbusch, 1991; Steinberg, Dornbusch, & Brown, 1992), "during the past twenty-five years, research based on Baumrind's conceptualization of parenting style has produced a remarkably consistent picture of the type of parenting conducive to the successful socialization of children into the dominant culture in the United States. Authoritative parenting—a constellation of parent attributes that includes emotional support, high standards, appropriate autonomy granting, and clear, bidirectional communication—has been shown to help children and adolescents develop an instrumental competence characterized by the balancing of societal and individual needs and responsibilities" (Darling & Steinberg, 1993, p. 487).

Research Linking Parenting Styles to Instrumental Competence Among Children and Adolescents

Substantial research supports relationships between authoritative parenting styles and instrumental competence among children and adolescents. For example, Mauro and Harris (2000) found that authoritative parenting was positively related to successful delay of gratification in preschool children, whereas permissive parenting was negatively related to it. In contrast to authoritarian and indifferent parenting, authoritative parenting has been positively associated with higher levels of psychosocial competence, maturity, and moral reasoning in fourteen- to eighteen-year-olds (Baumrind, 1991; Boyes & Allen, 1993; Lamborn et al., 1991;

Mantzicopoulos & Oh-Hwang, 1998). Dominguez and Carton (1997) found that authoritative parenting was related to self-actualization among college students.

In addition to responsible behaviors, authoritative parenting is related to independence among children of all ages. In ethnically diverse samples of students from fourth through tenth grades, authoritative parenting was positively associated with, whereas authoritarian and neglectful parenting were inversely related to, self-esteem, self-control, conflict resolution, and resistance to peer pressure (Carlson, Uppal, & Prosser, 2000; Jackson et al., 1998). In other research with high school students, authoritarian parenting was related to obedience, conformity, and lower self-conceptions, whereas indulgent parenting was related to high levels of self-confidence (Lamborn et al., 1991; Steinberg, Lamborn, Darling, Mounts, & Dornbusch, 1994). Moreover, Strage and Brandt (1999) found that authoritative parenting qualities were related to college students' confidence levels.

Authoritative parenting style has also been linked to children's interpersonal relationships. For example, white and African American children aged nine through twenty-two with authoritative parents reported better interpersonal relationships with parents, peers, and teachers when compared to those with authoritarian or permissive parents (Hall & Bracken, 1996; Hein & Lewko, 1994; Hill, 1995; Jackson et al., 1998; Strage & Brandt, 1999). Durbin, Darling, Steinberg, and Brown (1993) found that high school students with authoritative parents were more likely to be involved in well-rounded crowds that reward adult- and peer-supported norms (for example, "populars" and "brains"). In contrast, teens with uninvolved parents were involved in crowds with anti-adult values (for example, "druggies"), and boys with indulgent parents were oriented toward fun-culture crowds (for example, partyers). In other research (Fischer & Crawford, 1992), having an authoritarian father was linked to higher codependency in college students than was having a permissive or uninvolved father.

Much research focuses on the authoritative parenting style and children's achievement orientations. Authoritative parenting was positively associated with school engagement in fourteen- to eighteen-year-olds (Steinberg, Lamborn, Dornbush, & Darling, 1992), academic aspirations in graduating seniors (Slicker, 1998), and organization, achievement, and intellectual orientation in African American high school and college students (Morrongiello, Hillier, & Bass, 1995). Hein and Lewko (1994) found that authoritative parenting was related to higher levels of achievement motivation in adolescents from twelve to twenty-two years of age. In other research, effective achievement and learning strategies among urban and suburban students in middle school, high school, and college were related positively to authoritative parenting and inversely to nonauthoritative parenting (Aunola, Stattin, & Nurmi, 2000; Boveja, 1998; Glasgow, Dornbusch, Troyer, Steinberg, & Ritter, 1997; Onatsu-Arvilommi, Nurmi, & Aunola, 1998; Strage & Brandt, 1999).

In addition, authoritative parenting is related to children's school performance. Authoritarian and neglectful parenting show inverse relationships with, whereas authoritative parenting shows positive relations with, school adjustment in children from elementary school to college (Jackson et al., 1998; Hickman, Bartholomae, & McKenry, 2000). In other research, authoritative parenting was related to school grades and academic achievement in ethnically diverse students from fourteen to twenty-eight years of age (Cohen & Rice, 1997; Dornbusch et al., 1987; Hein & Lewko, 1994; Paulson, 1994; Steinberg, Lamborn et al., 1992; Strage & Brandt, 1999; Taylor, Hinton, & Wilson, 1995).

Research Linking Parenting Styles to Health-Risk Behaviors Among Children and Adolescents

In addition to instrumental competence, more and more research shows inverse relationships between authoritative parenting and health-risk behaviors among children and adolescents. For example, research has indicated that authoritative parenting is related inversely, whereas authoritarian, neglectful, and permissive parenting is related positively, to tobacco and alcohol use in children from grades four through twelve (Cohen & Rice 1997; Fletcher & Jefferies, 1999; Jackson et al., 1998; Lamborn et al., 1991; Slicker, 1998; Steinberg et al., 1994). In addition, authoritative parenting is inversely related to drug use in high school students (Baumrind, 1991; Lamborn et al., 1991; Mounts & Steinberg, 1995; Slicker, 1998; Steinberg et al., 1994).

Authoritative parenting is conversely related to other problem behaviors among adolescents as well. In contrast to authoritarian, indulgent, and indifferent parenting, authoritative parenting was shown to be inversely related to anger and alienation in seventh and eighth graders (Fletcher & Jefferies, 1999; Jackson et al., 1998) and to aggression, psychological distress, delinquency, and school misconduct in high school students (Lamborn et al., 1991; Slicker, 1998; Steinberg et al., 1994). In addition, authoritative parenting was related inversely, whereas indulgent, authoritarian, and neglectful parenting was related positively, to weapon-carrying and interpersonal violence in ninth- and tenth-grade students (Jackson et al., 1998).

Moreover, Steinberg and colleagues (Steinberg et al., 1994) followed adolescents from fourteen to eighteen years of age over a year to determine if differences in adjustment outcomes related to parenting styles are upheld. They found that differences in achievement and problem behaviors were either maintained or increased over time. The authors suggested that adolescents with continued authoritative parenting maintain previous levels of high adjustment, whereas teenagers with neglectful parenting may continue to accumulate deleterious effects.

Application of Authoritative Parenting to Adolescent Health Behavior

It is clear that authoritative parenting is associated with positive adolescent outcomes. Given its advantages, researchers have been attempting to apply authoritative parenting concepts in intervention studies to address adolescent health behavior. Adolescence, however, is a complex developmental period. Adolescents are changing physically, socially, psychologically, and cognitively. Also, parenting roles change during adolescence (Holmbeck, Paikoff, & Brooks-Gunn, 1995). When children are young, parenting attempts to nurture, protect, and establish values. As children age into adolescents, parenting aims to guide, direct, and support growing autonomy and independence. In addition, parent-child relations during this time are commonly characterized by increased conflict, emotional distancing, strained communication, and fewer shared activities (Csikszentmihalyi & Larson, 1984; Paikoff & Brooks-Gunn, 1991; Steinberg, 1987, 1989, 1990). Even if family relationships are not distressed, adolescents have more freedom, more responsibilities, and more life experiences with less parental supervision (Holmbeck et al., 1995).

By adolescence, some aspects of the parent-child relationship are well established. Teens should have a fairly good understanding of how their parents will react to their behavior, and parents may employ a limited number of parenting practices that have worked well in the past. Although qualitative changes in parent-child relationships may occur during adolescence, aspects of the emotional climate of the parent-teen relationship established during childhood are likely to carry over into adolescence, providing the context for how amenable to parental influence teens are and how effective specific parenting practices are likely to be.

Although it is clear that authoritative parenting is beneficial, it is not as clear what comprises authoritative parenting. Parenting is a complex activity for socializing children that involves numerous facets, including overall qualities of the parent-child relationship, parenting goals to promote certain child qualities, and parenting practices specific to parent-child interactions. Traditionally, authoritative parenting style refers to the emotional climate between parent and child, but that seems to include aspects of all these parenting dimensions. Adding to the confusion, researchers have employed various measures for authoritative parenting ranging from overall parent-child interaction climate (for example, parents' responsiveness, demandingness, and autonomy granting) to more specific parenting behaviors (for example, amount of parental monitoring or communication). While operational definitions of each parenting style can be expected to differ depending on social context, developmental period, and method of assessment (Baumrind, 1991), the variability and overlap in definitions of style and behavior makes it difficult to determine the extent to which general parenting style and specific parenting practices contribute to child outcomes.

Moreover, substantial research on specific parenting practices, apart from parenting style but related to authoritative parenting (for example, high parental monitoring, high parental involvement), shows significant relations with instrumental behaviors, including academic achievement and lower rates of health-risk behaviors such as substance use and delinquency (Dishion, Patterson, & Kavanagh, 1992; Dishion, Patterson, & Reid, 1988; Patterson, 1995; 1996; Patterson, Reid, & Dishion, 1992; Taylor & Biglan, 1998). Simons-Morton and colleagues found that clear parental expectations against drinking protected early adolescents against early initiation of drinking (Simons-Morton et al., 1999). In addition, involved parents protected girls against smoking, whereas a combination of parental involvement, support, and regard protected boys against smoking initiation (Simons-Morton, Crump, Haynie, Eitel, Saylor, & Yu, 1999). In a separate analysis of these data contrasting peer and parent influences on smoking and drinking, Simons-Morton and colleagues (Simons-Morton, Haynie, Crump, Eitel, & Saylor, 2001) found that clear expectations, high involvement, and positive regard protected teens from smoking and drinking, even in the presence of negative peer influences. Ary and colleagues (1999) demonstrated in prospective research with adolescents that inadequate parental monitoring and increased parent-child conflict, within a context of poor family relationships, contributed to the development of adolescent problem behavior.

A Useful Model for Applying Authoritative Parenting to Interventions

Darling and Steinberg (1993) have cleverly conceptualized possible relationships between parenting goals, parenting styles, parenting practices, and adolescent outcomes. Their conceptualization recognizes that parenting starts with values and goals for socializing children. Socialization goals include specific child skills and behaviors such as appropriate manners, social skills, and self-control, as well as the development of more global qualities including critical thinking, achievement, and independence. These goals and values, in turn, influence both parenting style and parenting practices. For Darling and Steinberg, parenting practices are overt behaviors defined by specific content and socialization goals (for example, monitoring behavior to promote responsibility or applying consequences for aggressive behavior). Parenting style "is a constellation of attitudes toward the child that are communicated to the child and create an emotional climate in which the parent's behaviors are expressed" (p. 493). Thus, parenting style includes behaviors within parenting practices, as well as more subtle behaviors that communicate emotional attitude (for example, tone of voice or body language).

Darling and Steinberg (1993) suggest that parenting style influences adolescent outcomes in two important ways. First, it influences the effectiveness of specific parenting practices. For example, in contrast to the emotional climate created by authoritarian parents, the generally positive emotional climate between parents and youth created by authoritative parenting increases the likelihood of success of a parent behavior. Second, parenting style influences the adolescent's willingness to be socialized. Being responsive to children and having high standards for their behavior are beneficial not just at the time of interactions. Parents' long-term commitment to authoritative parenting may elicit in their children a willingness or receptiveness to parental demands. Hence, parent effectiveness in promoting appropriate behavior is the product of a positive emotional climate and consistent application of positive parenting practices.

Most parent education programs attempt to improve both emotional climate and parenting practices as they relate to specific parenting goals. Ample evidence exists for the effectiveness of parent intervention programs for what are commonly called behavioral family interventions, which focus on increasing the effective application of authoritative parenting practices. These interventions attempt to increase the following behaviors: (1) positive parent-child interactions, (2) parental reinforcement of appropriate behavior with praise and rewards, (3) establishing and communicating clear limits, and (4) applying consistent consequences and effective discipline (Taylor & Biglan, 1998). For example, the primary goal of intervention programs for child rearing in distressed families and families with disruptive children is to identify and reduce coercive behaviors, primarily by teaching parents noncoercive parenting practices (Patterson, 1982).

A few programs have systematically trained parents in nondistressed families in the development of behavioral parenting skills such as communicating, monitoring, and discipline. These programs have shown improvements in actual parenting practices that lead to reductions in problem behaviors among adolescents (Taylor & Biglan, 1998). For example, Irvine, Biglan, Smolkowski, Metzler, and Ary (1999) randomly assigned parents of at-risk middle school students in eight small communities to group education or wait-list conditions. Compared to wait-list parents, those in group education reported improved problem-solving interactions, more appropriately timed reactions to their children, better attitudes toward their children, and improvements in child antisocial behavior (Dishion et al., 1992; Patterson, 1995, 1996; Patterson et al., 1992). Relatedly, Hawkins and colleagues reported successful intervention with families of preadolescents, including improved communication (Catalano, Kosterman, Haggerty, Hawkins, &

Spoth, 1998; Kosterman, Hawkins, Spoth, Haggerty, & Zhu, 1997) and positive intervention effects on parent behaviors such as increased involvement, monitoring, and rule enforcement (Hawkins, Catalano, & Kent, 1991). Hence, it appears from research with distressed and nondistressed families that it may be possible to increase the use of authoritative parenting practices, reduce coercion and conflict, prevent adolescent problem behavior, and improve other adolescent outcomes.

Using the principles of authoritative parenting seems to be a promising approach to improving important adolescent health behaviors among targeted families. However, research may benefit from expanding and clarifying the concept of authoritative parenting. Based on Darling and Steinberg's (1993) conceptualization, it appears that there are three levels of parenting—goals, style, and practices—that should be addressed in parent intervention programs to affect positive outcomes. From the literature, parents who are considered to be authoritative have characteristic goals, style, and practices. Figure 5.2 shows the conceptual framework for our proposed overall approach to authoritative parenting. Under this model, programs wishing to improve parenting should specify adolescent outcomes of interest; define aspects of authoritative parenting goals, style, and practices desired to affect adolescent outcomes; and direct intervention materials accordingly.

There are three levels of parenting—goals, style, and practices—that should be addressed in parent intervention programs to affect positive outcomes.

Applying Authoritative Parenting to Parental Management of Teen Driving

The privilege of driving is a nominal rite of passage for American teens. Driving confers adult status and represents new opportunities for independence. Although parents express concern about teens' driving, many are also glad to reduce their burden of responsibility for transporting teenagers. However, driving is a dangerous endeavor; motor vehicle crashes are the leading cause of death and injury among adolescents (Committee on Injury, 1996; National Highway Traffic Safety Administration, 2000). Oddly, driving skill does not seem to be a particularly important factor in driving risk, and training teens to be more skillful does not seem to reduce teen crashes (Vernick et al., 1999). The factors that do seem to relate to teen crash risk are age, experience, and the amount and conditions under which teens drive. Hence, parents may be able to reduce their teen's risk of driving-related crashes by managing teen driving using authoritative parenting principles that are consistent with what is known about teen driving risk.

FIGURE 5.2. CONCEPTUALIZATION OF AUTHORITATIVE PARENTING IN TERMS OF GOALS, STYLE, AND PRACTICE.

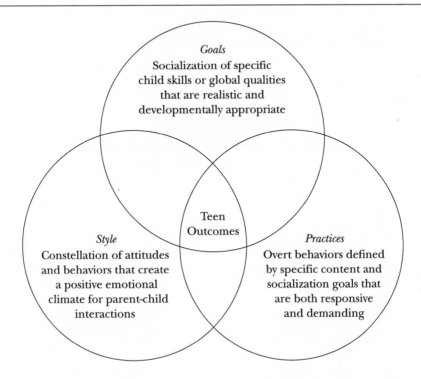

Goals
Socialization of specific
child skills or global qualities
that are realistic and
developmentally appropriate

Teen
Outcomes

Style
Constellation of attitudes
and behaviors that create
a positive emotional
climate for parent-child
interactions

Practices
Overt behaviors defined
by specific content and
socialization goals that
are both responsive
and demanding

Improving parental management of teen driving is an exciting and important target for intervention research for a number of reasons: (1) teen driving is dangerous, (2) teens are highly motivated to drive, (3) parents are somewhat ambivalent about their teens' starting to drive, and (4) clear guidelines for parents on why and how to manage teen driving are not generally available. Hence, teen driving provides an excellent focus for testing the effects of authoritative parenting on adolescent health behavior applied on a population-wide basis.

Reducing Teen Driving Risk

Motor vehicle crashes are the leading cause of death and injury among teenagers between the ages of sixteen and nineteen. Teen crash rates are higher than those of any other age group (Centers for Disease Control and Prevention, 1999; Jonah, 1986; Ulmer, Williams, & Preusser, 1997; Williams, 1985) and disproportionately high on weekends, with teen passengers, and at nighttime (Chen, Baker, Braver,

& Li, 2000; Doherty, Andrey, & MacGregor, 1998; Farrow, 1987; Preusser, Ferguson, & Williams, 1998; Ulmer et al., 1997; Williams, 1985). High crash rates among teens are attributed to their lack of driving experience and propensity for risky driving (Jonah, 1986; Romanowicz & Gebers, 1990). When compared to older drivers, teenagers report more risky driving behaviors such as speeding, following too closely, rapid accelerations, and other aggressive maneuvers that heighten the likelihood of crashes (Jonah, 1986; Jonah & Dawson, 1987).

In an effort to reduce high crash rates among teenage drivers, many states are implementing graduated driver licensing (GDL) programs. GDL programs increase the safety of teen drivers by delaying teen licensure and restricting high-risk teen driving in various ways: raising the ages for permit and licensure, increasing the amount of practice driving required during the learner's phase, lengthening the time periods for learners and provisional phases, increasing parental supervision of teen early driving, implementing nighttime driving curfews, establishing a zero-tolerance policy for alcohol or other drugs, restricting teen driving with teen passengers or on high-speed roads, and requiring seat belt use (Williams, 1993, 1996). Research indicates that certain components of GDL programs have resulted in reduced rates of teen risky driving behaviors, crashes, violations, and overall amount of driving. These include raised ages at permit and provisional license, increased supervised driving, and nighttime driving curfews (Doherty & Andrey, 1997; Ferguson, Leaf, Williams, & Preusser, 1996; Preusser, 1988; Preusser, Zador, & Williams, 1993; Williams & Preusser, 1997).

State-imposed delay and restriction of teen driving has been successful in increasing teen safety, but parent-imposed delay and restriction of teen driving may be equally successful for various reasons. GDL programs vary from state to state. As of November 2001, all but nine states have adopted or incorporated core elements of a three-stage GDL program (Insurance Institute for Highway Safety, 2001); however, no jurisdiction has all the elements of an optimal graduated licensing system as identified by the Insurance Institute for Highway Safety. In addition, although states mandate restrictions, parents are responsible for imposing and maintaining them. Whereas political and public support is needed before states can implement teen driving restrictions, parents are in a prime position to take such measures on their own and to enforce them at an individual level.

Research on the Relationship Between Parenting and Teen Driving Risks

Parents have a substantial opportunity to affect safe teen driving because they are involved in their teenagers' driving from the beginning, teaching them to drive and governing their access to vehicles. Teenagers also report that parents set driving rules such as "don't drink and drive," "tell parents where you are going and with whom," and "be home at a certain time" (Preusser, Williams, & Lund, 1985). The little research that has addressed the relationships between parenting and teen driving suggests that authoritative parenting practices are associated with reduced risky driving, traffic violations, and crashes among teenagers (Beck, Shattuck, & Raleigh, 2001; Hartos, Eitel, Haynie, & Simons-Morton, 2000; Hartos, Eitel, & Simons-Morton, 2001). For example, Hartos, Eitel, Haynie, and Simons-Morton (2000) interviewed three hundred adolescents licensed two years or less about risky driving behaviors, parenting practices, and other variables. Parental restrictions on teen driving were inversely related to teen risky driving behaviors. In addition, traffic violations were four times more likely and crashes seven times more likely among adolescents whose parents had lenient driving restrictions.

Parents have a substantial opportunity to affect safe teen driving because they are involved in their teenagers' driving from the beginning, teaching them to drive and governing their access to vehicles.

In prospective research, Hartos et al. (2002) found that when compared to adolescents with low risky driving over time, adolescents with high risky driving over time were about three times more likely to report low parental monitoring and two times more likely to report low parental restrictions on driving. In addition, Beck, Shattuck, and Raleigh (2001) found that more frequent parental supervision and less unrestricted teen access to a car were associated with less likelihood of teens' speeding and more likelihood of their using seat belts when driving.

Although parents are in a prime position to influence their teens' driving behaviors, research indicates that many parents are less involved than they could be. Beck and colleagues (Beck et al., 1999, 2001) found that for the majority of incidents, parents were not aware that their teens drove under the influence of alcohol, rode with other drinking drivers, were distracted by friends or other passengers while driving, did not wear seat belts, drove aggressively, or ran stop signs and traffic lights. Other studies (Beck, 1990; Beck, Scaffa, Swift, & Ko, 1995) also document a tendency of parents to underpersonalize risks related to teen driving and to attribute impaired driving to their teens' friends rather than to their own teens.

In addition, an alarming number of teens do not report having driving rules or restrictions for high-risk driving conditions, including driving at night and with teen passengers (Beck et al., 2001; Hartos et al., 2000). Despite the high prevalence of motor vehicle crashes among adolescents and research linking teen passengers with crashes (Aldridge, Himmler, Aultman-Hall, & Stamatiadis, 1999; Chen et al., 2000; Doherty et al., 1998; Williams, 1985; Williams, Ferguson, Leaf, & Preusser, 1998), Hartos and others (2000) found that adolescents reported that they were allowed to have "many" teens as passengers "most of the time. " And Beck et al. (2001) found that only a little more than half (55 percent) of the teen drivers in their survey reported any restrictions on the total number of passengers allowed in the car when they were driving, and only 25 percent reported being restricted to no teenage passengers.

Increasing Parental Management of Teen Driving: Checkpoints Program

Effective parent education to improve child and adolescent behavior has proven to be complicated and difficult to implement. Population-based programs face the unique challenges of identifying parents and delivering timely and appropriate motivational messages and instruction in a dose sufficient to cause an effect. Instructional materials for parents on how to teach and manage young drivers are widely available from public agencies, private groups, and insurance companies, but few materials have been evaluated and none are embedded in what might be considered a comprehensive, planned, theory-based educational program.

We are conducting the Young Drivers Intervention Study, a randomized trial that will test the effectiveness of a program of interventions, the Checkpoints Program, on parental management of teen driving and teen driving experience. The Checkpoints Program aims to reduce teen motor vehicle crashes and traffic violations by increasing parental management of teens' early driving and reducing the amount teens drive under higher-risk conditions. This is the first randomized trial targeting parental management of teen driving.

The Checkpoints Program is being implemented in Connecticut, a state without restrictions on teen driving after the permit period. Parents and teens ($n = 4,000$ parent-teen dyads) are recruited at local offices of the Department of Motor Vehicles when teens receive a learner's permit. After baseline data collection, families are randomly assigned to the Checkpoints Program or a general traffic safety education group and followed for two years. Teens and parents are interviewed by telephone on recruitment, within a few weeks of teen licensure, and at three months, six months, and twelve months postlicensure. Driving records will be reviewed for crashes and citations at age eighteen. Families assigned to the safety education group periodically receive by mail informational newsletters that focus on various aspects of driving, including car maintenance, safety belts, and alcohol and drugs.

The overall goal for families assigned to the Checkpoints Program is for parents to establish, and teens to adhere to, appropriate driving restrictions during the first two years of driving. During the teen driving permit period, specific parenting goals are to increase parent participation in practice driving and establish the expectation and intent to restrict teen driving after teen licensure. Specific Checkpoints Program goals for families during the first two years of teen licensure are to (1) adopt and maintain the Checkpoints Parent-Teen Driving Agreement, (2) establish appropriate restrictions on driving, (3) monitor teen driving, (4) apply appropriate consequences for deviations from the provisions of the agreement, and (5) modify the agreement over time, granting additional driving privileges consistent with teens' demonstrated responsible behaviors including driving. Hence, the Checkpoints Program aims to promote parental management of teen driving consistent with teen driving safety.

Strategies to Increase Authoritative Parenting

The Checkpoints Program includes mediated persuasive communications administered during the prelicensure and postlicensure phases and a parent-teen driving agreement. The persuasive communications are in the form of a video entitled *So Who Wants to Be a Driver?* and newsletters delivered by mail on a regular basis before and after teens receive their driver's license. The parent-teen driving agreement is a tool that families can use to establish teen driving privileges and restrictions and identify the conditions that teens must meet to gain additional privileges. As shown in Figure 5.3, these intervention materials are designed to incorporate and promote authoritative parenting in terms of goals, style, and practices to affect the safety of young drivers.

Introductory Video. Within a few weeks of recruitment, right after baseline assessment, families receive a package from the Checkpoints Program that includes a welcome letter and video that describe the Checkpoints Program, the risks of teen driving, and the benefits of adopting the Checkpoints Parent-Teen Driving Agreement. The video, which is less than ten minutes in length, includes expert and family accounts of experiences related to teen driving, and it follows two families as they negotiate the Checkpoints Driving Agreement and establish initial teen driving expectations.

Newsletters. During the time teens have their learner's permit, parents receive eight newsletters—one every three weeks. Each deals with risks associated with a specific driving condition: nighttime driving; teen passengers; high-speed roads; adverse weather; seat belt nonuse; and drugs, alcohol, and driving. Each includes recommended actions parents and families can take to reduce these risks, including talking with teens, setting clear expectations and standards for safe driving, and limiting driving under high-risk conditions until teens gain more driving experience. The ninth newsletter summarizes teen driving risks and ways parents can reduce these risks, and it emphasizes the advantages of adopting the parent-teen driving agreement.

FIGURE 5.3. INTERVENTION MATERIALS IN THE CHECKPOINTS PROGRAM.

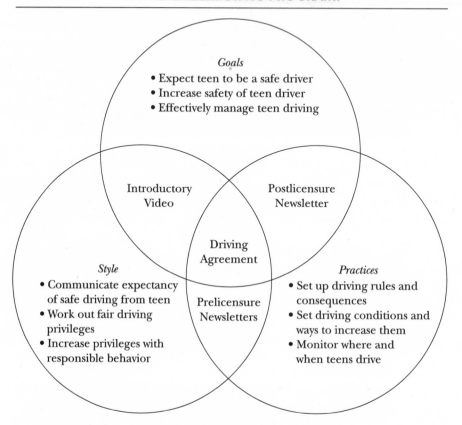

Postlicensure Newsletters. During the first six months that teens have a driver's license, families receive additional newsletters that remind and encourage them to maintain the Checkpoints Driving Agreement and renegotiate the terms of the agreement at the appropriate times. Each newsletter focuses on a specific aspect of teen driving, including the need for continued parental supervision, the lower risk of purposeful driving such as going to work or school compared with cruising, the types of distractions that increase teen crashes, and choosing a car. The spacing of the newsletters increases over time, with the first delivered a few weeks after licensure and the latter ones several months apart.

Checkpoints Parent-Teen Driving Agreement. The Checkpoints video and newsletters are designed to increase the likelihood that families will adopt and maintain the Checkpoints Driving Agreement, the primary behavior management tool by which families can establish clear guidelines and parameters for teen driving. Numerous parent-teen driving agreements have been developed and are distributed by insurance companies and other groups; however, none has been evaluated.

The features of the Checkpoints Driving Agreement include establishing the following: (1) a process of negotiation between parents and teens; (2) driving rules related to traffic safety and being responsible; (3) restrictions on teen driving, including driving curfews, teen passenger limits, types of roads on which they are allowed to drive, and the weather conditions necessary for them to drive; (4) the period each set of restrictions is to be in place before they can be reconsidered and new privileges can be awarded; (5) the requirements the teen must meet to qualify for additional privileges; and (6) the consequences for violating terms of the agreement.

The agreement is organized into four checkpoints that cover three- to six-month periods. At agreed-on times, families evaluate teens' responsible behavior and driving performance and renegotiate any additional driving privileges. The driving agreement provides recommendations that encourage the adoption and maintenance of relatively strict limitations on initial unsupervised teen driving that become relaxed over time, but families are free to adopt restrictions as they see fit. In addition, the driving agreement encourages families to adopt "check-in" procedures whereby the teen is responsible for informing a parent about the specifics of all trips, including destination, any passengers, return time, and other information as necessary before taking the car. This places responsibility on the teen for conforming to the requirements of the driving agreement. Parents are encouraged to, even if they grant exceptions, maintain the restrictions for the agreed-upon time period.

Checkpoints Program Evaluation

Several pilot studies have been conducted to assess the immediate impact of exposure to Checkpoint Program materials. To test the effect of exposure to Checkpoints newsletters on parental attitudes toward teen driving restrictions, we recruited ninety-eight parents of teens holding learner's permits and randomly assigned them to pretest-posttest or posttest-only groups (Hartos & Simons-Morton, 2001). Each group was mailed two newsletters about risks of teen driving and benefits of restrictions. In follow-up telephone interviews, most parents indicated that they had read the newsletters and found them useful. Exposure to the newsletters significantly increased parents' attitudes toward the risks of teen driving and the benefits of parental restrictions.

To assess how families would react and use the Checkpoints Driving Agreement, we recruited forty-seven volunteer families at driver school locations as teens received their driver's licenses and asked them to pilot-test the Checkpoints Driving Agreement (Hartos & Simons-Morton, 2000). Within three months after receiving the agreement, parent and teen participants were interviewed by telephone about their experience with the driving agreement. Most families (thirty-eight of forty-seven) adopted the driving agreement and indicated that they liked its organization and content. Most parents and teens indicated that it was not difficult to reach agreement and would recommend the driving agreement to other families. Most families adopted the recommended strict initial driving restrictions, including restrictions on number of teen passengers, nighttime curfew, and road conditions. Exposure to the driving agreement led many parents to adopt significantly stricter initial limits on teen driving than they had originally intended. Hence, it appears preliminarily that exposure to the Checkpoints Driving Agreement, even without being exposed to persuasive communications, is acceptable to families and serves as a useful tool for adopting and structuring teen driving restrictions.

This is the first controlled evaluation of the facilitated use of a parent-teen driving agreement, and it will assess the feasibility of altering authoritative parenting in terms of parental management of teen driving (see Figure 5.3). The Checkpoints video is designed to address authoritative parenting goals and style by promoting appropriate expectations and standards for teen driving by introducing ways parents can increase teen safety. The prelicensure newsletters address authoritative parenting style and practices by encouraging parents to talk to their teens, set up clear and fair driving privileges for them, and monitor teen driving. The postlicensure newsletters address authoritative parenting practices and goals by encouraging parents to continue to manage teen driving over time to increase the safety of their teens. The driving agreement addresses authoritative parenting overall by providing guidelines for parental management of teen driving. It is hoped that these methods will facilitate not only appropriate family goals for teen driving, but also a positive climate for families to negotiate teen driving privileges and consistent application of authoritative parenting practices as they relate to teen driving.

Future Directions

Further refinements to the conceptualization of authoritative parenting are inevitable and necessary. Despite much research showing consistent patterns of relations between authoritative parenting and child outcomes, issues continue to be raised. For example, research shows differing patterns of agreement and relations among parent and child and adolescent reports of parenting styles and child outcomes (Cohen & Rice, 1997; Paulson, 1994). In addition, more than four parenting styles emerge when considering mixed and middle-of-the-road parenting (Baumrind 1991; Mantzicopoulos & Oh-Hwang, 1998; Slicker, 1998). Also, various measures continue to be employed for authoritative parenting, ranging from overall parent-child interaction climate (for example, parents' responsiveness, demandingness, and autonomy granting) to more specific parenting behaviors (for example, amount of parental monitoring or communication). More research is needed to address the hypothesis of Darling and Steinberg (1993) that parenting styles moderate the effects of parenting practices; apply the conceptualization of the relations among authoritative parenting goals, style, and practices to adolescent behavior (see Figure 5.2); and evaluate the effects of interventions to increase authoritative parenting on adolescent outcomes.

Little is known about how best to reach and intervene with a broad range of families to increase authoritative parenting and improve adolescent outcomes. Studies have intervened with families dealing with difficult children or other specific populations, but only recently has this work been extended to broader populations. The Young Drivers Intervention Study addresses a population of middle adolescents and seeks to alter a target behavior, teen driving. Teen driving is common to all youth in this age group, but this group does not aggregate naturally for any period of time. More research is needed in the area of delivery and effectiveness of intervention materials within broad-range populations.

Given the changes in family relations during adolescence and the history of parent-child relations in the family, research needs to focus on ways to increase positive family goals, emotional climate, and practices to promote a variety of target adolescent outcomes.

Similarly, more needs to be learned about the extent to which authoritative parenting can be fostered among parents of adolescents. Given the changes in family relations during adolescence and the history of parent-child relations in the family, research needs to focus on ways to increase positive family goals, emotional climate, and practices to promote a variety of target adolescent outcomes.

Other applications and extensions of authoritative parenting are likely and warranted. One example is to promote authoritative teaching styles in continuing education for middle and high school teachers. Our group has been exploring this extension by conducting workshops with middle school teachers that include instruction on authoritative teaching. Substantial research on teacher training focuses on outcomes such as improved time on task or student test scores. The concept of authoritative teaching as we have been presenting it is not a way of improving teaching of content so much as a way of motivating students to try harder. In our school-based work on adolescent problem behavior (Simons-Morton et al., 1999), we have found that many teachers become discouraged with poor student performance and begin to expect less of students, which reinforces students' lack of motivation. So we encourage teachers to be demanding, that is, to keep expecting that their students will do well rather than giving up on them, and responsive, that is, monitoring and acknowledging student performance and giving feedback in a warm and personal way to encourage them. More research on applying authoritative teaching may be a promising approach to fostering students' academic achievement potential.

Authoritative parenting is a compelling conceptualization for how parents can best deal with child and adolescent development and behavior. Substantial research links authoritative parenting goals, style, and behaviors to positive adolescent development and behavior outcomes. The Young Drivers Intervention Study will test the extent to which increased parental management of teen driving, within the bounds of authoritative parenting, reduces teens' exposure to high risk driving situations and teen crashes. It will also provide evidence for the effectiveness of our (Figure 5.2) and Darling and Steinberg's (1993) conceptualizations of authoritative parenting in promoting adolescent health.

References

Aldridge, B., Himmler, M., Aultman-Hall, L., & Stamatiadis, N. (1999). Impact of passengers on young driver safety. In *Transportation research record 1693* (pp. 25–30). Washington, DC: National Academy Press.

Ary, D. V., Duncan, T. E., Biglan, A., Metzler, C. W., Noell, J. W., & Smolkowski, K. (1999). Development of adolescent problem behavior. *Journal of Abnormal Child Psychology, 27,* 141–150.

Aunola, K., Stattin, H., & Nurmi, J. (2000). Adolescents' achievement strategies, school adjustment, and externalizing and internalizing problem behaviors. *Journal of Youth and Adolescence, 29,* 289–306.

Baumrind, D. (1967). Child care practices anteceding three patterns of preschool behavior. *Genetic Psychology Monographs, 75,* 43–88.

Baumrind, D. (1971). Current patterns of parental authority. *Developmental Psychology Monograph, 4,* 1–103.

Baumrind, D. (1978). Parental disciplinary patterns and social competence in children. *Youth and Society, 9,* 239–276.

Baumrind, D. (1991). The influence of parenting style on adolescent competence and substance use. *Journal of Early Adolescence, 11,* 56–95.

Beck, K. H. (1990). Monitoring parent concerns about teenage drinking: A random digit dial telephone survey. *American Journal of Drug and Alcohol Abuse, 16,* 109–124.

Beck, K. H., Scaffa, M., Swift, R., & Ko, M. (1995). A survey of parent attitudes and practices regarding underage drinking. *Journal of Youth and Adolescence, 24,* 315–334.

Beck, K. H., Shattuck, T., Haynie, D. L., Crump, A. D., & Simons-Morton, B. G. (1999). Associations between parent awareness, monitoring, enforcement and adolescent involvement with alcohol. *Health Education Research, 14,* 765–775.

Beck, K. H., Shattuck, T., & Raleigh, R. (2001). Parental predictors of teen driving risk. *American Journal of Health Behavior, 25,* 10–20.

Boveja, M. E. (1998). Parenting styles and adolescents' learning strategies in the urban community. *Journal of Multicultural Counseling and Development, 26,* 110–119.

Boyes, M. C., & Allen, S. G. (1993). Styles of parent-child interaction and moral reasoning in adolescence. *Merrill-Palmer Quarterly, 39,* 551–570.

Carlson, C., Uppal, S., & Prosser, E. C. (2000). Ethnic differences in processes contributing to the self-esteem of early adolescent girls. *Journal of Early Adolescence, 20,* 44–67.

Catalano, R. F., Kosterman, R., Haggerty, K., Hawkins, J. D., & Spoth, R. (1998). A universal intervention for the prevention of substance abuse: Preparing for the drug free years. In R. S. Ashery, E. B. Robertson, & K. L. Kumpfer (Eds.), *Drug abuse prevention through family intervention* (Washington, DC: U.S. Government Printing Office.

Centers for Disease Control and Prevention. (1999). Motor vehicle safety—a twentieth century public health achievement. *Morbidity and Mortality Weekly Report, 48,* 369–374.

Chen, L., Baker, S. P., Braver, E. R., & Li, G. (2000). Carrying passengers as a risk factor for crashes fatal to sixteen- and seventeen-year-old drivers. *Journal of the American Medical Association, 283,* 1578–1618

Cohen, D. A., & Rice, J. (1997). Parenting styles, adolescent substance use, and academic achievement. *Journal of Drug Education, 27,* 199–211.

Committee on Injury and Poison Prevention and Committee on Adolescence. (1996). The teenage driver. *Pediatrics, 98,* 987–990.

Csikszentmihalyi, M., & Larson, R. (1984). *Being adolescent: Conflict and growth in the teenage years.* New York: Basic Books.

Darling, N., & Steinberg, L. (1993). Parenting style as context: An integrative model. *Psychological Bulletin, 113,* 487–496.

Dishion, T. J., Patterson, G. R., & Kavanagh, K. A. (1992). An experimental test of the coercion model: Linking theory, measurement, and intervention. In J. McCord & R. E. Tremblay (Eds.), *Preventing antisocial behavior: Interventions from birth through adolescence* (pp. 253–282). New York: Guilford Press.

Dishion, T. J., Patterson, G. R., & Reid, J. R. (1988). Parent and peer factors associated with drug sampling in early adolescence: Implications for treatment. In *Adolescent drug abuse: Analyses of treatment research.* Rockville, MD: National Institute on Drug Abuse: Research Monograph Series. Mono 77, 69–93.

Doherty, S. T., & Andrey, J. C. (1997). Young drivers and graduated licensing: The Ontario case. *Transportation, 24,* 227–251.

Doherty, S. T., Andrey, J. C., & MacGregor, C. (1998). The situational risks of young drivers: The influence of passengers, time of day and day of week on accident rates. *Accident Analysis and Prevention, 30,* 45–52.

Dominguez, M. M., & Carton, J. S. (1997). The relationship between self-actualization and parenting style. *Journal of Social Behavior and Personality, 12,* 1093–1100

Dornbusch, S. M., Ritter, P. L., Leiderman, H., Roberts, D. F., & Fraleigh, M. J. (1987). The relation of parenting style to adolescent school performance. *Child Development, 58,* 1244–1257.

Durbin, D. L., Darling, N., Steinberg, L., & Brown, B. B. (1993). Parenting style and peer group membership among European-American adolescents. *Journal of Research on Adolescence, 3,* 87–100.

Farrow, J. A. (1987). Young driver risk taking: A description of dangerous driving situations among sixteen- to nineteen-year-old drivers. *International Journal of Addictions, 22,* 1255–1267.

Ferguson, S. A., Leaf, W. A., Williams, A. F., & Preusser, D. F. (1996). Differences in young driver crash involvement in states with varying licensure practices. *Accident Analysis and Prevention, 28,* 171–180.

Fischer, J. L., & Crawford, D. W. (1992). Codependency and parenting styles. *Journal of Adolescent Research, 7,* 352–363.

Fletcher, A. C., & Jefferies, B. C. (1999). Parental mediators of associations between perceived authoritative parenting and early adolescent substance use. *Journal of Early Adolescence, 19,* 465–487.

Glasgow, K. L., Dornbusch, S. M., Troyer, L., Steinberg, L., & Ritter, P. L. (1997). Parenting styles, adolescents' attributions, and educational outcomes in nine heterogeneous high schools. *Child Development, 68,* 507–529.

Gray, M. R., & Steinberg, L. (1999). Unpacking authoritative parenting: Reassessing a multidimensional construct. *Journal of Marriage and the Family, 61,* 574–587.

Hall, W. N., & Bracken, B. A. (1996). Relationship between maternal parenting styles and African-American and white adolescents' interpersonal relationships. *School Psychology International, 17,* 253–267.

Hartos, J. L., Eitel, P., Haynie, D. L., & Simons-Morton, B. G. (2000). Can I take the car? Relations among parenting practices and adolescent problem driving practices. *Journal of Adolescent Research, 15,* 352–367.

Hartos, J. L., Eitel, P., & Simons-Morton, B. G. (2001). Do parent-imposed delayed licensure and restricted driving reduce risky driving behaviors among newly-licensed teens? *Prevention Science, 2*(2), 111–120.

Hartos, J. L., Eitel, P., & Simons-Morton, B. G. (2002). Parenting practices and adolescent risky driving: A three-month prospective study. *Health Education and Behavior, 29*(1), 71–82.

Hartos, J. L., & Simons-Morton, B. G. (2000). *Using persuasive communications in the CHECKPOINTS program to change parents' attitudes about teen driving restrictions.* Submitted for publication.

Hartos, J. L., & Simons-Morton, B. G. (2001). *Pilot results: Use of the CHECKPOINTS parent-teen driving agreement.* Submitted for publication.

Hawkins, J. D., Catalano, R. F., Kent, L. A. (1991). Combining broadcast media and parent education to prevent teenage drug abuse. In L. Donohew, P. Palmgreen, & W. J. Bukoski (Eds.), *Persuasive communication and drug abuse prevention* (pp. 283–294). Hillsdale, NJ: Erlbaum.

Hein, C., & Lewko, J. H. (1994). Gender differences in factors related to parenting style: A study of high performing science students. *Journal of Adolescent Research, 9,* 262–281.

Hickman, G. P., Bartholomae, S., & McKenry, P. C. (2000). Influence of parenting styles on the adjustment and academic achievement of traditional college freshmen. *Journal of College Student Development, 41,* 41–54.

Hill, N. E. (1995). The relationship between family environment and parenting style: A preliminary study of African American families. *Journal of Black Psychology, 21,* 408–423.

Holmbeck, G. N., Paikoff, R. L., Brooks-Gunn, J. (1995). Parenting Adolescents. In M. H. Bornstein (ed). *Handbook of parenting: Vol. 1: Children and parenting.* Hillsdale, NJ, Erlbaum.

Insurance Institute for Highway Safety. (2001). *U.S. licensing systems for young drivers.* Available: www.highwaysafety.org/safety_facts/state_laws/grad_license.htm.

Irvine, A. B., Biglan, A., Smolkowski, K., Metzler, C. W., & Ary, D. V. (1999). The effectiveness of a parenting skills program for parents of middle school students in small communities. *Journal of Consulting and Clinical Psychology, 67,* 811–825.

Jackson, C., Henriksen, L., & Foshee, V. A. (1998). The authoritative parenting index: Predicting health risk behaviors among children and adolescents. *Health Education and Behavior, 25,* 319–337.

Jonah, B. A. (1986). Accident risk and risk-taking behavior among young drivers. *Accident Analysis and Prevention, 18,* 255–271.

Jonah, B. A., & Dawson, N. E. (1987). Youth and risk: Age differences in risky driving, risk perception, and risky utility. *Alcohol, Drugs, and Driving, 3,* 13–29.

Kosterman, R., Hawkins, J. D., Spoth, R., Haggerty, K. P., & Zhu, K. (1997). Effects of a preventive parent-training intervention on observed family interactions: Proximal outcomes from Preparing for the Drug Free Years. *Journal of Community Psychology, 25,* 337–352.

Lamborn, S. D., Mounts, N. S., Steinberg, L., & Dornbusch, S. M. (1991). Patterns of competence and adjustment among adolescents from authoritative, authoritarian, indulgent and neglectful families. *Child Development, 62,* 1049–1065.

Maccoby, E. E., & Martin, J. A. (1983). Socialization in the context of the family: Parent-child interaction. In P. H. Mussen (Series Ed.) & E. M. Hetherington (Volume Ed.), *Handbook of child psychology: Vol. 4. Socialization, personality and social development* (4th ed., pp. 1–101) New York: Wiley.

Mantzicopoulos, P. Y., & Oh-Hwang, Y. (1998). The relationship of psychosocial maturity to parenting quality and intellectual ability for American and Korean adolescents. *Contemporary Educational Psychology, 23,* 195–206.

Mauro, C. F., & Harris, Y. R. (2000). The influence of maternal child-rearing attitudes and teaching behaviors on preschoolers' delay of gratification. *Journal of Genetic Psychology, 161,* 292–306.

Morrongiello, B. A., Hillier, L., & Bass, M. (1995). What I said versus what you heard: A comparison of physicians and parents reporting of anticipatory guidance on child safety issues. *Injury Prevention, 1,* 223–227.

Mounts, N. S., & Steinberg, L. (1995). An ecological analysis of peer influence on adolescent grade point average and drug use. *Developmental Psychology, 31,* 915–922.

National Highway Traffic Safety Administration. (2000). *Motor vehicle traffic crashes as a leading cause of death in the U.S., 1997.* Springfield, VA: National Technical Information Service.

Onatsu-Arvilommi, T., Nurmi, J., & Aunola, K. (1998). Mothers' and fathers' well-being, parenting styles, and their children's cognitive and behavioral strategies at primary school. *European Journal of Psychology of Education, 13,* 543–556.

Paikoff, R. L., & Brooks-Gunn, J. (1991). Do parent-child relationships change during puberty? *Psychological Bulletin, 110,* 47–66.

Parish, T. S., & McCluskey, J. J. (1994). The relationship between parenting styles and young adults' self-concepts and evaluations of parents. *Family Therapy, 21,* 223–226.

Patterson, G. R. (1982). *Coercive family process.* Eugene, OR: Castalia.

Patterson, G. R. (1995). Coercion as a basis for early age of onset for arrest. In J. McCord (Ed.), *Coercion and punishment in long-term perspectives* (pp. 81–105). Cambridge: Cambridge University Press.

Patterson, G. R. (1996). Some characteristics of a developmental theory for early-onset delinquency. In M. F. Lenzenweger & J. J. Haugaard (Eds.), *Frontiers of developmental psychopathology* (pp. 81–124). New York: Oxford University Press.

Patterson, G. R., Reid, J. B. Dishion, T. J. (1992). *Antisocial boys: A social interactional approach* (Vol. 4). Eugene, OR: Castalia.

Paulson, S. E. (1994). Relations of parenting style and parental involvement with ninth-grade students' achievement. *Journal of Early Adolescence, 14,* 250–267.

Preusser, D. F. (1988). Delaying teenage licensure. *Alcohol, Drugs and Driving, 4,* 283–295.

Preusser, D. F., Ferguson, S. A., & Williams, A. F. (1998). The effect of teenage passengers on the fatal crash risk of teenage drivers. *Accident Analysis and Prevention, 30,* 217–222.

Preusser, D. F., Williams, A. F., & Lund, A. K. (1985). Parental role in teenage driving. *Journal of Youth and Adolescence, 14,* 73–84.

Preusser, D. F, Zador, P. L., & Williams, A. F. (1993). The effect of city curfew ordinances on teenager motor vehicle fatalities. *Accident Analyses and Prevention, 25,* 641–645.

Romanowicz, P. A., & Gebers, M. A. (1990). *Teen and senior drivers.* Sacramento: California Department of Motor Vehicles.

Simons-Morton B. G., Crump, A. D., Haynie, D., Eitel, P., Saylor, K., & Yu, K. (1999). Psychosocial, school, and parent factors associated with recent smoking among early adolescent boys and girls. *Preventive Medicine, 28,* 138–148.

Simons-Morton, B. G., Crump, A. D., Haynie, D. L., & Saylor, K. (1999). Student-school bonding and adolescent problem behavior. *Health Education Research, 14,* 99–107.

Simons-Morton, B. G., Haynie, D. L., Crump, A. D., Saylor, K. E., Eitel, P., & Yu, K. (1999). Expectancies and other psychosocial factors associated with alcohol use among early adolescent boys and girls. *Addictive Behaviors, 24,* 229–238.

Simons-Morton, B. G., Haynie, D., Crump, A. D., Eitel, P., & Saylor, K. (2001). Peer and parent influence on smoking and drinking among early adolescents. *Health Education and Behavior, 28,* 95–107.

Slicker, E. K. (1998). Relationship of parenting style to behavioral adjustment in graduating high school seniors. *Journal of Youth and Adolescence, 27,* 345–372.

Steinberg, L. D. (1987). Impact of puberty on family relations: Effects of pubertal status and pubertal timing. *Developmental Psychology, 23,* 451–460.

Steinberg, L. D. (1989). Pubertal maturation and parent-adolescent distance: An evolutionary perspective. In G. R. Adams, R. Montemayor, & T. P. Gullotta (Eds.), *Biology of adolescent behavior and development: Advances in adolescent development* (Vol. 1, pp. 71–97). Thousand Oaks, CA: Sage.

Steinberg, L. D. (1990). Autonomy, conflict, and harmony in the family relationship. In S. Feldman & G. Elliot (Eds.), *At the threshold: The developing adolescent* (pp. 255–276). Cambridge, MA: Harvard University Press.

Steinberg, L., Dornbusch, S. M., & Brown, B. B. (1992). Ethnic differences in adolescent achievement: An ecological perspective. *American Psychologist, 47* (6), 723–729.

Steinberg, L., Lamborn, S. D., Darling, N., Mounts, N. S., & Dornbusch, S. M. (1994). Over-time changes in adjustment and competence among adolescents from authoritative, authoritarian, indulgent, and neglectful families. *Child Development, 65,* 754–770.

Steinberg, L., Lamborn, S. D., Dornbusch, S. M., & Darling, N. (1992). Impact of parenting practices on adolescent achievement: Authoritative parenting, school involvement, and encouragement to succeed. *Child Development, 63,* 1266–1281.

Strage, A., & Brandt, T. S. (1999). Authoritative parenting and college students' academic adjustment and success. *Journal of Educational Psychology, 91,* 146–156.

Taylor, T. K., & Biglan, A. (1998). Behavioral family interventions for improving child-rearing: A review of the literature for clinicians and policy makers. *Clinical Child and Family Psychology Review, 1,* 41–60.

Taylor, L. C., Hinton, I. D., & Wilson, M. N. (1995). Parental influences on academic performance in African-American students. *Journal of Child and Family Studies, 4,* 293–302.

Ulmer, R. G., Williams, A. F., & Preusser, D. F. (1997). Crash involvements of sixteen-year-old drivers. *Journal of Safety Research, 28,* 97–103.

Vernick, J. S., Li, G., Ogaitis, S., MacKenzie, E. J., Baker, S. P., & Gielen, A. C. (1999). Effects of high-school driver education on motor vehicle crashes, violations, and licensure. *American Journal of Preventive Medicine, 16,* 40–46.

Williams, A. F. (1985). Nighttime driving and fatal crash involvement of teenagers. *Accident Analysis and Prevention, 17,* 1–5.

Williams, A. F. (1993). *Society confronts the young driver problem.* Arlington, VA: Insurance Institute for Highway Safety.

Williams, A. F. (1996). *Protecting new drivers: Ten components of graduated licensing that make sense.* Arlington, VA: Insurance Institute for Highway Safety.

Williams, A. F., Ferguson, S. A., Leaf, W. A., & Preusser, D. F. (1998). Views of parents of teenagers about graduated licensing systems. *Journal of Safety Research, 29,* 1–7.

Williams, A. F., & Preusser, D. F. (1997, January). Night driving restrictions for youthful drivers. *Journal of Public Health Policy,* pp. 1–12.

CHAPTER SIX

NATURAL HELPER MODELS TO ENHANCE A COMMUNITY'S HEALTH AND COMPETENCE

Eugenia Eng
Edith Parker

The folks down in my area . . . may not know that Mrs. Smith and Jones are "health advisers." They may not know to call them that. . . . But if you got a problem, you call Mrs. Smith and you call Mrs. Jones, and they are going to help you. You can call it whatever you want, but they get the job done. They meet the needs.

A COMMUNITY HEALTH ADVISER IN THE MISSISSIPPI DELTA, 1992

This statement was made during our evaluation of a health promotion project that applied a natural helper model to improve community competence and health (Eng & Parker, 1994). Mrs. Smith and Mrs. Jones are doing what they have always done in their communities because they are natural helpers. Natural helpers are particular individuals to whom others naturally turn for advice, emotional support, and tangible aid. They provide informal, spontaneous assistance, which is so much a part of everyday life that its value is often not recognized (Israel, 1985). Consequently, their work with a project as community health advisers can be invisible to others and frequently to the community health advisers themselves. Being unobtrusive, natural helping can be difficult to demonstrate, operationalize, and capture empirically.

Natural helpers are particular individuals to whom others naturally turn for advice, emotional support, and tangible aid.

In recent years, public health professionals have introduced a number of approaches, loosely referred to as lay health adviser interventions, that include a parallel but separate line of work with natural helpers. The Centers for Disease Control and Prevention (U.S. Department of Health and Human Services, 1994) compiled a two-volume directory of lay health adviser projects and programs in the United States, as well as a computerized database that is regularly updated. A few examples illustrate the wide range of settings, health issues, and populations involving natural helpers and other types of lay health advisers.

Barbers (Wilkinson, 1992) and church members nominated by their pastors in North Carolina (Eng & Hatch, 1992) served as lay health advisers to improve hypertension screening, management, and control among African Americans. Migrant farmworker women served as *promotores* (promoters) to address the maternal and child health needs of families traveling in the Midwest (Booker, Robinson, Kay, Najera, & Stewart, 1997) and East Coast migrant streams (Watkins et al., 1994). In a small southern town with big-city rates of sexually transmitted diseases (STD), a community resource group identified twenty-five natural helpers willing to serve as advisers. Known as Respect and Protect, advisers helped people they know to use condoms with their main partners and helped people seek screening when they had unprotected sex (Thomas, Eng, Clark, Robinson, & Blumenthal, 1998). A network of 160 lay health advisers, called Save Our Sisters, was established across North Carolina across five rural counties to assist older African American women in breaking the silence about breast cancer screening (Eng & Smith, 1995; Earp et al., 1997). Village Health Workers in Detroit have undertaken activities in their neighborhoods to improve the health of women and children (Parker, Israel, Schulz, & Hollis, 1998). Students in suburban high schools can seek confidential health counseling at a designated room during specified class periods from peer educators who were nominated by the student body and the adults they trust (Berkley-Patton, Fawcett, Paine-Andrews, & Johns, 1997). Health centers in the San Francisco Bay Area (Love, Gardner, & Legion, 1997) and a health coalition in rural Massachusetts (Baker et al., 1997) selected local residents and paid them to work as community health advisers.

In short, lay health adviser interventions have emerged as an important approach in health promotion. Implicit in this approach is the exchange of social support, such as information, advice, tangible aid, and referrals to external resources (House, 1981). From a public health perspective, the associations found between social support and health (Nuckolls, Cassel, & Kaplan, 1972; Cassel, 1976; Kaplan, Cassel, & Gore, 1977; Broadhead et al., 1983) hold substantial potential for translating the health-enhancing effects into social support interventions (Heaney & Israel, 1997). The common feature of lay health adviser interventions is to enlist indigenous members of a given population in channeling health-enhancing social support to individuals and groups (Eng & Young, 1992; Israel, 1985; Service & Salber, 1979). At the same time, important conceptual and methodological distinctions among lay health adviser interventions have been viewed as falling along a continuum (Eng, Parker & Harlan, 1997). At one end are interventions in which lay health advisers serve as paid employees of an agency, such as a paraprofessional or outreach worker, and seek to deliver social support, such as information and assistance to individuals that protect the health of those individuals. At the other end are interventions for which lay health advisers are natural helpers with expertise and knowledge that contribute to the health and competence of their community through information distribution, assistance, and organization of community-building activities within their social networks. This emphasis on natural helpers working within their own social network, defined as person-centered webs of relationships that connect individuals to other individuals or groups (Israel, 1982; Israel & Rounds, 1987), differs from the lay health adviser who provides social support to individuals who may or may not be part of his or her social network, such as outreach workers.

Lay health adviser interventions that explicitly intend to collaborate with natural helpers to enhance a community's health and competence are the focus of this chapter.

The Genesis and Emergence of Natural Helper Interventions in Public Health

"In lesser degree than the family, but with similar dynamics, the primary friendship group may prove to be an epidemiological unit of some significance" (Steuart & Kark, 1993, p. 41). With this observation, a group of South African researchers began their pioneering work of uncovering the structure and function of a community's natural helping system, examining associations between social relationships and health, and recognizing that health is a social concern. Their initial studies were conducted from 1945 to 1959 in communities of various incomes and ethnicities in South Africa that were served by seven primary health care centers. Their methodology and broad inclusion of social factors as determinants of health have been acknowledged as the fundamental work of the twentieth century in social epidemiology (Trostle, 1986).

Sidney Kark, the group's leader, credited Guy Steuart, the psychologist in the group, with calling their attention to the importance of social networks and primary groups for their work in community health education (Israel, Dawson, Steckler, Eng, & Steuart, 1993). Steuart developed a unique procedure for recording the structure and functions of a community's natural helping system. His findings revealed sophisticated and complex skill sets and expertise on how communities manage with life, deal with its frustrations, and strive to ensure the conditions for the good health for its members (Steuart, 1978). Natural helping was a part of everyday living even for communities whose life conditions, such as apartheid policy or rural poverty, would be expected to exert an undeniably harmful influence on health.

The staff of the seven health centers in South Africa were trained at the South African Institute of Family and Community Health to conduct research on the connection between social relationships and health. The significant feature of their work was that they developed techniques that incorporated the findings into the daily practice of the health centers (Kark, 1951). Staff began working with social groupings of people as a natural extension of their interviews with individuals receiving medical care and guidance. That is, by entering into a functional relationship with the presumed natural helpers in a social group, health center staff intended a two-way flow of communication and influence that would be mutually beneficial. They found that by engaging natural helpers and their social networks in a ten-week mutual exchange of discussion and decision making, changes in infant feeding practices were achieved in the desired direction (Steuart & Kark, 1993). Of equal significance, health center staff increased their own understanding of individuals in terms of their family situation, of families in their life situation within a community, and of what it is like to live in a community in relation to the social structure of South Africa (Kark, 1951).

The process of working through natural helpers' social networks, ranging from formalized groups to only two or three intimate friends gathered together in a home, was considered by this group of South African researchers to be among the institute's most important learning experiences (Steuart & Kark, 1993). Their research came to an abrupt end in South Africa in 1959, when the new government began to apply apartheid policy to the medical professions. Individual members of the group dispersed to Israel, Kenya, and the United States, where they continued to develop their methods and ideas on the social determinants of health.

Those who relocated to North Carolina refined their ideas and methods for engaging a community's natural helping system in behavioral and social change interventions. Steuart (1969b, 1977) introduced the action-oriented community diagnosis procedure into the curriculum for the master's degree in public health in the Department of Health Education at the University of North Carolina (Eng & Blanchard, 1991). He used the term *diagnosis* to indicate that the purpose of the analysis is to result in action, change, and improvement that meet a community's needs (Steuart, 1969a). The procedure drew on methods of inquiry from the disciplines of epidemiology and anthropology to reveal the following information:

- The nature of a community's power structure and the lay groups that might participate in both planning and implementing an intervention
- The appropriate unit of practice, such as the individual, family, social groups, or neighborhood
- The interpersonal and nonpersonal methods most appropriate to the tasks of behavior and social change
- The informal opinion leaders and influential persons in social networks through whom influence may be brought to bear on a health issue

Eva Salber, a colleague of Steuart in South Africa, conducted such a diagnosis in a rural community of North Carolina while at Duke University's Department of Family and Community Medicine. She and a small team of health educators documented the detailed procedures they used to identify social networks and their natural helpers, and they recruited these individuals to complete training sessions on the needs and issues that had emerged from the community diagnosis (Salber, Beery, & Jackson, 1976; Service & Salber, 1979; Jackson & Parks, 1997). They linked these natural helpers to the resources of the local health care system and called them lay health advisers. For many public health scholars, Salber's systematic application of the principles and methods developed in South Africa to a rural community in the United States marks the beginning of our field's conceptualization of natural helper interventions in the field of public health (Eng & Young, 1992; Jackson & Parks, 1997; Earp et al., 1997; Watkins et al., 1994, Parker et al., 1998).

At the University of North Carolina, John Hatch designed and implemented the first church-based lay health adviser intervention by building on the skills and expertise of natural helpers in congregations of rural black churches (Hatch & Lovelace, 1980). Before joining Steuart's faculty, Hatch had been applying the principles and methods developed in South Africa with rural African American communities in the Mississippi Delta. His collaborator in Mississippi was Jack Geiger, who, as a medical student at Case Western, had completed a one-year clerkship with Steuart and his colleagues at the South African Institute for Family and Community Health (Geiger, 1984; Trostle, 1986). Geiger and Hatch had received war-on-poverty federal funding to establish in Mississippi the first rural community health center in the United States, for which they clearly acknowledged the work of the South African institute (Hatch & Eng, 1983; Geiger, 1971; Israel et al., 1993).

The focal point of Hatch's body of work is the black church as a community-based institution with structures and functions that nurture leadership, accord rewards and recognition, mobilize social action, and ensure mutual aid for its members (Hatch & Lovelace, 1980; Eng, Hatch, & Callan, 1985; Eng & Hatch,

1992). His research on the health-enhancing effects of natural helping in the black church has opened up new space for developing lay health adviser interventions that are relevant and authentic to the everyday lives of African Americans. Hatch is now recognized nationally and internationally for promoting collaborative methods of inquiry and planning between health service delivery systems and African American communities' natural helping systems (Hatch, Moss, Saran, Presley-Cantrell, & Mallory, 1993).

Natural Helping Concepts and Public Health Practice

To recognize the relevance of natural helping to public health practice, it is essential to understand the following concepts: community support system, neighborhood attachment, informal helping networks, and community competence. Understanding these concepts and their relationship to public health practice is key to understanding the public health natural helper interventions.

Community Support System

The President's Commission on Mental Health (1978) defined a *community support system* as (1) natural helping networks to which people belong, (2) work site relationships, and (3) self-help or mutual aid groups. This commission's Community Support Systems Task Panel, chaired by June Jackson Christmas and directed by Marie Killilea, marked the first time that a prestigious nationwide study group afforded such prominence to the role of community and its support systems in mental health (U.S. Department of Health, Education and Welfare, 1979; Biegel & Naparstek, 1982). In addition, the commission devoted a separate section of its report to disease prevention and health promotion through improving coping and enabling people to realize their full potential. The surgeon general's report, *Healthy People* (U.S. Department of Health, Education and Welfare, 1979), provided further impetus for the field of public health to recognize the importance of life circumstances, such as housing or employment, life events, such as immigrant status or divorce, and lifestyles that may affect people's vulnerability to a wide range of disorders and disease (Cassel, 1976; Jessor & Jessor, 1981; Bloom, 1979).

The emphasis of these two national reports on community support systems and conditions of community life that enable people to be healthy signified a distinct departure from medical model theories (Biegel & Naparstek, 1982). First, these reports suggested that health promotion interventions do not need to stress the role of identifiable factors in the etiology of a particular class of disorders. Second, these reports suggested that health promotion interventions can have nonspecific preventive consequences. Moreover, as Caplan (1982) observed, routine intervention by health professionals done without recognition of natural support systems may weaken, instead of strengthen, the operation of a community's natural support systems and mutual help organizations. This recognition of the existence and power of community support systems to reduce people's vulnerability to disease and illness has continued to increase among public health professionals and is reflected in the recent popularity of such concepts as social capital in the field of public health.

The professional disciplines of public health and social work have drawn heavily from Roland Warren's (1963a) conceptualization of community as a social system with structures and functions that help its members adjust to social, political, and economic change. Donald Warren (1971) delineated the following five functions of a community: a center for interpersonal influence, a source of mutual aid, a base for formal and informal organizations, a reference group and social context, and an arena for according status. In the context of these functions, community members' adjustment to social, political, and economic change is viewed as a process of help seeking and help giving, as opposed to a discrete event or behavioral occurrence. Similarly, problems do not just happen; they are manifested through an accumulation of events, behaviors, and symptoms during a period of time. The point at which a problem begins is as indeterminate as the point at which help becomes effective, and the course between these two vague points is often a long one. This view that most people are engaged in help-seeking and help-giving processes opened up new space for health and human service professionals to examine how their programs could strengthen the natural helping networks of communities, workplaces, and associations (Gottlieb, 1982).

Neighborhood Attachment

The body of work on natural helping networks has offered strong evidence for the important role of neighborhood attachment to place, groups, and other individuals. These attachments, viewed as a proxy for adjustment to one's environment (Nuckolls et al., 1972; Lin, Simeone, Ensel, & Kuo, 1979), have been found to improve people's adaptive competence during times of life stress (Killilea, 1976; Caplan, 1974, 1976). Neighborhood attachment has also been shown to provide a sense of belonging, reduce alienation, and offer a reason for overcoming the frustrations of a changing world (D. Warren, 1977). Explanations have been attributed to communality of experience, collective willpower, sharing of information, constructive activity, and receiving help through giving it (Riessman, 1965; Plaut, 1982; Shanas, 1978; Cantor, 1979; Guttman, 1979).

Furthermore, natural helping has been found to flourish when the issues were either of little interest to professionals or involved considerable numbers of people who did not have access to the services of professionals (Tracy & Gussow, 1976). Ethnic communities with disproportionately more members who are elderly and low income, for example, may have stronger neighborhood attachment and patterns of natural helping than that of the general population (Mann, 1965; Gans, 1961; Lee, 1968; Biegel, Naparstek, & Khan, 1982; Stack, 1974). Scholars have therefore emphasized taking into account communities' social and cultural backgrounds (Hamburg & Killilea, 1979; Biegel et al., 1982; Lin et al., 1979) when developing health promotion programs aimed at strengthening natural helping networks.

Informal Helping Networks

Informal helping networks are those indirect ties to resources that one may have access to through the different social groupings to which one belongs (for example, family, neighborhood, work, and voluntary associations). Through interactions with persons in one's social groupings, one may gain access to information, resources, people, and pathways for help that are outside one's intimate circles (Warren, 1963b). The social groupings may themselves be linked and thereby can tie people indirectly to a variety of helping networks simultaneously. For example, a woman confides a recent concern to her daughter-in-law, who mentions relevant information she had gained from one of her coworkers. Although the woman never needs to be in contact with the coworker, she is part of a viable helping network through a helping transaction with one person. Furthermore, being part of a helping network can direct her attention to the needs of others in her community (D. Warren, 1982).

These informal helping transactions are relatively spontaneous and may involve mutual exchanges of support for a variety of large and small stresses of everyday life. Health and human service professionals have long recognized that for most people, their principal sources of help for a wide range of problems are family, friends, neighbors, coworkers, and other personal relationships (Gourash, 1978; Litwak & Szelenyi, 1969; Pancoast & Chapman, 1982). The focus of agency services on delivering care to an identified patient or client population represents only a small proportion of the support, crisis intervention, and problem solving that occur in communities. Agencies have consequently recognized the potential of forming partnerships with informal helpers and have developed different intervention strategies for cooperating with and reinforcing a community support system's natural helping networks.

The body of work by Froland (1980) on the interface between formal and informal helping systems generated a valuable typology of informal helping network interventions observed to be the most relevant and accessible to health and human service professionals (see Table 6.1). The interventions are based on six types of relationships found in informal helping networks of communities:

- *Family and friends.* These are the most intimate of helping relationships and are characterized as being long standing through preexisting ties and involving equality of exchange over the long term. In informal helper interventions involving family and friends, agencies usually ask only for commitment to help, without requiring special skills or knowledge, and the intervention is short term.

- *Neighbors.* Those who live next door or very close are the most likely to be involved in helping, but when encouraged by an agency, they may also live in an area beyond the geographical boundaries of a neighborhood. Their helping relationship is characterized as being long standing through preexisting ties, involves equality of exchange over the long term, and is locality based. Informal interventions involving helping from neighbors need to consider that the forms of helping from neighbors are not based on obligation of kinship or friendship and have defined limits on level of involvement and what is appropriate to ask for and offer.

- *Natural helpers.* These are individuals to whom people naturally turn for advice, emotional support, and tangible aid. They may be known in a neighborhood context or in a wider network. Their helping relationship is characterized as being long standing through preexisting ties, is locality based, and is a central part of their activities. Helping from natural helpers is based on personal motivation to help others and skills that have earned them respect and confidence. Although they share many of the same sociodemographic characteristics as those they help, their coping abilities are superior. In interventions with natural helpers, agencies usually link these helpers to appropriate formal services and provide them with social, emotional, and material resources.

- *Role-related helpers.* These are individuals in such positions as hairstylists, shopkeepers, and clergy who come in contact with a large number of people through the positions they hold. Their helping relationship is characterized as being long standing through preexisting ties and is locality based. In addition, they are often active on agency-sponsored task forces, boards, and committees created to improve services. In their agency-defined role as informal helpers, they are more likely to be a source of information and referral and to work to make the agency more responsive than they are to provide friendship and emotional support.

- *People with similar problems.* These are helping relationships that are usually fostered by an agency or program that brings together people with similar problems to share their experiences and support one another. The help involves equality of exchange over time but seldom occurs in the homes of participants. Helping

TABLE 6.1. TYPOLOGY OF INFORMAL HELPER INTERVENTIONS.

Type of Informal Helper	Examples of Activities Conducted by Agencies
Family and friends	Elicit commitment from clients' personal networks to share tasks during clients' short-term limitation in functioning
	Reinforce preexisting helping relationships by providing counseling or training on how to be more supportive to clients
	Identify and train focal person to mobilize and maintain helping relationships
Neighbors	Broker help for individual clients from their neighbors
	Create helping relationships by creating opportunities for neighbors to interact, such as by organizing block groups to help residents in need or reviving old acquaintances
Natural helpers	Identify natural helpers by conducting reputational method
	Reinforce preexisting helping relationships to provide improved advice, assistance, material resources, and referrals
	Link appropriate formal agency services to informal helping network
	Support natural helpers in implementing short- and long-term self-help action in response to local needs
Role-related helpers	Make contact with individuals who are influential and visibly located at a crossroads, such as storekeepers and pharmacists
	Create helping relationships in which they can be a source of information and referral to people they encounter in their positions
	Encourage them to make their institutions and businesses more responsive to needs of agency clients
People with same problems	Legitimate groups' learning from one another using experiential rather than professional knowledge
	Create helping relationships by facilitating groups' meeting each other
	Mobilize agency resources
	Share skills in group dynamics and group process
Volunteers	Recruit willing individuals by advertisement, referral, or from client group
	Create, initiate, and sustain helping relationships for isolated people
	Heavy investment of agency resources for more specialized problem solving

Source: Based on Pancoast & Chapman (1982).

usually takes place within a self-help group, and short-term returns are often expected. The role of agencies varies from being proactive by taking the initiative in establishing these groups to being responsive when approached by one or more persons with similar problems requesting resources.

• *Volunteers.* These individuals are the most familiar informal helpers to most professionals because volunteers require considerable input from professionals. They are usually recruited, trained, and channeled through a formal organization's programs to offer help, on a stranger-to-stranger basis, to persons who do not have a helping network of their own. The volunteer is clearly defined as the helper, and therefore, this type of helping relationship is the most likely to involve inequality in social status and coping ability.

Acknowledging that informal helping network interventions do not all engage the natural helping networks of a community's support system has important implications for public health practice (Eng et al., 1997). It is important to distinguish between interventions that are embedded within ongoing networks of relationships, such as interventions working with family and friends, neighbors, or natural helpers, and those helping relationships that are created by an agency, such as volunteers and people with similar problems (Pancoast & Chapman, 1982). Although the latter type of interventions are formed to meet a specific need on a short-term basis, helping relationships based on kinship, friendship, residential proximity, and natural helping are long term, highly individualized, flexible, and likely to be meeting some basic needs. Agencies that want to interface with embedded helping relationships such as these must be willing to be flexible and spend time in the beginning to identify natural helpers, analyze their networks, and understand the particular culture of their community support system. Interventions that create helping relationships, such as those that use volunteers or people with similar problems, will require a substantial investment of agency resources to sustain them.

Interventions that create helping relationships, such as those that use volunteers or people with similar problems, will require a substantial investment of agency resources to sustain them.

Recruitment methods of programs that intend to certify and employ local residents as lay health advisers, but without consideration of the origin of helping relationships, may use eligibility criteria according to qualifications set by personnel policies. The natural helpers to whom people in a community turn therefore may not necessarily be among the local residents recruited because they are not seeking employment or do not fit the agency's qualifications for a lay health adviser. In contrast, the qualifications for a natural helper have been established by the community rather than an agency. Other programs, which intend to accept all willing volunteers, may cast as wide a recruitment net as possible through posters, windshield leaflets, and media advertising. Natural helpers, however, may not respond because they are already too busy helping people and groups in their communities or do not self-identify as natural helpers.

The nature and level of influence or impact that can be expected from natural helper interventions may also differ from those based on agency-created helping relationships. Although all informal helper interventions are generally aimed at enhancing the health and well-being of individuals through peer-to-peer dynamics, natural helper interventions operate through a community's political dynamics and neighborhood attachment. Because natural helping networks are part of a community support system, natural helper interventions can bring people together and set a political dynamic in motion to transform and secure improved quality of community life (Labonte, 1989; McKnight, 1991; Heller, 1989). In addition to securing well-being for members of a community, natural helper interventions also give attention to changing policies and practices of organizations and acting on environmental factors that impede the health and development of a community (Ketterer, Bader, & Levy, 1980; Plaut, 1982; Eng & Parker, 1994). Therefore, one important outcome from natural helper interventions is a more competent community.

Community Competence

The term *community competence* was first codified in social psychiatry by Cottrell (1976). His conceptualization of a community's being competent was strongly influenced by George Herbert Mead's body of work on the process of social interaction (Cottrell, 1980). Cottrell's description of a competent community is one in which its various component parts are able to (1) collaborate effectively in identifying collective problems and needs, (2) achieve a working consensus on goals and priorities, (3) agree on ways and means to implement the agreed-on goals, and (4) collaborate effectively in the required actions. He observed that the more competent a community is, the more mentally healthy are its members. From these observations, he defined eight dimensions of community competence that represent social interactions among community members as well as between a community and the larger society (see Table 6.2).

A few empirical studies of community competence have attempted to operationalize its dimensions (Denham, Quinn, & Gamble, 1998) and develop measures to evaluate community development programs (Hurley, Barabrin, & Mitchell, 1981; Gatz et al., 1982) and related health promotion programs (Goeppinger & Baglioni, 1985; Knight, Johnson, & Holbert, 1991). With regard to applying the concept to natural helper interventions, only one study evaluated changes in community

TABLE 6.2. COMMUNITY COMPETENCE DIMENSIONS.

Dimensions	Definitions	Illustrative Quotes from a Natural Helper
Participation in community life	Process by which a community member commits himself or herself to a community and contributes to the definition of goals as well as to ways and means for their implementation	"I've always been the type to want to help, but just didn't know how to go about doing it. So, that way, this health adviser program has helped me to do things I always wanted to do."
Commitment to the collective	Commitment to a community as a relationship worth enhancing and keeping	"One of the things is the pulling together of the community to get things done. And we found out that we had to do that in order to get things done. We were not going to get things done apart. The more of us that come together and shared ideas, we realized the problems we were having were about the same."
Self-other awareness and clarity of situational definitions	Clarity with which each part of a community can perceive its own identity and position on issues in relationship to other parts of a community	"And the people are now beginning to realize who the power brokers are. Well, they were aware before, but they didn't know how it impacts their lives. They didn't realize the role an election plays in getting things done."
Articulateness	Ability of a community to articulate involvement in community collective views, attitudes, needs, and intentions	"Health advisors talked to people to tell people that might need some of the things that they could do. In fact, that very day, just in conver-
Communication	Process by which information is exchanged in a community and ability to amass common meanings from different parts of a community	sation, they learned about some- body that needed some food. They didn't have any food in their house. And health advisers were able to make a contact there."
Conflict containment and accommodation	Ability to establish procedures by which open conflicts may be accommodated and interaction between different parts of a community will continue	"I think the health adviser program as a whole is probably our best bet to get a racial community effort. An interracial, biracial. And since the program has been here, I say I could see greater unity with people working together to try to improve their conditions."

Dimensions	Definitions	Illustrative Quotes from a Natural Helper
Management of relations with the wider society	Ability to use resources and supports that the larger society makes available and to act to reduce the threats to community life posed by a larger social pressure	"As far as actual person-to-person contact, one of the strongest points of the health adviser program was this working together and knowing where services can be provided and people willing. And people will channel things to us now that would not have ever been addressed."
Machinery for facilitating participant interaction and decision making	Ability of a community to establish more formal means for ways to ensure representative input in decision making as size of community increases	"The health advisers have gone to the county board of supervisors and their representatives to talk about housing. They are now building two new housing projects."
Social support	Community members know and care about neighbors; show willingness to lend a hand in cognitive, instrumental, and emotional support	"Health advisers have helped in terms of going into the patient's home to teach or render some kind of care, if it's nothing other than companionship."

Source: Based on Cottrell (1976); Eng & Parker (1994).

competence as an outcome and will be described later in this chapter (Eng & Parker, 1994).

The Natural Helper Intervention Model and Applications

The field of health promotion has realized that a partnership with natural helpers can interweave formal services with the help provided by a community support system and result in a more appropriate response to the needs of clients and communities (Pancoast & Chapman, 1982; Service & Salber, 1979; Eng & Hatch, 1991; Eng & Young, 1992). Natural helpers provide a community-based system of care and social support that complements, but does not extend or serve as a replacement for, the more specialized services of health professionals (Eng & Smith, 1995). Through a wide spectrum of associations in a community, as formal as a church or guild (Eng et al., 1985) or as informal as a neighbor's kitchen (Heaney & Israel, 1997), natural helpers are linked to individuals, groups, and the wider society that no health professional could begin to reach alone.

Outcomes and intermediate benefits from the various roles and social action arenas through which natural helpers and health professionals can collaborate are presented in Figure 6.1. As shown, professionals can form a partnership with natural helpers to achieve three levels of outcomes: improved health practices, improved coordination of agency services, and improved community competence.

Improved Health Practices

Health professionals can offer training to natural helpers so the helpers can assist individuals with information and referral needs that are difficult for professionals to provide directly. For example, a natural helper intervention to reduce transmission of STDs in a small southern town conducted in-depth interviews with young African American women. The findings revealed that the principal barriers to seeking STD screening and care were confusion about the services offered by local health agencies and apprehension about interacting with the predominantly white staff at the local health department (Schuster, Thomas, & Eng, 1995). To overcome these barriers, staff from the STD clinic and local health center were invited to participate in training natural helpers. Staff listened to their concerns, explained how their respective agencies operated, and offered to be a contact person for referrals from the natural helpers (Thomas, Earp, & Eng, 2000). In turn, the natural helpers could demystify the agencies for members of their helping networks. After eighteen months, evaluation showed a 60 percent increase in the number seeking

FIGURE 6.1. NATURAL HELPER INTERVENTION MODEL.

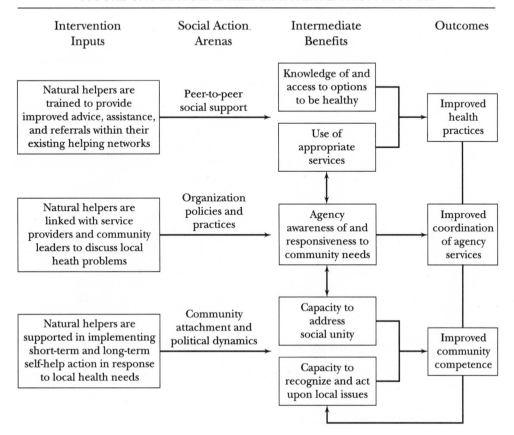

| Intervention Inputs | Social Action Arenas | Intermediate Benefits | Outcomes |

STD care within three days of symptoms among the African American women who reported experiencing symptoms. An increase of 26 percent was found for those who said they sought care when they thought they had an STD but did not report symptoms (Thomas et al., 2000).

A natural helper intervention implemented with migrant farmworker families reported that between 50 percent and 82 percent of maternal and child health patients at two migrant health centers interacted with a trained natural helper (Watkins et al., 1994). Mothers who had contact with a trained natural helper were significantly more likely to bring their children for sick care and had significantly greater knowledge of health practices. Moreover, a significantly higher proportion of pregnant migrant farmworker women who had contact with a trained natural helper reported completing the recommended number of prenatal visits. These findings indicated that Latinas in this migrant farmworker population were connected to one another through natural helping relationships that can bridge cultural diversity in language and health beliefs between farmworkers and health providers.

Improved Coordination of Agency Services

A second partnership opportunity is for health professionals to link their formal service delivery system with the informal helping networks of natural helpers, with the benefit being that agencies can become more aware of and responsive to community needs. A statewide program in North Carolina, for example, offered subsidized breast cancer screening to low-income women. The number of forms to be completed and the number of documents required to determine eligibility proved to be a barrier for older African American women, particularly for those with low literacy and who were embarrassed by the questions about income and onset of menopause. Natural helpers, who were recruited and trained through an intervention, negotiated with the clinic to cosponsor two breast cancer screening days and organize a campaign, called Days of Our Lives, in which they assisted women with the paperwork in the privacy of their homes before going to the clinic.

Improved Community Competence

A third opportunity for health professionals to collaborate with natural helpers is to mobilize the resources of community associations to implement self-help action in response to local health needs. The benefit is to increase a community's social unity and problem-solving capacity. For example, older African American women in rural North Carolina who participated in focus group interviews revealed that they delayed or avoided annual breast cancer screenings largely due to their memories of a segregated health care system (Tessaro, Eng, & Smith, 1994). In addition, the stigma of the fatal and hereditary nature of cancer imposed a prevailing silence in their communities about discussing cancer. Given older African American women's sense of modesty about their bodies, they would discuss concerns and questions about breast cancer only with women they knew. Natural helpers, recruited and trained as part of the Save Our Sisters program, shared this same history, thereby placing them in a position of trust to overcome the barriers to mammography screening that older women discerned (Eng & Smith, 1995).

To break this silence, natural helpers used their existing channels of influence and communication to show an educational video they had produced, as well as to raise funds from churches to cover the cost of bringing a mobile mammography unit to housing projects (Eng & Smith, 1995). The intervention appears to have had an impact on reducing disparity between African Americans and whites in mammography use, particularly with lower-income women, among whom the racial gap has been very nearly eliminated (Earp, Rauscher, & O'Malley, 2000). In the first two and a half years of the project period, mammography use increased by 42 percent (from 41 percent to 58 percent) from the past two years among African American women, compared to a rise of 11 percent in white women (67 percent to 74 percent). Among lower-income women (those with family incomes below $12,000 a year), African American women's use of mammography increased from just 37 percent to 59 percent, nearly overtaking white women, whose mammography use rose from 54 percent to 60 percent.

The intervention inputs of training natural helpers, linking them to service providers, and supporting their actions in a community are typically coordinated by a community outreach coordinator. Hiring a coordinator, who is active in a range of local social groups and associations of the participating community, is the critical first step toward identifying and gaining entry to the various natural helping networks. The coordinator's initial task is to form a community advisory group (CAG) with contacts to additional groups and organizations, such as churches and community-based organizations, to increase the intervention's reach to natural helping networks. The CAG offers entry to these groups and guidance on collecting and interpreting data during the formative phase of the intervention. For the breast cancer intervention, for example, the focus group interviews with older African American women were arranged through CAG members (Tessaro et al., 1994). The CAG also provided technical assistance in interpreting the findings and using them to develop the learning objectives for training natural helpers, determine the characteristics of natural helpers, develop strategies for recruiting natural helpers, and identify potential trainers (Eng & Smith, 1995).

◆ ◆ ◆

In sum, natural helpers can do much more than counsel and assist individuals to change their behaviors. They can build a partnership with the formal service delivery system, which acknowledges that a community's natural helping system is different and would enable both systems to develop. Natural helpers can also work as a group with the coordinator and CAG members to recognize a problem, plan a solution, and take action that strives for structural change in the health system and social change in their communities.

Case Study: Partners for Improved Nutrition and Health Project

This case study illustrates how the natural helper intervention model and concepts have been applied in a health promotion project. A more detailed description of intervention activities, evaluation methods, and specific program recommendations can be found elsewhere (Eng, 1993; Eng & Parker, 1994; Bressler & Lingafelter, 1995).

In a rural Mississippi county that typified many of the conditions found in the Delta Region, the Partners for Improved Nutrition and Health (PINAH) Project began with the guiding principles of health promotion and community empowerment (Wallerstein, 1992). In following these principles, fifty-two community health advisers from three communities tailored the agenda to their own unique circumstances and vision for change. The agenda for the natural helper intervention did not include a categorical health problem, predetermined by the funding agency, for PINAH's partners to address. The partners were the Mississippi Cooperative Extension Agency, a district health office of the Mississippi State Health Department, the county's Interagency Council, and, joining later, the County Union for Progress.

During the year prior to initiating the project, the funding agency completed an analysis similar to Steuart's action-oriented community diagnosis (1969a), from which the project partners were identified, and they then decided to introduce a natural helper intervention. Project staff and evaluators contracted by the funding agency began the planning process with local providers and citizens by conducting a series of workshops on community health development. Members of the Interagency Council (a body of representatives from county health and human service agencies) and the County Union for Progress (an African American civil rights action group) attended. These workshops offered an opportunity for PINAH staff and people in the county to examine their understanding of health-related decisions made by the service delivery system and communities, identify desired outcomes attainable by exerting influence over such decisions, and explore potential actions for achieving these desired outcomes. The workshops also served to introduce PINAH to the communities. A number of products stemmed from these workshops—for example:

- PINAH's long-term goal and premises
- A printed directory of local agencies and their services for the Interagency Council to distribute

- The "characteristics of communities that can pull it together" (participants' terminology for dimensions of community competence)
- The names and ranking of communities in the county from most to least competent

Drawing on the results from these workshops, PINAH staff selected three communities for the intervention, hired a local resident to be the community outreach coordinator, formed a CAG, and with evaluators constructed a questionnaire to measure community competence. The three project communities, with unique characteristics and moderate levels of competency, were the African American neighborhoods of three incorporated towns. PINAH's coordinator and staff recruited fifty-two natural helpers from the three communities, who completed thirty hours of training, and then served as unpaid community health advisers (CHA). The CAG and PINAH staff agreed on the following natural helper intervention inputs and outcomes (Eng & Parker, 1994):

1. PINAH will train CHAs to help improve the health-promoting practices of individuals by providing a) interpersonal and small group counselling on health information and referral to services, b) emotional support, and c) direct assistance.
2. PINAH will link CHAs to the county's Interagency Council to help improve coordination of outreach and referral patterns of local health and human service agencies by communicating community needs to service providers.
3. PINAH will support CHAs to function as a community action group to identify community-wide problems and mobilize residents to undertake community-based responses to those needs, thereby improving community competence of local communities.

Six months were needed to complete the community health development workshops and recruit the first group of CHAs. During this time, the evaluators met three times with project staff to identify intermediate outcomes, design the evaluation, and develop the instruments. The Interagency Council assisted staff and evaluators with pretesting and revising the instruments. Evaluators then met with PINAH's CAG to approve the evaluation plan and select comparison counties. Finally, a specific session on evaluation was included in the thirty-hour training for CHAs so that they could review and discuss expected outcomes and data collection methods with the evaluators. PINAH's staff, CAG, and CHAs worked closely with the evaluators to articulate and frame their respective definitions of "effective" in ways that could be assessed during the five-year project period.

For the next five years, each community's group of CHAs met monthly with PINAH staff and the coordinator to develop and implement action plans for intermediate changes based on their respective communities' long-term goals. Examples of CHA collaborative activities with agencies included community cleanup campaigns, health fairs, drug awareness and teen pregnancy workshops, and creation of a mobile library that could serve outlying communities. On a countywide level, the three communities' CHA groups met together twice a year to plan and mobilize residents for a combined project, such as the establishment and maintenance of an emergency food pantry called Helping Hands. With assistance from PINAH, the CHAs founded the Community Health Adviser Network, which distributed a quarterly newsletter throughout the county, to reinforce solidarity among the three communities and coordinate community actions. This network would eventually serve as an organizational structure for CHAs and their communities to mediate with external institutions and agencies for new resources or partnerships.

The evaluation found strong evidence that PINAH facilitated improved interagency coordination among agencies as well as between agencies and CHAs from the three communities (referred to as North, Center, and South). The evaluation monitored referrals and was specifically interested in monitoring the change, if any, in the number of referrals from agencies to community-based organizations as an indicator of how well the project was increasing coordination between service agencies and community-based organizations. Over seven reporting periods, providers of health and social services in the intervention county showed an increase in mean number of referrals (fifteen); of these referrals, the proportion to community-based organizations increased from 9 percent to 30 percent. In the comparison county, the increase in mean number of referrals was six, and the proportion to community-based organizations increased from 0 percent to 13 percent. With regard to improved coordination between agencies and CHAs, CHA self-reports indicated that their referral rate to agencies increased from one referral per week per CHA to two agency referrals per week per CHA. Moreover, analysis of total agency referrals made by all CHAs, reporting for a given week, revealed that half were to health and social agencies and half to community-based organizations such as schools, churches, legal agencies, and the food pantry.

From the evaluation's analysis of qualitative responses from providers and residents, four improvements in agencies' service delivery (access, availability, quality, and utilization) were attributed specifically to natural helping from CHAs. With regard to improving access to services, for which nearly all staff and facilities were located in North, the county seat, CHAs in Center and South served as important links between residents and agencies by calling providers on the behalf of residents, arranging transportation for residents, or simply making referrals.

Regarding service availability, CHAs in Center and South organized tutoring programs, arranged for a mobile library, and solicited funding to build a park rather than sending local children to services and facilities located in North. CHAs in North, however, provided services that agency staff could not normally offer but their clients needed, such as grocery shopping for home health patients and assisting welfare clients with household management. CHAs were also requested by agencies to participate in planning new services. To improve service quality, CHA assistance enabled agencies to be more efficient about regulations and eligibility requirements, which frequently restricted agency responsiveness. For example, when agencies encountered difficulties with determining a client's eligibility to entitlement programs, providers called on CHAs as credible and quick sources of information about clients. Another way that CHAs improved the quality of services was to provide feedback to agencies about client satisfaction, as well as to inform agencies on the extent to which community needs were met. Agencies solicited CHA opinions through personal communication and meetings of the Interagency Council. To encourage service utilization, CHAs played an important role by eliciting community support and participation in events and programs such as health fairs sponsored by local agencies. CHAs also encouraged and referred individuals who were reticent about using agency services, such as teens in need of prenatal care or family members who were eligible for Medicaid but not enrolled.

Reports from health department clients, interviewed over a three-year period, indicated that those reporting CHA assistance increased from 17 percent to 42 percent. For this same three-year period, CHAs reported on their helping activities for ten seven-day periods. CHA assistance nearly doubled from four people helped per CHA per week to seven people. Themes from the qualitative data revealed that assisting individuals to use health department services was only a part of CHAs' natural helping because the CHAs also worked with populations for whom there were no services at the health department. In all three communities, youth were described as the beneficiaries of CHA assistance. The focus of CHA activities with youth was to keep them from straying toward "the wrong track" by enriching their lives. A few examples of youth projects undertaken by CHAs included workshops and individual counseling to prevent drug abuse, violence, and teen pregnancy; recreational activities; library services; and after-school tutoring. In addition, CHAs in North and Center were noted for their work with elderly residents, particularly those who were homebound or otherwise isolated. South CHAs were recognized for their assistance to flood victims. These results suggested that natural helping from CHAs provided services to a wide spectrum of people and met diverse needs that included, but were not limited to, linking individuals to the formal helping system.

The evaluation also found evidence for effects from PINAH's natural helper intervention on the community competence of the three communities. In each community, fifteen key informants were interviewed annually, using a questionnaire of twenty-six open-ended items and forty-one scale items to measure eight dimensions of community competence. The median score, calculated from key informants' responses (ranging from a score of 4 for highest competence to 0 for lowest competence) to items for a specific dimension, was used as the indicator for each dimension.

Among the three communities, Center demonstrated the most improvement in community competence. Center's scores increased over time, and by the final year, they surpassed those of North and South for the following four dimensions: participation in community life, social support, commitment to the collective, and management of relations with the wider society. Although no change was observed in Center's scores for articulateness and communication, conflict containment and accommodation, and self/other awareness by the final year, neither North nor South surpassed Center on these three dimensions. The only decrease observed was in Center's scores over time for machinery for facilitating participant interaction and decision making.

Overall, the dimension of community competence for which all three communities' scores increased was participation in community life. Moreover, the three communities either sustained or increased their scores for social support and conflict containment and accommodation over the four-year period. A slight decline was observed in the scores of all communities for machinery for facilitating participant interaction and decision making. For the remaining four dimensions of community competence, the scores for Center and North either increased or stayed the same.

The scores for South showed the least improvement over time. From examining the final year's scores only, differences by community revealed that South did not surpass North or Center on any dimension, showing at most a comparable score for social support. Analysis of the qualitative data on community competence revealed some explanations for the difficulties that South experienced. South was described as the community in the county with the least concentration of internal resources, the weakest access to external resources, low community pride, and frustration with lack of initiation of community action. These conditions were attributed to the nonresponsiveness of elected officials, regardless of their race. Moreover, no theme linked any effect, positive or negative, from South's CHAs to the following three dimensions of community competence: conflict containment and accommodation, self/other awareness, and machinery for facilitating participant interaction and decision making.

From the analysis of qualitative responses from North, these same three dimensions of community competence were linked with negative forces that affected the work of North's CHAs. The negative forces referred to resistance from traditional power holders who perceived PINAH and CHAs to be espousing a political agenda. Although political organizing was neither an explicitly stated objective nor a CHA role defined by PINAH, the involvement of some CHAs in black voter registration drives raised controversy in North on the appropriateness of including a political agenda in health promotion.

Very different themes emerged from the qualitative responses from Center about self/other awareness and conflict containment and accommodation. These two dimensions were associated with a boycott by African American residents of white merchants, which predated PINAH. The boycott confronted racial tensions and stimulated the community's progress toward improving race relations. No mention was made about CHA's involvement in Center's current progress toward improving race relations.

During PINAH's first three years of implementation, no natural helper who is white would accept the invitation to serve as a CHA. Gaining trust from white residents required PINAH to demonstrate that its mission was to improve health and nutrition for all residents, regardless of race. PINAH provided "proof" by supporting self-help actions that offered a range of concrete, easy, and short-term ways for all residents to participate and experience tangible results. Specifically cited activities were the health fairs, cleanup campaigns, food pantry, and an interagency council. From the one-time donation of canned goods to assembling a budget for a grant proposal, the actions were entirely voluntary and open to everyone. No commitment to PINAH was needed. No political values were espoused.

In its final year, PINAH's successful recruitment and training of white CHAs from North was described by white and African American residents alike as an important milestone for improved race relations in the county. Nevertheless, PINAH's capacity to address social unity was viewed by traditional power holders as an unanticipated side effect rather than an integral part of health promotion. As involvement in and support for health promotion increased among traditional power holders, so did their voices and opinions on the issues to be addressed by CHAs. Power holders contended that the involvement of CHAs in political organizing activities, such as voter registration drives or campaigning for a particular candidate, was inappropriate for a health promotion program. Yet CHAs, many of whom had been involved in their community's political dynamics long before they were recruited and trained by PINAH, considered it natural to continue to apply the community organizing skills they learned during the civil rights movement to their current work in health promotion.

Analysis of qualitative responses from CHAs revealed three effects from their involvement with PINAH. CHAs from North reported being influenced by PINAH in two ways. First, they experienced greater satisfaction with the assistance they provided because they were directly informed about and connected to local services. Second, they indicated they felt a stronger commitment to what they could do for their communities because training had inspired them to recognize their potential as a network of natural helpers. Finally, CHAs from all three communities indicated they experienced an affirmation of their accountability to their community. That is, their work with PINAH as CHAs helped them to understand the importance of the reputation and trust they hold among community people as natural helpers. The implication is that PINAH was able to identify natural helpers, whose roles were often invisible to others as well as to themselves, and engage them in three arenas of action and change: (1) improving individuals' health practices through appropriate use of services, (2) improving coordination of services through agencies' awareness of and responsiveness to community needs, and (3) improving a community's competence through addressing social unity and acting on locally recognized issues.

Future Directions for Research and Practice

The natural helper intervention model presented in Figure 6.1 is a distillation of concepts, theories, and findings from descriptive and applied studies in social epidemiology, mental health, community psychology, social work, and organization development. Although the intervention model represents a planned attempt to induce behavioral, organizational, and social changes, the actual design and implementation of natural helper interventions almost always depend on unplanned or natural determinants of stability and change (Steuart, 1969a; Parker, Eng, Schulz, & Israel, 1999). A growing body of research on the social ecology of health promotion (McLeroy, Bibeau, Steckler, & Glanz, 1988; Stokols, 1992), community assessments (Centers for Disease Control, 1992), social diagnosis (Green & Kreuter, 1991), and action-oriented community diagnosis (Eng & Blanchard, 1991) highlights the importance of uncovering the range of natural determinants of stability and change that exist in each community's social and physical environment.

The challenge for natural helper interventions is to enable the structure and functions of community support systems and their natural helping networks to understand and respond to unplanned determinants of stability and change. At the same time, a fair number of examples, including the PINAH case study described in this chapter, suggest that a generic natural helper intervention model is unlikely to exist. Comprehensive recruitment and training of natural helpers is necessary but not sufficient for an intervention to engage them in multiple arenas of social action and achieve multiple levels of outcomes (Blumenthal, Eng, & Thomas, 1999; Altpeter, Earp, Bishop, & Eng, 1999). Natural helper interventions that deserve the greatest attention for future research and practice are those for which (1) the natural helpers and health educators are equally active in designing and adapting the intervention and the evaluation to unplanned determinants, (2) defining and monitoring intervention effects on community competence is as important to the evaluation as monitoring the effects on health practices, and (3) intervention activities to recognize and address power differentials between the formal and informal helping systems are carefully described.

A key asset of a natural helper intervention is that it builds on and is responsive to the particular characteristics and resources of a local community support system. The features that make a natural helper intervention effective in one community may be different in another. Such variations in interventions will likely require evaluation measures and study designs that differ. For example, there has been increased recognition that embedded support systems are moving beyond geographically defined neighborhoods and communities to locations such as work sites, special interest clubs, and even the Internet. Given these evolving sources of social support, future research will need to explore the feasibility of newly emerging informal helping networks, such as chatrooms at a Web site, for possible natural helping interventions. The research and practice reviewed in this chapter suggest that although the challenges are substantial, the potential health benefits obtained from a natural helper intervention model are considerable given that efforts are structured around people who are trusted, address organizational change, and build community competence.

A key asset of a natural helper intervention is that it builds on and is responsive to the particular characteristics and resources of a local community support system.

References

Altpeter, M., Earp, J. A., Bishop, C., & Eng, E. (1999). Lay health adviser activity levels: Definitions from the field. *Health Education and Behavior, 26,* 495–512.

Baker, E. A., Bouldin, N., Durham, M., Lowell, M. E., Gonzalez, M., Jodaitis, N., Cruz, L. N., Torres, I., Torres, M., & Adams, S. T. (1997). The Latino health advocacy program: A collaborative lay health adviser approach. *Health Education and Behavior, 4,* 495–509.

Berkley-Patton, J., Fawcett, S. B., Paine-Andrews, A., & Johns, L. (1997). Developing capacities of youth as lay health advisers: A case study with high school students. *Health Education and Behavior, 24,* 481–494.

Biegel, D. E., & Naparstek, A. J. (Eds). (1982). *Community support systems and mental health.* New York: Springer.

Biegel, D. E., Naparstek, A. J., & Khan, M. M. (1982). Social support and mental health in urban ethnic neighborhoods. In D. E. Biegel & A. J. Naparstek (Eds.), *Community support systems and mental health.* New York: Springer.

Bloom, B. L. (1979). Prevention of mental disorders: Recent advances in theory and practice. *Community Mental Health Journal, 15,* 179–191.

Blumenthal, C., Eng, E., & Thomas, J. C. (1999). STEP sisters, sex, and STDs: A process evaluation of the recruitment of lay health advisers. *American Journal of Health Promotion, 14,* 4–6.

Booker, V. K., Robinson, J. G., Kay, B. J., Najera, L. G., & Stewart, G. (1997). Changes in empowerment: Effects of participation in a lay health promotion program. *Health Education and Behavior, 4,* 452–464.

Bressler, M., & Lingafelter, T. (1995). Neighbor Helping Neighbor for Health Care: Rural community health adviser program. In J. P. Troxel (Ed.), *Government works: Profiles of people making a difference.* Alexandria, VA: Miles River.

Broadhead, W. E., Kaplan, B. H., James, S. A., Wagner, E. H., Schoenbach, V. J., Grimson, R., Heydon, S., Tibblin, G., & Gehlbech, S. H. (1983). The epidemiologic evidence for a relationship between social support and health. *American Journal of Epidemiology, 117,* 521–537.

Cantor, M. H. (1979). The informal support system of New York's inner city elderly: Is ethnicity a factor? In D. E. Gelfand & A. J. Kutzik (Eds.), *Ethnicity and aging: Theory, research, and policy.* New York: Springer.

Caplan, G. (1974). *Support systems and community mental health: Lectures on concept development.* New York: Behavioral Publications.

Caplan, G. (1976). *Support systems and mutual help.* New York: Grune & Stratton.

Caplan, G. (1982). Foreword. In D. E. Biegel & A. J. Naparstek (Eds.), *Community support systems and mental health.* New York: Springer.

Cassel, J. C. (1976). The contribution of the social environment to host resistance. *American Journal of Epidemiology, 104,* 107–123.

Centers for Disease Control and Prevention, National Center for Chronic Disease Prevention and Health Promotion. (1992). PATCH: Planned approach to community health. *Journal of Health Education, 23,* 129–192.

Cottrell, L. S. (1976). The competent community. In B. H. Kaplan, R. N. Wilson, & A. H. Leighton (Eds.), *Further explorations in social psychiatry.* New York: Basic Books.

Cottrell, L. S. (1980). George Herbert Mead, the legacy of social behaviorism. In R. K. Merton & M. W. Riley (Eds.), *Sociological traditions from generation to generation.* Norwood, NJ: Ablex.

Denham, A., Quinn, S. C., & Gamble, D. (1998). Community organizing for health promotion in the rural South: An exploration of community competence. *Journal of Family and Community Health, 21,* 1–21.

Earp, J. A., Rauscher, G., & O'Malley, M. S. (2000, November). *Closing the black-white gap in mammography use.* Paper presented at the 128th Annual Meeting of the American Public Health Association, Boston.

Earp, J. A., Viadro, C., Vincus, A., Altpeter, M., Flax, V., Mayne, L., & Eng, E. (1997). Lay health advisors: A strategy for getting the word out about breast cancer. *Health Education and Behavior, 24,* 432–451.

Eng, E. (1993). *Partners for improved nutrition and health: Did the partnership make a difference.* Davis, CA: Freedom from Hunger Foundation.

Eng, E., & Blanchard, L. (1991). Action-oriented community diagnosis: A health education tool. *International Quarterly of Community Health Education, 11,* 93–110.

Eng, E., & Hatch, J. W. (1991). Networking between black churches and agencies: The lay health adviser model. *Journal of Prevention and Human Services, 10,* 123–146.

Eng, E., & Hatch, J. W. (1992). Networking between agencies and black churches: The lay health adviser model. In K. I. Pargament, K. I. Maton, & R. E. Hess (Eds.), *Religion and prevention in mental health: Research, vision, and action.* New York: Haworth Press.

Eng, E., Hatch, J. W., & Callan, A. (1985). Institutionalizing social support through the church and into the community. *Health Education Quarterly, 12,* 81–92.

Eng, E., & Parker, E. A. (1994). Measuring community competence in the Mississippi Delta: The interface between program evaluation and empowerment. *Health Education Quarterly, 21,* 199–220.

Eng, E., Parker, E. A., & Harlan, C. (1997). Lay health advisor intervention strategies: A continuum from natural helping to paraprofessional helping. *Health Education & Behavior, 24,* 413–417.

Eng, E., & Smith, J. (1995). Natural helping functions of lay health advisers in breast cancer education. *Breast Cancer Research Treatment, 35,* 23–29.

Eng, E., & Young, R. (1992). Lay health advisers as community change agents. *Family Community Health, 15,* 24–40.

Froland, C. (1980). Formal and informal care: Discontinuities in a continuum. *Social Service Review, 54,* 572–587.

Gans, H. (1961). *The urban villagers.* New York: Free Press.

Gatz, M., Barbarin, O., Tyler, F., Mitchell, R., Moran, J., Wirzbicki, P., Crawford J., & Engelman, A. (1982). Enhancement of individual and community competence: The older adult as community worker. *American Journal of Community Psychology, 10,* 291–303.

Geiger, H. J. (1971). A health center in Mississippi—A case study in social medicine. In L. Corey, S. E. Saltman, & M. F. Epstein (Eds.), *Medicine in a changing society.* St. Louis, MO: Mosby.

Geiger, H. J. (1984). Community health centers: Health care as an instrument of social change. In V. W. Sidel & R. Sidel (Eds.), *Reforming medicine: Lessons of the past quarter century.* New York: Pantheon Books.

Goeppinger, J., & Baglioni, A. J. (1985). Community competence: A positive approach to needs assessment. *American Journal of Community Psychology, 13,* 507–523.

Gottlieb, B. H. (1982). Social support in the workplace. In D. E. Biegel & A. J. Naparstek (Eds.), *Community support systems and mental health.* New York: Springer.

Gourash, N. (1978). Help-seeking: A review of the literature. *American Journal of Community Psychology, 6,* 413–423.

Green, L. W., & Kreuter, M. W. (1991). *Health promotion planning: An educational and environmental approach* (2nd ed.). Mountain View, CA: Mayfield.

Guttman, D. (1979). Use of informal and formal supports by the ethnic aged. In D. E. Gelfand & A. J. Kutzik (Eds.), *Ethnicity and aging: Theory, research, and policy.* New York: Springer.

Hamburg, B., & Killilea, M. (1979). Relation of social support, stress, illness and use of health services. In U.S. Department of Health, Education, and Welfare, *Surgeon General's Report: Background Papers.* Washington, DC: U.S. Government Printing Office.

Hatch, J. W., & Eng, E. (1983). Health worker role in community oriented primary care. In E. Connor & F. Mullan (Eds.), *Community oriented primary care.* Washington, DC: National Academy Press.

Hatch, J. W., & Lovelace, K. (1980). Involving the southern rural church and students of the health professions in health education. *Public Health Report, 95,* 23–25.

Hatch, J. W., Moss, N., Saran, A., Presley-Cantrell, L., & Mallory, C. (1993). Community research: Partnerships in black communities. *American Journal of Preventive Medicine, 9,* 27–31.

Heaney, C. A., & Israel, B. A. (1997). Social networks and social support. In K. Glanz, F. M. Lewis, & B. K. Rimer (Eds.), *Health behavior and health education: Theory, research, and practice.* San Francisco: Jossey-Bass.

Heller, K. (1989). The return to community. *American Journal of Community Psychology, 17,* 1–15.

House, J. (1981). *Work stress and social support.* Reading, Mass: Addison-Wesley.

Hurley, D., Barbarin, O., & Mitchell, R. (1981). An empirical study of racism in community functioning. In O. Barbarin, P. Good, M. Pharr, & J. Suskind (Eds.), *Institutional racism and community competence.* Rockville, MD: National Institute of Mental Health.

Israel, B. A. (1982). Social network and health status: Linking theory, research, and practice. *Patient Counselling and Health Education, 4,* 65–79.

Israel, B. A. (1985). Social networks and social support: Implications for natural helper and community level interventions. *Health Education Quarterly, 12,* 65–80.

Israel, B. A., Dawson, L., Steckler, A. B., Eng, E., & Steuart, G. W. (1993). The person and his works. *Health Education Quarterly* (Suppl. 1), S137-S146.

Israel, B. A., & Rounds, K. A. (1987). Social networks and social support: A synthesis for health educators. *Advances in Health Education and Promotion, 2,* 311–351.

Jackson, E. J., & Parks, C. P. (1997). Recruitment and training issues from selected lay health adviser programs among African Americans: A 20-year perspective. *Health Education and Behavior 24,* 418–431.

Jessor, R., & Jessor, S. (1981). *Problem behavior and psycho-social development: A longitudinal study on youth.* New York: Plenum Press.

Kaplan, B. H., Cassel, J. C., & Gore, S. (1977). Social support and health. *Medical Care, 15,* 47–58.

Kark, S. (1951). Health center service. In E. H. Cluver (Ed.), *Social medicine.* Johannesburg, South Africa: Central News Agency.

Ketterer, R. F., Bader, B. C., & Levy, M. R. (1980). Strategies and skills for promoting mental health. In R. H. Price, R. F. Ketterer, B. C. Bader, & J. Monahann (Eds.), *Prevention in mental health.* Thousand Oaks, CA: Sage.

Killilea, M. (1976). Mutual help organizations: Interpretations in the literatures. In G. Caplan & M. Killilea (Eds.), *Prevention in mental health.* Thousand Oaks, CA: Sage.

Knight, E., Johnson, H. H., & Holbert, D. (1991). Analysis of the competent community: Support for the community. *International Quarterly of Community Health Education, 11,* 145–154.

Labonte, R. (1989). Community empowerment: The need for political analysis. *Canadian Journal of Public Health, 80,* 87–88.

Lee, T. (1968). Urban neighborhood as a socio-spatial schema. *Human Relations, 21,* 241–268.

Lin, N., Simeone, R., Ensel, W., & Kuo, W. (1979). Social support, stressful life events and illness: A model and an empirical test. *Journal of Health and Social Behavior, 20,* 108–119.

Litwak, E., & Szelenyi, I. (1969). Primary group structures and their functions: Kin, neighbors, and friends. *American Sociological Review, 34,* 465–481.

Love, M. B., Gardner, K., & Legion, V. (1997). Community health workers: Who they are and what they do. *Health Education and Behavior, 24,* 510–522.

Mann, P. (1965). *An approach to urban sociology.* New York: Routledge.

McLeroy, K. R., Bibeau, D., Steckler, A., & Glanz, K. (1988). An ecological perspective on health promotion programs. *Health Education Quarterly, 15,* 351–377.

McKnight, J. (1991). Comments made at Leadership and Model Development Meeting for Community-Based Public Health Initiative, W. K. Kellogg Foundation, Chicago.

Nuckolls, K. B., Cassel, J. C., & Kaplan, B. H. (1972). Psycho-social assets, life crisis and the prognosis of pregnancy. *American Journal of Epidemiology, 95,* 431–441.

Pancoast, D. L., & Chapman, N. J. (1982). Roles for informal helpers in the delivery of human services. In D. E. Biegel & A. J. Naparstek (Eds.). *Community support systems and mental health.* New York: Springer.

Parker, E. A., Eng, E., Schulz, A. J., & Israel, B. A. (1999). Evaluating community-based health programs that seek to increase community capacity. *New Directions for Evaluation, 83,* 37–54.

Parker, E. A., Israel, B. A., Schulz, A. J., & Hollis, R. (1998). East Side Detroit village health worker partnership: Community-based lay health adviser intervention in an urban area. *Health Education and Behavior, 25,* 24–45.

Plaut, T. (1982). Primary prevention in the 80s: The interface with community support systems. In D. E. Biegel & A. J. Naparstek (Eds.). *Community support systems and mental health.* New York: Springer.

President's Commission on Mental Health. (1978). *Report to the President from the President's Commission on Mental Health* (Vol. 2). Washington DC: U.S. Government Printing Office.

Riessman, F. (1965). The "helper" therapy principle. *Social Work, 10,* 27–32.

Salber, E. J., Beery, W. B., & Jackson, E. J. (1976). The role of the health facilitator in community health education. *Journal of Community Health, 2,* 5–20.

Schuster, J., Thomas, J. C., & Eng, E. (1995). Bridging the culture gap in sexually transmitted disease clinics. *North Carolina Medical Journal, 56,* 256–269.

Service, C., & Salber, E. J. (Eds). (1979). *Community health education: The lay health adviser approach.* Durham, NC: Health Care Systems.

Shanas, E. (1978). The family as a social system in old age. *Gerontologist, 18,* 169–174.

Stack, C. B. (1974). *All our kin.* New York: HarperCollins.

Steuart, G. W. (1969a). Planning and evaluation in health education. *International Journal of Health Education, 2,* 65–76.

Steuart, G. W. (1969b). Scientist and professional: The relations between research and action. *Health Education Monograph, 29,* 1–10.

Steuart, G. W. (1977, November). *The world is not round: Innovation and the medical wheel.* Paper presented at the Annual Meeting of the American Public Health Association, Washington, DC.

Steuart, G. W. (1978, February). Social and cultural perspectives: Community intervention and mental health. In *Perspectives in primary prevention: Proceedings of the Fourteenth Annual John W. Umstead Series of Distinguished Lectures.* Raleigh: North Carolina Division of Mental Health and Mental Retardation Services.

Steuart, G. W., & Kark, S. L. (1993). Community health education. *Health Education Quarterly* (Suppl. 1), S29-S47. (Originally published 1962)

Stokols, D. (1992). Establishing and maintaining healthy environments: Toward a social ecology of health promotion. *American Psychologist, 47,* 6–22.

Tessaro, I., Eng, E., & Smith, J. (1994). Breast cancer screening in older African-American women: Qualitative research findings. *American Journal of Health Promotion, 8,* 286–293.

Thomas, J. C., Earp, J. A., & Eng, E. (2000). Evaluation and lessons learned from a lay health adviser programme to prevent sexually transmitted diseases. *International Journal of STD & AIDS, 11,* 812–818.

Thomas, J. C., Eng, E., Clark, M., Robinson, J., & Blumenthal, C. (1998). Lay health advisors: Sexually transmitted disease prevention through community involvement. *American Journal of Public Health, 88,* 1252–1253.

Tracy, G. S., & Gussow, Z. (1976). Self-help groups: A grassroots response to a need for services. *Journal of Applied Behavioral Science, 12,* 381–396.

Trostle, J. (1986). Anthropology and epidemiology in the twentieth century: A selective history of collaborative projects and theoretical affinities, 1920 to 1970. In C. R. Janes, R. Stall, & S. M. Gifford (Eds.), *Anthropology and Epidemiology.* Boston: D. Reidel.

U.S. Department of Health, Education and Welfare. (1979). *Healthy people: The surgeon general's report on mental promotion and disease prevention.* Washington, DC: U.S. Government Printing Office.

U.S. Department of Health, Education, and Welfare Task Force. (1979). *Report to the president from the President's Commission on Mental Health.* Washington DC: U.S. Government Printing Office.

U.S. Department of Health and Human Services. (1994). *Community health advisers: Models, research and practice selected annotations—United States.* Atlanta, GA: Centers for Disease Control and Prevention.

Wallerstein, N. (1992). Powerlessness, empowerment, and health: Implications for health promotion programs. *American Journal of Health Promotion, 6,* 197–205.

Warren, D. I. (1971). Neighborhoods in urban areas. In *Encyclopedia of social work* (Vol. 1). New York: National Association of Social Workers.

Warren, D. I. (1977). Neighborhoods in urban areas. In *Encyclopedia of social work* (Vol. 1). New York: National Association of Social Workers.

Warren, D. I. (1982). Using helping networks: A key social bond of urbanites. In D. E. Biegel & A. J. Naparstek (Eds.), *Community support systems and mental health.* New York: Springer.

Warren, R. L. (1963a). *Social research consultation: An experiment in health and welfare planning.* New York: Russell Sage Foundation.

Warren, R. L. (1963b). *The community in America.* Skokie, IL: Rand McNally.

Watkins, E. L., Harlan, C., Eng, E., Gansky, S. A., Gehan, D., & Larson, K. (1994). Assessing the effectiveness of lay health advisers with migrant farmworkers. *Family and Community Health, 16,* 72–87.

Wilkinson, D. Y. (1992). Indigenous community health workers in the 1960s and beyond. In R. L. Braithwaite & S. E. Taylor (Eds.), *Health issues in the black community.* San Francisco: Jossey-Bass.

CHAPTER SEVEN

TOWARD A COMPREHENSIVE UNDERSTANDING OF COMMUNITY COALITIONS

Moving from Practice to Theory

Frances D. Butterfoss
Michelle C. Kegler

Communities, organizations, businesses, and even nations today form alliances, joint ventures, and public-private partnerships. One type of strategic relationship, a coalition, develops when different sectors of the community, state, or nation join together to create opportunities that will benefit all of the partners. Community coalitions are a specific type of coalition defined as a group of individuals representing diverse organizations, factions, or constituencies within the community who agree to work together to achieve a common goal (Feighery & Rogers, 1990).

The development of coalitions escalated rapidly over the past two decades. Thousands of coalitions anchored by government or community-based organizations formed to support community-based, health-related activities across the United States. For example, coalitions of health-related agencies, schools, and community-based action groups have formed to reduce, and eventually to eliminate, the use of tobacco among youth. Advocates for environmental issues such as asthma and lead contamination have rallied to highlight their issue or enable favorable policy and legislation. Civic and faith-based groups developed coalitions to ensure adequate housing for the elderly and health insurance for the poor. Community coalitions

Community coalitions bring people together, expand available resources, and focus on a problem of community concern to achieve better results than any single group or agency could have achieved alone.

bring people together, expand available resources, and focus on a problem of community concern to achieve better results than any single group or agency could have achieved alone.

Unfortunately, not every coalition has been successful, and not every coalition has achieved its results without having its members pay a high price for its success (Dowling, O'Donnell & Wellington Consulting Group, 2000; Wolff, 2001). Although coalitions are usually built from unselfish motives to improve communities, they still may experience difficulties that are common to many types of organizations, as well as some that are unique to collaborative efforts. With the initiation of a coalition, frustrations often arise. Promised resources may not be made available, conflicting interests may prevent the coalition from having its desired effect in the community, and recognition for accomplishments may be slow in coming. Coalitions are not a panacea. Because coalition building involves a long-term investment of time and resources, a coalition should not be established if a simpler, less complex structure will get the job done or if the community does not embrace this approach.

The premise of this chapter is that public health professionals have eagerly embraced the practice of coalition building. They have looked for an effective, inclusive approach to complex health issues and coalitions fit the bill. The time has come to step back from the practice of building coalitions and forge a comprehensive theory of community coalitions. This theory, complete with constructs and propositions, will lead to an increased understanding of how community coalitions work in practice.

Origins and Roots of the Theory

The underlying theoretical basis for the development and maintenance of community coalitions borrows from many arenas, including community development, citizen participation, political science, interorganizational relations, and group process. Community development and related approaches such as community organization, community empowerment, and citizen participation provide much of the philosophy that underlies community coalition approaches. Coined by the United Nations in 1955, *community development* was designed to create conditions of economic and social progress for the whole community with its active participation and the fullest possible reliance on the community's initiative (Brager, Sprecht, & Torczyner, 1987). This approach is based on assumptions that communities can develop the capacity to deal with their own problems; people should participate in making, adjusting, or controlling the major changes taking place in their communities; and changes in community living that are self-imposed or self-developed have a meaning and permanence that imposed changes do not have. Additional assumptions underlying community approaches to problem solving are that holistic approaches can deal successfully with problems where fragmented approaches cannot, democracy requires cooperative participation and action in the affairs of the community, and people must learn the skills that make this possible.

In a similar vein, *community participation* is the process of involving people in the institutions or decisions that affect their lives (Checkoway, 1989). Citizen participation is the mobilization of citizens for the purpose of undertaking activities to improve conditions in the community. Much of the initial coalition research in the 1990s was based on two significant research efforts in the area of citizen participation. The Neighborhood Participation Project examined the process of citizen participation through a systematic study of block organizations in a Nashville, Tennessee, neighborhood (Florin & Wandersman, 1990; Prestby, Wandersman, Florin, Rich, & Chavis, 1990; Prestby & Wandersman, 1985; Giamartino & Wandersman, 1983). Researchers posed questions similar to those posed in coalition research: Who participates, who does not, and why? What are the effects of citizen participation in block organizations? What are the characteristics of organizations that are active and successful versus those that are inactive (Florin & Wandersman, 1990)? Research questions asked in the Block Booster Project in New York City also helped shape the coalition research agenda (Perkins, Florin, Rich, Wandersman, & Chavis, 1990). This project assessed the role of block associations in encouraging community development and increasing a sense of community (Florin & Wandersman, 1990).

Community-based coalitions differ from block organizations. Although some coalition members can be characterized as interested citizens (or volunteers), many of the members represent organizations. Thus, research and conceptual work done in the field of interorganizational relations is also relevant to coalition theory. Much of the early research on interorganizational relations focused on the formation of collaborative relationships in an effort to understand why organizations join collaborative alliances (Gray & Wood, 1991; Berlin, Barnett, Mischke, & Ocasio, 2000; Provan & Milward, 1995).

Gray and Wood (1991) discussed several theoretical perspectives that help to inform interorganizational collaboration. For example, resource dependence theory posits that acquiring resources and reducing uncertainty are the primary forces underlying collaboration (Sharfman, Gray, & Yan, 1991; Mizruchi & Galaskiewicz, 1994). Institutional theory suggests that organizations adjust to institutional directives and norms in an attempt to achieve legitimacy (Gray & Wood, 1991; Gulati, 1995). Finally, political science emphasizes the negotiation of potential conflict through coalitions and power distribution within coalitions (Bazzoli et al., 1997).

Each of these perspectives sheds insight into the formation of community coalitions. For example, community coalitions often form in response to an opportunity, such as new funding exemplified by the tobacco settlement funds made available for coalition building around preventing youth tobacco use. Coalitions may form because of a threat such as a national story about rising asthma prevalence or a local event such as an outbreak of bacterial meningitis on a college campus. Local health organizations may voluntarily form or join coalitions to augment their limited resources of staff, time, talent, equipment, supplies, materials, contacts, and influence. Joining with other agencies and individuals can benefit an organization, giving it expanded access to printing and postage services, media coverage, marketing services, meeting space, community residents, influential people, personnel, community and professional networks, and expertise (Whitt, 1993). In addition, coalition formation may be mandatory or required by a funding source, such as the Robert Wood Johnson Allies Against Asthma initiative.

Another major contribution of the field of interorganizational relations to coalition theory is the fact that organizations decide to join collaborative relationships when the benefits outweigh the costs (Gray, 1989; Prestby et al., 1990; Roberts-DeGennaro, 1986; Whetten, 1981). Ultimately, collaboration is possible when a perceived need exists and an organization anticipates deriving a benefit that is contingent on mutual action (Wood & Gray, 1991). Coalitions offer such benefits by serving as effective and efficient vehicles for the exchange of knowledge, ideas, and strategies. Through coalitions, individuals and organizations can become involved in new, broader issues without assuming sole responsibility. Coalitions can also demonstrate and develop community support or concern for issues; maximize the power of individuals and groups through collective action; improve trust and communication among community agencies and sectors; mobilize diverse talents, resources, and strategies; build strength and cohesiveness by connecting individual activists; build a constituency for a given issue; reduce the social acceptability of health-risk behaviors; and change community norms and standards (Whitt, 1993). Additional benefits include the potential to minimize duplication and use resources efficiently; the opportunity to gain access to new information, ideas, materials, and other resources; the opportunity to reduce uncertainty in the environment; and the sharing of costs and associated risks (Alter & Hage, 1993; Gray, 1989; Whetten, 1981; Zapka et al., 1992; Wandersman & Alderman, 1993; Butterfoss, Goodman, & Wandersman, 1993; Penner, 1995).

The costs associated with coalition membership may include loss of autonomy and the ability to control outcomes unilaterally, conflict over goals and methods, loss of resources (time, money, information, and status), risk of losing competitive position, and possible delays in solving problems (Alter & Hage, 1993).

Community coalitions that survive over time must provide ongoing benefits that outweigh the costs of membership.

Finally, the field of interorganizational relations has contributed to our understanding of the stages of collaboration that community coalitions often experience. Gray (1989), for example, proposed three stages: problem setting, direction setting, and implementation. Similarly, Alter and Hage (1993) suggested a model of network development whereby networks evolve through three stages: from exchange networks to action networks to fully developed systemic networks. According to their model, action networks result when organizations can no longer meet a goal alone due to environmental conditions. A network shifts from an exchange to an action network when members contribute private resources for access to collective output, depend on the collective output, and feel a normative obligation to comply with the coordinating mechanism. An action network shifts to a systemic network when it begins to produce together, with specialized roles.

Although clear and definite theoretical underpinnings exist for community coalitions, the practice of coalition building has outpaced the development of coalition theory. The rise of coalitions as a prominent health promotion strategy parallels the growth of communitywide health promotion over the past two decades. This growth is partially due to the widespread dissemination of strategies employed in the National Heart, Lung and Blood Institutes' community demonstration projects (Mittelmark, 1999). These projects, which include the Stanford Three Community and Five City Projects and the Minnesota and Pawtucket Heart Health Programs, used community advisory boards to plan and implement communitywide cardiovascular disease prevention strategies (Shea & Basch, 1990; Carlaw, Mittelmark, Bracht, Luepker, 1984; Mittelmark et al., 1986; Lefebvre, Lasater, Carleton, & Peterson, 1987; Farquhar et al., 1990). Additionally, the Centers for Disease Control and Prevention (CDC) advocated forming community coalitions in the Planned Approach to Community Health, which was widely adopted by state and local health departments in the late 1980s and early 1990s (Kreuter, 1992; Green & Kreuter, 1992).

In contrast to traditional, individual-focused behavior change efforts, community approaches, including those that build coalitions, attempt to alleviate community problems by organizing the community to bring about change. These communitywide approaches recognize that behaviors are inextricably tied to the environment (Milio, 1989; Thompson & Kinne, 1990; Stokols, 1992; Tesh, 1988). In theory, no single approach for community change is as effective as a broad-based coalition effort

The general focus of community organizing for health promotion is on changing systems, rules, social norms, or laws in order ultimately to change the social acceptability of certain behaviors.

that provides the means for multiple strategies and involves key community individuals (McLeroy, Kegler, Steckler, Burdine, & Wisotzky, 1994). The general focus of community organizing for health promotion is on changing systems, rules, social norms, or laws in order ultimately to change the social acceptability of certain behaviors. The venue for community organizing is often the policy arena and can often involve community elected officials, businesses, community groups, media, and local and state legislatures to create positive community change.

Community coalitions have the potential to involve multiple sectors of the community and to conduct multiple interventions that focus on both individuals and their environments. The pooling of resources and the mobilization of talents and diverse approaches inherent in a successful coalition approach make it a logical strategy for disease prevention based on a social ecological model that acknowledges the significance of the environment on health. The fact that individuals and organizations apply their skills and resources in collective efforts to meet their own needs is also the basis of *community empowerment.* Community empowerment enjoyed a resurgence of interest and also fueled the formation of community coalitions in the early 1990s (Israel, Checkoway, Schultz, & Zimmerman, 1994; Labonte, 1994; Minkler, 1994; Perkins, 1995; Rappaport, 1987; Robertson & Minkler, 1994; Wallerstein, 1992; Zimmerman & Rappaport, 1988).

Finally, interest in how well community coalitions develop the capacity of communities to address future critical health issues is growing. Community coalitions are a promising strategy for building capacity and competence among member organizations and, ultimately, in the communities they serve (Chavis, 2001; Kegler, Steckler, McLeroy, & Malek, 1998b). Associated increases in community participation and leadership, skills, resources, social and interorganizational networks, sense of community, and community power may contribute to future successful community problem-solving efforts (Goodman et al., 1998).

To summarize, coalitions are excellent vehicles for consensus building and active involvement of diverse organizations and constituencies in addressing community problems. They enable communities to build capacity and intervene using a social ecological approach. By involving community members, coalitions help to ensure that interventions meet the needs of the community and are culturally sensitive. Community participation through coalitions also facilitates ownership, which is thought to increase the chances of successful institutionalization into the community (Bracht, 1990). These advantages of community coalition approaches are widely accepted by government agencies and foundations, and, as a result, the majority of prevention initiatives over the past decade required the formation of community coalitions.

Description of Theory, Constructs, and Assumptions

Certain theoretical underpinnings and assumptions form the framework on which most community coalitions are, or should be, built. A wealth of practice-proven propositions have arisen that provide the basis for grounded theories about the development and maintenance of coalitions, as well as how they result in successful actions and health outcomes. The propositions presented in Tables 7.1 and 7.2 are the rationale behind the Community Coalition Action Theory; Figure 7.1 depicts the theory visually.

The theory applies primarily to community coalitions. A community coalition is different from other types of community entities in that a structured arrangement for collaboration by organizations exists in which all members work together toward a common purpose. If a group is composed solely of individuals and not organizations, then it is not a coalition in its truest form. As an action-oriented partnership, a coalition usually focuses on preventing or ameliorating a community problem by (1) analyzing the problem, (2) gathering data and assessing need, (3) developing an action plan with identified solutions, (4) implementing those solutions, (5) reaching community-level outcomes, such as health

FIGURE 7.1. COMMUNITY COALITION ACTION THEORY.

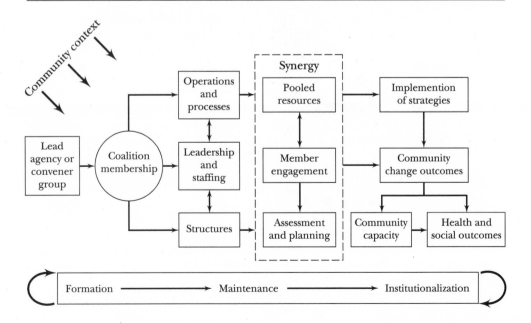

TABLE 7.1. CONSTRUCTS AND PROPOSITIONS RELATED TO COMMUNITY COALITION FORMATION, STRUCTURE, AND PROCESSES.

Constructs	Propositions
Stages of development	*Proposition 1.* Coalitions develop in specific stages and recycle through these stages as new members are recruited, plans are renewed, and new issues are added.
	Proposition 2. At each stage, specific factors enhance coalition function and progression to the next stage.
Community context	*Proposition 3.* Coalitions are heavily influenced by contextual factors in the community throughout all stages of development.
Lead agency/ convener group	*Proposition 4.* Coalitions form when a lead agency or convening group responds to an opportunity, threat, or mandate.
	Proposition 5. Coalition formation is more likely when the lead agency or convening organization provides technical assistance, financial or material support, credibility, and valuable networks and contacts.
	Proposition 6. Coalition formation is likely to be more successful when the convener group enlists community gatekeepers who thoroughly understand the community to help develop credibility and trust with others in the community.
Coalition membership	*Proposition 7.* Coalition formation usually begins by recruiting a core group of people who are committed to resolving the health or social issue.
	Proposition 8. More effective coalitions result when the core group expands to include a broad constituency of participants who represent diverse interest groups, agencies, organizations, and institutions.
Coalition operations and processes	*Proposition 9.* Open and frequent communication among staff and members helps to create a positive organizational climate, ensures that benefits outweigh costs, and makes pooling of resources, member engagement, and effective assessment and planning more likely.
	Proposition 10. Shared and formalized decision-making processes help create a positive organizational climate, ensure that benefits outweigh costs, and make pooling of resources, member engagement, and effective assessment and planning more likely.
	Proposition 11. Conflict management helps to create a positive organizational climate, ensures that benefits outweigh costs, and achieves pooling of resources, member engagement, and effective assessment and planning.
	Proposition 12. The benefits of participation must outweigh the costs to make pooling of resources, member engagement, and effective assessment and planning more likely.
	Proposition 13. Positive relationships among members are likely to create a positive coalition climate.

Constructs	Propositions
Leadership and staffing	*Proposition 14.* Strong leadership from a team of staff and members improves coalition functioning and makes pooling of resources, member engagement, and effective assessment and planning more likely.
	Proposition 15. Paid staff who have the interpersonal and organizational skills to facilitate the collaborative process improve coalition functioning and increase pooling of resources, member engagement, and effective assessment and planning.
Structures	*Proposition 16.* Formalized rules, roles, structures, and procedures make pooling of resources, member engagement, and effective assessment and planning more likely.

TABLE 7.2. CONSTRUCTS AND PROPOSITIONS RELATED TO COMMUNITY COALITION INTERVENTIONS AND OUTCOMES.

Constructs	Propositions
Pooled member and external resources	*Proposition 17.* The synergistic pooling of member and community resources prompts effective assessment, planning, and implementation of strategies.
Member engagement	*Proposition 18.* Satisfied and committed members will participate more fully in the work of the coalition.
Assessment and planning	*Proposition 19.* Successful implementation of strategies is more likely when comprehensive assessment and planning occur.
Implementation of strategies	*Proposition 20.* Coalitions are more likely to create change in community policies, practices, and environment when they direct interventions at multiple levels.
Community change outcomes	*Proposition 21.* Coalitions that are able to change community policies, practices, and environment are more likely to increase capacity and improve health and social outcomes.
Health and social outcomes	*Proposition 22.* The ultimate indicator of coalition effectiveness is the improvement in health and social outcomes.
Community capacity	*Proposition 23.* As a result of participating in successful coalitions, community members and organizations develop capacity and build social capital that can be applied to other health and social issues.

behavior changes, and (6) creating social change (Whitt, 1993). This theory does not apply to short-term grassroots coalitions that form for a specific purpose, such as opposing a landfill, and then disband when the goal is achieved.

Community coalitions are characterized as formal, multipurpose, and long-term alliances (Butterfoss, Goodman, & Wandersman, 1993). The scope of community coalition work tends to be local or regional, and coalitions usually have some paid staff whose time is dedicated to coalition efforts. The size of its membership varies, as does the diversity of professional and grassroots organizations and the individuals who represent these organizations. The degree of formalization of working relationships and role expectations ranges from very formal, with strict adherence to by-laws and contractual relationships, to rather informal.

According to the proposed theory depicted in Figure 7.1, coalitions progress through stages from formation to institutionalization, with frequent loops back to earlier stages as new issues arise or as planning cycles are repeated (see Propositions 1 and 2, Table 7.1). The theory also acknowledges contextual factors of the community, such as the sociopolitical climate, geography, history, and norms surrounding collaborative efforts that will have an impact on each stage of coalition development from formation to institutionalization (Proposition 3, Table 7.1).

Coalitions progress through stages from formation to institutionalization, with frequent loops back to earlier stages as new issues arise or as planning cycles are repeated.

In the formation stages, a convener or lead agency, with strengths and linkages to the community, brings together core organizations that recruit an initial group of community partners to initiate a coalition effort focusing on a health or social issue of concern (Propositions 4 through 8, Table 7.1). The coalition identifies key leaders and staff, who then develop structures (such as committees and rules) and operating procedures (processes) that promote coalition effectiveness (Propositions 9 through 16, Table 7.1). Structural elements in the coalition ensure that the coalition will adequately assess the community, develop an action plan, and select and implement strategies based on best practices. This stage requires balancing benefits associated with membership to ensure they outweigh any costs of participation.

The maintenance stage involves sustaining member involvement and taking concrete action steps to achieve the goals of the coalition. In public health, these steps usually are assessing, planning, selecting, and implementing strategies (Propositions 19 and 20, Table 7.2). Success in this stage also depends on the mobilization and pooling of member and external resources (Proposition 17, Table 7.2). The coalition relies on resources from members and external sources to design and then implement the planned strategies. Acquisition of resources, combined with a competent planning and implementation process, are precursors to successful transition to the institutionalization stage. With adequate resources, members become engaged in assessment, planning, and implementing strategies and experience increased levels of commitment, participation, and satisfaction (Proposition 18, Table 7.2). By implementing strategies of sufficient duration and intensity according to the action plan, shorter-term outcomes such as changes in individual knowledge, beliefs, self-efficacy, and behavior, as well as changes in community systems, policies, practices, and environment, should occur (Proposition 20 and 21, Table 7.2). These intermediate changes should lead to long-term outcomes, such as reductions in morbidity and mortality, or substantive progress toward other social goals (Proposition 22, Table 7.2).

In the institutionalization stage, successful strategies result in outcomes. If resources have been adequately mobilized and strategies effectively address an ongoing need, coalition strategies may become institutionalized in a community as part of a long-term coalition, or they may be adopted by some organizations within the community. The coalition itself may or may not be institutionalized in a community. Both maintenance and institutionalization stages have the potential to increase community capacity to solve problems. Progress in ameliorating one community problem can potentially increase the capacity of local organizations to apply these skills and resources to address additional issues that resonate with the community (Proposition 23, Table 7.2).

Empirical Support for the Theory

This section describes the practice-proven propositions that accompany the model presented in Figure 7.1 and the empirical evidence that supports the propositions. Each box (or construct) in the model is sustained by one or more propositions. Table 7.1 contains sixteen propositions related to community coalition formation, structure, and processes, and Table 7.2 focuses on Propositions 17 through 23, which are related to community coalition interventions and outcomes. The twenty-three propositions are supported by empirical evidence (Table 7.3) and material from the "wisdom literature" (how-to manuals and guidelines) when empirical evidence is limited.

The studies cited in Table 7.3 are not intended to be a comprehensive review of the coalition literature on each construct in the model. Several recent reviews offer a more comprehensive summary of recent coalition and community partnership research (Roussos & Fawcett, 2000; Foster-Fishman, Berkowitz, Lounsbury, Jacobson, & Allen, 2001; Holden, Pendergast, & Austin, 2000; Lasker, Weiss, & Miller, 2000). Rather, the studies listed in Table 7.3 are those that most heavily influenced development of the theory described here. For each of these studies,

TABLE 7.3. EMPIRICAL EVIDENCE SUPPORTING THE COMMUNITY COALITION ACTION THEORY.

	Butterfoss et al. (1996)	Chinman et al. (1996)	Center for Substance Abuse and Prevention (1998)	Fawcett et al. (1997)	Florin et al. (1993)	Kegler et al. (1998a, 1998b)	Kumpfer et al. (1993)	Mayer et al. (1998)	McMillan et al. (1995)	Nelson (1994)	Reininger et al. (1999)	Rogers et al. (1993)
Description of the study												
Number of coalitions[a]	3	3	24	1	35	10	1	2	35	1	3	61
Methods[b]	S,D	S	S,I, D,O	S,I, D,L	S,I, D	S,I, D,O	S,D	F	S,I	D,O	S,I, D,O	S
Stages of development		X				X						
Community context					X	X				X	X	
Lead agency/ convener group			X									
Coalition membership			X	X		X						X
Operations and processes												
Communication						X						X
Decision making	X					X		X				
Conflict management			X			X		X				
Benefits and costs	X	X				X		X	X			
Climate	X					X			X			
Leadership	X			X		X	X				X	X
Staffing	X		X	X		X					X	X

	Butterfoss et al. (1996)	Chinman et al. (1996)	Center for Substance Abuse and Prevention (1998)	Fawcett et al. (1997)	Florin et al. (1993)	Kegler et al. (1998a, 1998b)	Kumpfer et al. (1993)	Mayer et al. (1998)	McMillan et al. (1995)	Nelson (1994)	Reininger et al. (1999)	Rogers et al. (1993)
Structures												
Organizational structure						X						
Formalization						X		X			X	X
Pooled resources				X		X						X
Member engagement												
Satisfaction	X			X		X	X					X
Participation	X	X		X		X		X				
Commitment									X			X
Assessment and planning	X		X	X	X	X	X	X				
Implementation of strategies			X	X		X		X			X	
Community change outcomes				X				X		X	X	
Health and social outcomes			X	X								
Community capacity						X						

[a] In several of these studies, the unit of analysis was at the subcommittee level.

[b] Methods codes: S: member survey, I: interviews, D: document review/archival records, 0: observation, L: logs, F: focus groups.

Table 7.3 lists the number of coalitions studied and the major data collection methods employed: surveys of members or the general population, interviews with key informants, review of documents and/or archival data, observation, logs, and focus groups. The table also lists the major constructs in the theory and identifies which of the studies examined each construct.

Stages of Development

Researchers and practitioners agree that effective coalitions develop over a period of time. In Table 7.1, Proposition 1 states that coalitions develop in stages and recycle through these stages as new members are recruited, plans are renewed, and new issues are added. Thus, the process of building and maintaining coalitions is not linear, but rather cyclical, with coalitions returning to earlier stages as community situations dictate (McLeroy et al., 1994). The naming of those stages and specific tasks that should be accomplished at each stage differ. Several different series of stages have been proposed, including formation, implementation, maintenance, and outcomes (Butterfoss et al., 1993); planning, intervention, and outcomes (Fawcett, Paine, Francisco, & Vliet, 1993); and mobilizing, establishing structure and function, building capacity for action, planning for action, implementation, refinement, and institutionalization (Florin, Mitchell, & Stevenson, 1993).

Researchers and practitioners agree that the following tasks must occur at some stage to ensure coalition effectiveness: recruiting and mobilizing coalition members, establishing organizational structure, building capacity and planning for action, selecting and implementing strategies, evaluating outcomes, refining strategies and approaches, and institutionalizing those strategies or the coalition itself (McLeroy et al., 1994). McLeroy and his colleagues agree that at each stage, certain factors enhance coalition function and progression to the next stage (Proposition 2). Finally, those who study or work in coalition settings agree that to accomplish their objectives, attention must be paid to maintaining coalitions and constantly recruiting new organizations in order to increase their impact (Kreuter, Lezin, & Young, 2000; Kaye & Wolff, 1995; Dowling et al., 2000; Butterfoss et al., 1998a). Most of the research to date focuses on the early stages of coalition development; consequently, less is known about the factors related to coalition success in the later stages of development (Table 7.3).

Community Context

Coalitions are embedded in communities, and as a result, factors in the community environment can have a significant impact on a coalition (Butterfoss et al., 1993; McLeroy et al., 1994; Lasker, Weiss, & Miller, 2000). Proposition 3 asserts that coalitions are heavily influenced by contextual factors throughout all stages of development. Several studies support this proposition. For example, Reininger, Dinh-Zarr, Sinicrope, and Martin (1999) discuss tension and mistrust between groups and how the lack of trust affected a coalition. Others have documented the impact of political and administrative contexts on coalitions (Dill, 1994; Clark, Baker, & Chawla, 1993; Nelson, 1994). Kegler et al. (1998a) noted the impact of tobacco-related politics on tobacco control coalitions in several stages of coalition development, from recruitment in the formation stage to the types of activities conducted in the maintenance stage. History of collaboration is widely cited in the wisdom and theoretical literature as another contextual factor that can affect the formation of collaborative relationships, including coalitions (Gray, 1989), with positive norms for collaboration increasing the likelihood of future successful collaboration. Additional contextual factors that affect coalitions include social capital (see Chapter Nine, this volume), trust between segments of a community, geography, and community readiness (Wolff, 2001).

Lead Agency/Convener Group

Proposition 4 states that coalitions usually form when a lead agency or convener group responds to an opportunity, threat, or mandate. Propositions 5 and 6 state that a lead agency begins coalition formation by recruiting a core group of community leaders and providing initial support for the coalition. The lead agency or convener is the organization that has the vision or mandate to mobilize community members initially to form a coalition focused on a specific issue of concern. This organization may or may not have written a grant or otherwise procured funds for coalition operation. The convener does, however, accept responsibility to host an initial meeting and recruit prospective partners. The lead agency may also provide physical space for coalition operation and a part- or full-time staff person to manage the initiative.

Although the literature concerning coalition practice acknowledges that the convening agency must have sufficient organizational capacity, commitment, leadership, and vision to build an effective coalition, research on these and other factors that lead agencies should possess is sorely lacking (Butterfoss et al., 1993). In one of the few studies comparing coalitions with differing reasons for initiation, Mansergh, Rohrbach, Montgomery, Pentz, and Johnson (1996) found that researcher and community-initiated coalitions were similar in terms of perceived coalition efficiency, outcome efficacy, benefits of involvement, and interagency collaboration. The only difference between the two was that action committee effectiveness ranked higher in the researcher-initiated coalition. The researchers concluded that factors other than the impetus for initiation might be more critical for coalition effectiveness. A related area with little research is whether coalitions develop anew or simply evolve from other preexisting coalitions and networks in a community (Herman, Wolfson, & Forster, 1993; Nezlek & Galano, 1993).

Coalition Membership

Limited research has focused on the defining characteristics of the founding members of community coalitions. Common wisdom holds that previous experience with the health issue or experience with coalitions increases the commitment of these core members. Experience shows that members participate in coalitions with varying levels of intensity—what Brager et al. (1987) described as active, occasional, and supporting participants. Brager et al. noted that flexible participation is essential when working with volunteers.

Composition of the core group may affect its ability to engage a broad cross section of the community. Propositions 6, 7, and 8 state that the core group must recruit community gatekeepers, those committed to the issue, and a broad constituency of diverse groups and organizations. This pooling of diverse views, perspectives, and resources is one of the hallmarks of coalitions and gives them the potential to solve problems that individual agencies could not address alone. Effective coalitions make concerted efforts to recruit memberships that are diverse in terms of expertise, constituencies, sectors, perspectives, and backgrounds. In addition, funders are often concerned about increasing the diversity of coalition members as evidenced by the recent focus on reducing health disparities in such efforts as the Centers for Disease Control and Prevention's REACH initiative.

Coalition Operations and Processes

Coalitions must fulfill certain basic functions such as making decisions, communicating, and managing conflict (Propositions 9 through 11). Indeed, much of the research on coalitions has focused on internal processes and operations, with the assumption that effective internal functioning is necessary for progress toward achieving goals (see Table 7.3). The quality of interactions among member networks is demonstrated by the frequency and intensity of contacts and the benefits that members receive from them, such as emotional or tangible support and access to social contacts (Israel, 1982). Research suggests that the extent of regular contacts among community members can foster cooperation (Putnam, 1993). Similarly, members can be empowered by building networks and experiencing positive social relationships (Kumpfer, Turner, Hopkins, & Librett, 1993). Research has also suggested that frequent and productive communication and networking among members increase satisfaction, commitment, and implementation of strategies (Rogers et al., 1993; Kegler et al., 1998b). Similarly, staff members are most satisfied and committed when good communication exists between members and themselves (Rogers et al., 1993). Members who report an increase in the number and type of linkages with outside organizations tend to participate more in the coalition (Butterfoss et al., 1996; Mayer et al., 1998). Coalition studies have also examined decision making and shown that the influence that participants have in making decisions is vital to a partnership. In turn, influence in decision making is related to increased satisfaction and participation and reporting of more positive benefits (Butterfoss et al., 1996; Mayer et al., 1998).

Another internal process that must be initiated to ensure smooth internal functioning is conflict management. Mizrahi and Rosenthal (1992) argue that conflict is an inherent characteristic of partnerships. Conflict may arise between the partnership and its priorities for social change or among partners concerning issues such as loyalty, leadership, goals, benefits, contributions, and representation. Conflict has been shown to lead to staff turnover, avoidance of certain activities, and difficulty in recruiting members (Kegler et al., 1998a). Conflict transformation is the process whereby resolution of conflict strengthens the coalition and builds capacity. Research shows that conflict transformation results from effective coalition planning and contributes to coalition goal attainment (Mayer et al., 1998).

Proposition 12 posits that perceptions of benefits must outweigh perceived costs to ensure ongoing participation in assessment, planning, and resource development. The literature points out several examples in which member costs and benefits were related to the process of engagement. In general, providing incentives and reducing costs increased member participation in voluntary associations (Wandersman, Florin, Friedmann, & Meier, 1987; Prestby et al., 1990) and in coalition committees, especially during the formation and early maintenance stages (Butterfoss et al., 1996; Butterfoss et al., 1998a; Chinman et al., 1996; Mayer et al., 1998). The wisdom literature is consistent in encouraging coalition leaders to provide incentives for continued participation (Kaye & Wolff, 1995).

Another factor related to member engagement is the organizational climate of the coalition. Proposition 13 states that positive relationships among members are likely to create a productive coalition environment or climate. Organizational climate refers to members' perceptions of the personality of an organization and is typically measured by ten factors: cohesion, leader support, expression, independence, task orientation, self-discovery, anger and aggression, order and organization, leader control, and innovation (Moos, 1986). Organizational climate characteristics (such as leader support and leader control) are related to satisfaction with the work, participation in the partnership, and perceived costs and benefits (Butterfoss et al., 1996), as well as increased implementation of action plans (Kegler et al., 1998b). Researchers have found that task focus is related to satisfaction (Kegler et al., 1998b) and psychological and organizational empowerment (McMillan et al., 1995). Similarly, the wisdom literature points out the value of promoting positive group climate and relationships among members (Kaye & Wolff, 1995; Dowling et al., 2000).

Leadership and Staffing

Propositions 14 and 15 emphasize the importance of leadership and staffing in coalitions. Without these, coalitions are unlikely to move beyond the initial steps in the formation stage of development. Coalition leaders and staff organize the structure through which coalitions accomplish their work and are responsible for coalition processes such as communication and decision making that keep members satisfied and committed to coalition efforts. Effective coalition leadership requires a collection of qualities and skills that are typically not found in one individual but rather in a team of committed leaders. Thus, a common approach to leadership in coalitions is the formation of steering committees composed of leaders from action-focused work groups. Empirical research on coalitions shows a consistent relationship between leader competence and member satisfaction (see Table 7.3).

Leadership is complex, and researchers have examined many facets in addition to member perceptions of leader competence (Glidewell, Kelly, Bagby, & Dickerson, 1998). For example, Kumpfer et al. (1993) studied leadership style and found that an empowering style was related to action plan quality. Butterfoss and colleagues (1996) found that leader support and control were related to several member-related outcomes but not to quality of the action plan. Reininger et al. (1999) explored how leaders' being indigenous or not affected coalitions. In a study of ten rural coalitions formed to prevent drug abuse, Braithwaite, Taylor, and Austin (2000) noted that the most successful coalitions had strong leadership and a commitment to a common goal. Others have found that the ability of a coalition to develop a clear and shared vision, a likely result of good leadership, is associated with success (Kegler et al., 1998a; Center for Substance Abuse and Prevention, 1998).

In many coalitions, leadership and staffing are intertwined, with paid staff fulfilling many leadership functions, such as setting agendas and facilitating meetings. Staff often support the coalition, encourage membership involvement, and build community capacity (Sanchez, 2000). Some research suggests that coalitions with staff who play a supportive role for the coalition rather than a visible leadership role have higher levels of implementation (Kegler et al., 1998a).

Several studies of coalitions have examined how staffing is related to intermediate indicators of effectiveness, including member-related outcomes, action plan quality, resource mobilization, and implementation of planned activities (see Table 7.3). Two of these studies demonstrated relationships between staff competence and member satisfaction (Rogers et al., 1993; Kegler et al., 1998b). Furthermore, Butterfoss and colleagues (1996) found an association between staff competence and member benefits. Kegler et al. (1998b) also found a positive relationship between staff time devoted to coalition efforts and the amount of resources mobilized and level of implementation of planned activities, thereby lending support to the need for paid staff with sufficient time to devote to the coalition. Minimal or nondisruptive staff turnover has also been linked to positive outcomes (Center for Substance Abuse and Prevention, 1998; Kegler et al., 1998a).

Coalition Structures

Proposition 16 asserts that coalitions are more likely to engage members, pool resources, and assess and plan well when they have formalized rules, roles, structures, and procedures. Formalization is the degree to which rules, roles, and procedures are precisely defined. Examples of formal structures are committees, written memoranda of understanding, by-laws, policy and procedures manuals, clearly defined roles, mission statements, goals, objectives, and regular reorientation to the purposes, goals, and procedures of collaboration (Butterfoss et al., 1993; Goodman & Steckler, 1989). Formal structures often result in the routinization or persistent implementation of the partnership's operations. The more routinized operations become, the more likely it is that they will be sustained (Goodman & Steckler, 1989). Research shows that the existence of formal structural elements such as by-laws, agendas, and minutes is related to organizational commitment (Rogers et al., 1993). In addition, structuring a coalition to focus on action, such as creating task forces or action teams, is associated with increased resource mobilization and implementation of strategies (Kegler et al., 1998b).

Pooled Member and External Resources

A major premise underlying the widespread adoption of coalitions to address community problems is that working together creates a synergy that enables individuals and organizations to accomplish more than they could achieve independently (McLeroy et al., 1994). Proposition 17 in Table 7.2 asserts that this pooling of resources ensures more effective assessment, planning, and implementation of strategies. Resource sharing also gives coalitions unique advantages over less collaborative problem-solving approaches. Lasker, Weiss, and Miller (2000) pointed out that much of the research on coalitions focuses on internal functioning, but does not explicate the pathways through which collaboration increases the likelihood of achieving outcomes over traditional single-agency interventions. They proposed that synergy is the mechanism through which partnerships gain advantage over more traditional, less collaborative approaches. Furthermore, they hypothesized that synergy is the proximal outcome linking partnership functioning to achieved outcomes.

Resources, defined broadly, are one of the major determinants of synergy as conceptualized by Lasker and colleagues. Coalition members are the greatest asset in a coalition-based initiative. They bring energy, knowledge, skills, expertise, perspectives, connections, and tangible resources to the table. The pooling of these diverse resources enables coalition members to achieve together what they could not accomplish alone. Research has shown that staffing and structure of coalitions are related to resource mobilization, which is related to effective implementation of coalition strategies (Kegler et al., 1998b). Successful resource mobilization allows for more creative solutions and more practical, comprehensive approaches (Lasker et al., 2000).

Resources from outside the membership and the community are also helpful, as they often fund staff and pay costs associated with implementing planned activities. Such resources relieve some of the burden that communities with limited financial resources face. External resources may also provide additional expertise, meeting facilities, mailing lists, referrals, additional personnel for special projects, grant funding, loans or donations, equipment, supplies, and cosponsorship of events (Chavis, Florin, Rich, & Wandersman 1987; Prestby & Wandersman, 1985; Braithwaite et al., 2000).

Member Engagement

Member engagement is best defined as the process by which members are empowered and develop a sense of belonging to the coalition. Positive engagement is evidenced by commitment to the mission and goals of the coalition, high levels of participation both in and outside coalition meetings and activities, and satisfaction with the work of the coalition. Among the factors that enhance engagement are that the perceived benefits of membership outweigh the costs and that members experience a positive coalition environment (Propositions 12 and 13; Butterfoss et al., 1996).

Members who experience more benefits than costs participate more fully and are more satisfied with the work of the coalition. Proposition 18 asserts that satisfied and committed members will have higher levels of participation than less satisfied members. Research supports this assertion and consistently demonstrates that satisfied and committed members will also participate more in the work of the coalition (Butterfoss et al., 1996, 1993; Roberts-DeGennaro, 1986; Rogers et al., 1993; Mayer et al., 1998). Although satisfied and highly participating members are valued, the same studies failed to support the hypothesis that these factors lead to desired intermediate outcomes (for example, producing high-quality action plans) or long-term outcomes (reducing ATOD [alcohol, tobacco, and other drug] use). However, case examples of coalitions exist in which intermediate and long-range successes can be attributed to the commitment and satisfaction of their members (Butterfoss et al., 1998a).

Assessment and Planning

Achieving a coalition's goals involves assessing the situation and deciding what action to take. A coalition-based initiative, such as one that is a part of a state or national program, usually engages in an extensive assessment and planning process that can last as long as two years and is typically followed by an implementation phase of three to five years. Several coalition studies have examined the quality of the action plans produced by these types of coalition efforts. Analyses of activities selected by coalitions have shown a tendency toward activities that promote changes in awareness (Florin et al., 1993). Kreuter and colleagues (2000) note that despite a strong emphasis on needs assessment, written objectives, and logic models that depict cause-and-effect relationships between interventions and outcomes, many collaborative efforts fail to produce rigorous plans. Quality plans, associated with competent staffing, leadership, and resource mobilization, contribute to successful implementation (Butterfoss et al., 1996; Kumpfer et al., 1993; Kegler et al., 1998b). Proposition 19 states that successful implementation of strategies is more likely when comprehensive planning and assessment occur.

Implementation of Strategies

Successful implementation depends on numerous factors such as sufficient resources, completion of tasks on schedule, fidelity to the planned intervention strategies, and a supportive, or nonturbulent, organizational and community environment. Assuming the interventions link logically to planned outcomes, the likelihood of achieving these outcomes depends on the extent to which the strategies are implemented and reach the priority populations. Adaptations of interventions that have been previously evaluated (evidence based) or are commonly accepted as best practices increase the likelihood that interventions will result in community change and, ultimately, desired health and social outcomes (Green, 2001; Cameron, Jolin, Walker, McDermott, & Gough, 2001).

Focusing on best practices or evidence-based interventions may minimize the extent to which coalitions engage in community awareness activities. This tendency to focus on easier interventions and quick wins may help to maintain member interest, but it is unlikely to lead to more valued outcomes and may help explain why some coalition-based efforts are not able to achieve systems or health outcomes change (Kreuter et al., 2000). Most researchers and practitioners agree that effective health promotion efforts require change at multiple levels, including environmental and policy change (McLeroy, Bibeau, Steckler, & Glanz, 1988). Goodman, Wandersman, Chinman, Imm, and Morrisey (1996) further suggest that as coalition interventions become more complex and focus less on individual behavior change, the assessments of such coalitions should focus across multiple levels and take community readiness into account. Proposition 20 emphasizes the importance of implementing interventions at multiple levels in order to create change in community policies, practices, and environments.

As coalition interventions become more complex and focus less on individual behavior change, the assessments of such coalitions should focus across multiple levels and take community readiness into account.

Community Change Outcomes

By implementing interventions at multiple levels, coalitions are able to create change in communities that can reduce risk factors and increase protective factors. Fawcett and colleagues (1997) categorized these into changes in programs, changes in policies, and changes in practices of community agencies, businesses, and government entities. Coalitions can also create change in communities by developing the skills of individuals, increasing the sense of community, and providing new perspectives on community problem solving for residents. At other levels, coalitions can create changes in opportunities for civic participation, linkages between organizations, and the physical and social environment of a community (Kegler, Twiss, & Look, 2000). The Community Coalition Action Theory posits that coalitions that are able to create these types of community changes are more likely to increase community capacity to address other issues of concern and to realize their long-term goals (Proposition 21).

Health and Social Outcomes

Proposition 22 states that the ultimate indicator of coalition effectiveness is improvement in health and social outcomes. Several recent reviews have been published documenting only modest evidence of effective collaborative partnerships. Roussos and Fawcett (2000) reviewed thirty-four studies that represented 252 collaborative partnerships. The authors categorized the studies into those that provided evidence for more distant population-level outcomes, communitywide behavior change, and environmental change. The review stated that research is insufficient to make strong conclusions about the impact of partnerships on population-level outcomes largely due to design issues (most of the research consists of case studies). With respect to communitywide behavior change, Roussos and Fawcett concluded that partnerships could make modest contributions. Strongest evidence existed for partnerships' contributions to environmental change, broadly defined to include changes in programs, services, and practices.

Similarly, Kreuter and colleagues (2000) reviewed sixty-eight published descriptions of coalitions and consortia with evaluation protocols in place and found only six examples of documented health status or systems change. Numerous reasons have been discussed in the literature as possible explanations for the disappointing findings associated with collaborative initiatives (Roussos & Fawcett, 2000; Mittelmark, 1999; Kreuter et al., 2000; Berkowitz, 2001). For example, design issues and secular trends make the detection of community-level change challenging. Also, some note that coalitions tend to focus on quick wins and awareness activities. These strategies alone will not lead to significant changes in systems or health status.

Community Capacity

In addition to coalition outcomes associated with health or social issues, another set of outcomes is associated with increases in a community's capacity to solve problems (see Chapter Eight, this volume). Proposition 23 asserts that coalitions can develop community capacity, which has been discussed as both a possible prerequisite to community problem solving and an outcome of community health promotion efforts (Goodman et al., 1998). It includes dimensions that coalitions can theoretically affect (positively or negatively) such as participation and leadership, networks of individuals and organizations, skills and resources, and sense of community. Crisp, Swerissen, and Duckett (2000) identify the development of partnerships as one of four distinct approaches to building capacity, arguing that two-way communication between groups that previously have not worked together can result in more resources for planning and implementation. Little coalition research has focused on outcomes associated with community capacity, although current evaluation research is examining these issues (Norton, Kegler, & Aronson, 2000).

Application of the Model: Consortium for the Immunization of Norfolk's Children

In 1992, the Centers for Disease Control and Prevention's National Immunization Program selected Norfolk, Virginia, as a site to demonstrate how a community coalition could improve immunization rates for children under two years of age. Norfolk was selected due to its low immunization rates (49 percent of two-year-olds in 1993), ethnic diversity, and public, private, and military health care systems. By helping citizens develop and implement comprehensive, effective strategies, the Consortium for the Immunization of Norfolk's Children (CINCH) realized its goals and increased childhood immunization rates by 17 percent. This case example shows how CINCH followed the community coalition model presented in Figure 7.1.

Stages of Development

CINCH was in the formation stage for approximately six months. During this time, underimmunization was defined as a community problem, coalition members were recruited, and mission, rules, and roles were specified. The members were also trained during this stage. During the next stage, maintenance, coalition membership was sustained, and actual work began. Coalition members assessed needs, collected and analyzed data, developed a plan, initiated and monitored strategies, and supported and evaluated their group process. After three years, the coalition expanded geographically to include the Hampton Roads region and was renamed the Consortium for Infant and Child Health (with the same acronym). CINCH subsequently recycled through formation and maintenance stages as it engaged in a new recruitment and needs assessment process. In February 1997, CINCH released the *Report on the Health of Children in Hampton Roads*. After engaging in a priority-setting process, the coalition decided to focus on immunization and add perinatal issues (such as low birthweight, teen pregnancy, and infant mortality) to its mission. CINCH collaborated with and reenergized an existing perinatal council and eventually relinquished responsibility for this health issue (institutionalization stage).

In March 2000, the *Report on the Health of Children in Hampton Roads* identified childhood asthma as the number one diagnosis for hospital admission, as well as emergency room and physician visits in the region. CINCH then launched an asthma work group and applied for and received funding from the Robert Wood Johnson Foundation in 2001. The coalition recruited new members with asthma expertise and concern, and conducted an asthma-related needs assessment. CINCH recycled through the developmental stages three times during eight years as new issues arose, strategies were revised, and many new members were recruited.

Lead Agency/Convener Group

The Center for Pediatric Research, a joint program of a children's hospital and medical school, convened CINCH and serves as its lead agency. Although the center was new, the region valued collaborative efforts and embraced the concept of coalition building as proposed by the center staff, who were experienced with this strategy. The staff recruited a core group of organizations, which then recruited fifty-five service agencies; academic, civic, and faith-based institutions; health care providers; and parents.

Coalition Membership

Members from various grassroots and professional organizations provided diversity in age, occupation, race, and ethnicity. They willingly put aside differences in order to share responsibility for all of the community's children. Relying on new knowledge and core values, the coalition developed its mission to improve immunization rates for children under two years of age. This common mission and commitment to community improvement helped members overcome barriers that often stall new coalitions, such as lack of direction or turf battles (Kaye & Wolff, 1995; Butterfoss et al., 1996).

Coalition Operations and Processes

Members reported that they had either a great degree of influence (74 percent) or some influence (26 percent) in determining policies and actions of the consortium. When conflict arose, 82 percent reported that they were able to resolve it effectively. Content analysis of meetings showed that activities were balanced among tasks of orienting members, assessing needs, planning and revising coalition structure and functions, sharing information, and developing and evaluating products or services. Members evaluated meetings to identify successful elements (Goodman & Wandersman, 1994) and rated work group and general meetings as 88 percent and 92 percent effective, respectively. Leaders and staff debriefed about barriers to effective meetings and recommended improving agendas, attendance, tardiness, participation, leadership, and grassroots representation.

Leadership and Staffing

From the outset, CINCH had a full-time staff coordinator and part-time administrative assistant. The leaders of the coalition were community members who were elected by the membership. The steering committee, which consisted of coalition and work group chairs and vice chairs, as well as staff and other nonvoting honorary members, prepared the job description and advertised, interviewed, and hired the coalition coordinator. The coordinator had previously served as a coalition member and now worked for the coalition.

Leaders were sensitive to member needs by allowing varying levels of participation during each coalition stage. They reduced burnout and maximized resources by recognizing that some members are better planners and others are better doers. Staff supported members by preparing draft documents, minutes, rosters, meeting reminders, and mailings. They helped leaders set agendas, run effective meetings, and plan strategies to promote member retention. To engage members, lead agency staff provided training on a variety of issues related to immunization.

Membership and commitment may waiver as a coalition realizes that it takes time to accomplish its goals. To keep members involved, CINCH participated in health fairs, marches, and other community health efforts. Leaders worked to maximize member participation. Meetings provided opportunities to cultivate and renew relationships and celebrate incremental achievements. Members received written reminders and telephone calls about meetings and follow-up when they were absent. Member surveys measured satisfaction and participation and defined areas for improvement.

Coalition Structures

Members developed written rules of operation, criteria for membership, and roles for members, leaders, and staff. CINCH also developed work groups focused on specific tasks and populations that complemented each other. Chairs and vice chairs were elected for work groups and the coalition at large.

Pooled Member and External Resources

Each member brought individual skills to the coalition, but also represented an organization that brought resources to the table. Member organizations contributed financially or in-kind to implement strategies, since grant funds were earmarked only for research. When personal agendas were put aside, resources were more effectively pooled. Work group members invited health department and hospital directors, as well as professional and voluntary agencies from neighboring cities, to join them at the table. As previously competitive organizations learned the value of collaborating to accomplish tasks, the level of trust improved.

Funding restrictions prompted CINCH to develop community support for its activities and increased the likelihood of sustaining its efforts beyond the grant period. Private foundation funding enabled the coalition to hire an outreach coordinator, conduct a media campaign, and implement key strategies. In-kind contributions from CINCH members included the printing of posters, flyers, and brochures; arranging satellite teleconferences; and contributing parent incentives. In this way, the resources from the federal grant, local foundation, and member organizations complemented each other and created synergy.

Member Engagement

Training, defined roles, and ongoing contact with participating institutions were essential for member retention. Member involvement was bolstered by achievement of objectives and positive results. A clear vision of leadership and commitment to a quality process kept members interested. CINCH also made good use of each member's linkage with others. Members constantly recruited others, who provided resources or represented the priority population. New recruits stimulated creativity and renewed effort among founding members. Member surveys showed that 86 percent were satisfied with the work of the coalition (Butterfoss et al., 1998a). Average attendance over 130 CINCH meetings was 59 percent, considered acceptable by coalition research (Prestby & Wandersman, 1985).

Assessment and Planning

Following formation, CINCH's major tasks focused on needs assessment, data collection, analysis, feedback, and plan development. First, work group members participated in a needs assessment to diagnose local causes of underimmunization. Parent focus groups, patient exit interviews, and household and health care provider surveys were planned and conducted (Houseman, Butterfoss, Morrow, & Rosenthal, 1997; Butterfoss et al., 1998a).

Staff conducted workshops to train work group members to develop quality action plans. Once trained, each work group used data to identify a prioritized set of needs related to their priority group (for example, parents, health care providers). Goals, objectives, and strategies were developed to address each identified community need. The groups considered the strengths of their community and the resources they could draw on to implement various strategies. Linkages among community agencies were identified, and evaluation of strategies was planned. Work group leaders combined the individual plans into one overall two-year strategic immunization plan that focused on parent and provider education and support for at-risk families, thereby increasing access to immunizations and improving immunization delivery. The intrinsic negotiation involved in this process cemented relationships among group leaders and strengthened internal support for the plan. The planning process led to the creation of a steering committee that still meets regularly to share successes and challenges. Members also learned that planning is a continuous process and later developed timelines, management plans, and budgets.

Implementation of Strategies

During this time, new strategies were initiated, and others were maintained and monitored. Work groups collaborated on strategies and responsibilities and even merged to streamline operations. Some activities were initiated and finished quickly, while others were not achieved until after funding ended. CINCH had an impact on the Norfolk community by effectively implementing sixty-one of seventy-nine planned strategies (77 percent). An evaluation component for each strategy helped members decide whether it was based on need, implemented as planned, and could be improved. Action plans were revised annually.

Community Change and Health Outcomes

CINCH accomplished some of its more difficult objectives such as Women, Infants and Children (WIC) linkage, physician practice assessment and feedback, hospital birth reminder systems, and legislative action. Members not only directed the course of community events, but also wielded power to influence larger institutions such as hospitals and the state legislature. Although any change in immunization levels for two-year-olds could not be attributed to CINCH alone, rates rose from 48 percent in 1993 to 66 percent in 1996 (Morrow et al., 1998). Higher rates were reported among hospital and military clinics.

Community Capacity

Through training and practice in leadership, meeting facilitation, needs assessment, and planning, coalition members developed skills that improved their participation and could be generalized to other civic areas. Members and staff also provide technical assistance to other local partnerships that deal with tobacco use, child safety, and school health. CINCH collaborated with projects focused on case management, community policing, and neighborhood improvement. In addition, it fostered new state contracts and federal grants that promote environmental change. A contract between CINCH's lead agency and the state health department was forged to develop and manage a state immunization coalition, Project Immunize Virginia, which used the CINCH model to help other localities develop community partnerships to advocate for immunizing children across the state. Under an Association of Teachers of Preventive Medicine grant, the Coalition Training Institute was established in Norfolk in 1995 to train key health agency staff who coordinated immunization coalitions in eighty-eight urban, state, and territorial sites (Butterfoss, Webster, Morrow, & Rosenthal, 1998b).

Strengths and Limitations of the Theory

Any new theory is bound to have strengths and limitations and must be open to constructive criticism from practitioners and researchers who have a stake in the related work.

Any new theory is bound to have strengths and limitations and must be open to constructive criticism from practitioners and researchers who have a stake in the related work. The Community Coalition Action Theory is long overdue. The benefit of its delayed appearance, however, is that it is grounded in almost two decades of practice and research. Perhaps one reason that this theory has not been developed before is that the complexity of community coalitions and the multifaceted nature of their work overwhelm researchers and practitioners alike. The model that describes our theory is complex and takes into account the diverse factors that influence the formation, implementation, and maintenance of coalitions.

Although community coalitions are found in a variety of settings that range from urban to rural, the empirical research and subsequent findings have focused mostly in the area of alcohol, tobacco, and other drug abuse prevention. This is not surprising when one considers that the highest level of foundation and governmental agency funding for coalition work has centered on these health issues. Although coalitions exist for many other health issues, including cardiovascular disease, human immunodeficiency virus and acquired immunodeficiency syndrome, unintentional injury prevention, and immunization, large-scale evaluative research findings have not yet been reported for these issues. Similarly, much of the research that forms the basis of the Community Coalition Action Theory is from studies conducted in the early 1990s and tends to focus on coalition functioning and intermediate indicators of effectiveness, such as satisfaction, participation, action plan quality, and implementation. Because of the widely acknowledged difficulty in attributing health outcome change to community collaborative efforts, much of the more recent research uses case study methodology. Although very informative, case study findings are difficult to generalize from and focus less often on associations among constructs.

The constructs that are used in the Community Coalition Action Theory are informed by research, yet we have speculated on how they interrelate with one another. We have used a set of propositions to help us order the constructs in a logical sequence and develop reciprocal or directional linkages among them. But the research evidence does not totally ensure that these assumptions are correct. In addition, we have not weighted each variable in our model. How important are coalition processes, for example, as compared to coalition structures? The model does not quantify the resources needed to implement successful strategies or the level of member engagement that leads to effective assessment and planning. Further research should help clarify the constructs, their importance to the whole, linkage patterns, and directionality.

The model is complicated by the complexity of each of the constructs. For example, the operation and processes construct includes communication, decision making, and conflict management. All of these are likely related to organizational climate, but which are more important and in what situations and stages? Similarly, we identify several dimensions of community context and assert that context affects each construct in the model and each stage in coalition development. Yet much research remains to be done to understand how distribution of power in a community, for example, affects what organization serves as the lead agency, who makes up the core group, and whose needs are assessed.

Numerous types of collaborative relationships exist. We focused on community coalitions and defined them as long-term community structures that enable organizations and individuals to work collaboratively to address community problems. We were careful not to cite research done with other types of collaborative initiatives because in the past, careful distinctions have not been made when summarizing "coalition" findings. Different types of collaborative partnerships (for example, state level, grassroots, mandated, and voluntary) may function differently and be influenced by different factors in each stage of coalition development. Stages of coalition development may also need to be conceptualized differently for different types of partnerships. For example, a grassroots citizens' group formed to keep a landfill out of a neighborhood may not need to institutionalize anything once the landfill is sited elsewhere.

Future Directions

With the advent of evidence-based medicine and outcomes-based interventions, coalitions have recently been criticized as not meeting expectations for success (Green, 2000). Given the tremendous infusion of resources, both monetary and in donated volunteer time, some see this criticism as well deserved. The overall evidence for positive coalition outcomes is lacking; however, traditional scientific methodology may not be adequate to capture the outcomes of these complex collaborative organizations (Berkowitz, 2001). For example, we cannot underestimate the amount of time that it takes to create and sustain viable coalitions or the difficult task of identifying and implementing best practices. Similarly, evaluators and coalitions are often reluctant to accept qualitative methods of evaluation or to identify realistic intermediate- and long-term outcomes. Finally, communities may not always understand the long-term benefits and unintended positive outcomes of coalitions. However, we need to be careful lest we throw the baby out with the bathwater by criticizing coalitions for not achieving measurable outcomes.

Evaluators are beginning to argue for more research focusing on what coalitions contribute to community-based interventions above and beyond more traditional approaches (Lasker et al., 2001; Berkowitz, 2001; Butterfoss, Cashman, Foster-Fishman, & Kegler, 2001). For example, do coalition approaches develop more innovative strategies due to the pooling of expertise and resources? Do they reach previously untapped community assets? Are they better able to implement certain types of interventions than traditional public health and social service agencies, such as policy or media advocacy efforts? A logical future direction for research on coalitions, and this theory in particular, would be to document and describe what Lasker and colleagues term *partnership synergy*.

Unfortunately, community coalitions are in the same situation as almost all other community-level initiatives in facing the challenges associated with documenting long-term outcomes and attributing resulting changes to the initiative. Our contention is that by strengthening the theoretical base and developing a model of action for community coalitions, we will advance this area of scientific inquiry. We encourage theoreticians to test the logic of this model. We challenge researchers to use the model, at both the case study and large-scale level, to field-test our assumptions and advance the understanding of which coalition characteristics and interactions are most likely to fuel goal attainment. Finally, we ask practitioners, the front-line coalition pioneers, to determine whether this model is useful to increase local support and capacity for further coalition development.

This theoretical model is a starting point; we welcome all contributions that improve its validity, reliability, and utility.

References

Alter, C., & Hage, J. (1993). *Organizations working together: coordination in interorganizational networks.* Thousand Oaks, CA: Sage.

Bazzoli, G., Stein, R., Alexander, J., Conrad, D., Sofaer, S., & Shortell, S. (1997). Public-private collaboration in health and human service delivery: Evidence from community partnerships. *Milbank Quarterly, 75,* 533–561.

Berkowitz, B. (2001). Studying the outcomes of community-based coalitions. *American Journal of Community Psychology, 29,* 213–227.

Berlin, X., Barnett, W., Mischke, G., & Ocasio W. (2000). The evolution of collective strategies among organizations. *Organization Studies, 21,* 325–354.

Bracht, N. (Ed.). (1990). *Health promotion at the community level.* Thousand Oaks, CA: Sage.

Brager, G. A., Sprecht, H., & Torczyner, J. L. (1987). *Community organizing* (2nd ed.). New York: Columbia University Press.

Braithwaite, R., Taylor, S., & Austin, J. (2000). *Building health coalitions in the black community.* Thousand Oaks: Sage.

Butterfoss, F. D., Cashman, S., Foster-Fishman, P., & Kegler, M. (2001). Roundtable discussion of Berkowitz's paper. *American Journal of Community Psychology, 29,* 229–239.

Butterfoss, F. D., Goodman, R., & Wandersman, A. (1993). Community coalitions for prevention and health promotion. *Health Education Research, 8,* 315–330.

Butterfoss, F. D., Goodman R., & Wandersman, A. (1996). Community coalitions for prevention and health promotion: Factors predicting satisfaction, participation and planning. *Health Education Quarterly, 23,* 65–79.

Butterfoss, F. D., Morrow, A. L., Rosenthal, J., Dini, E., Crews, R. C., Webster, J. D., & Louis, P. A. (1998a). CINCH: An urban coalition for empowerment and action. *Health Education and Behavior, 25,* 213–225.

Butterfoss, F. D., Webster, J. D., Morrow, A. L., & Rosenthal, J. (1998b). Immunization coalitions that work: Training for public health professionals. *Journal of Public Health Management and Practice, 4,* 79–87.

Cameron, R., Jolin M., Walker, R., McDermott, N., & Gough, M. (2001). Linking science and practice: Toward a system for enabling communities to adopt best practices for chronic disease prevention. *Health Promotion Practice, 2,* 35–42.

Carlaw, R., Mittelmark, M., Bracht, N., & Luepker, R. (1984). Organization for a community cardiovascular health program: Experiences from the Minnesota Heart Health Program. *Health Education Quarterly, 11,* 243–252.

Center for Substance Abuse and Prevention. (1998). *National evaluation of the Community Partnership Demonstration Program.* Washington, DC: Substance Abuse and Mental Health Services Administration, U.S. Department of Health and Human Services.

Chavis, D. M. (2001). The paradoxes and promise of community coalitions. *American Journal of Community Psychology, 29,* 309–320.

Chavis, D. M., Florin, P., Rich, R., & Wandersman, A. (1987). *The role of block associations in crime control and community development: The Block Booster Project.* New York: Ford Foundation.

Checkoway, B. (1989). Community participation for health promotion. *Prescription for public policy* (Vol. 6).

Chinman, M., Anderson, C., Imm, P., Wandersman, A., & Goodman R. (1996). The perceptions of costs and benefits of high active versus low active groups in community coalitions at different stages in coalition development. *Journal of Community Psychology, 24,* 263–274.

Clark, N., Baker, E., & Chawla, A. (1993). Sustaining collaborative problem-solving: Strategies from a study in six Asian countries. *Health Education Research, 8,* 385–402.

Crisp, B., Swerissen, H., & Duckett, S. (2000). Four approaches to capacity building in health: Consequences for measurement and accountability. *Health Promotion International, 15,* 99–107.

Dill, A. (1994). Institutional environments and organizational responses to AIDS. *Journal of Health and Social Behavior, 35,* 349–369.

Dowling, J., O'Donnell, H. J., & Wellington Consulting Group (2000). *A development manual for asthma coalitions.* Northbrook, IL: CHEST Foundation and the American College of Chest Physicians.

Farquhar, J., Fortmann, S., Flora, J., Taylor, C., Haskell, W., Williams, P., Maccoby, N., & Wood, P. (1990). Effects of community-wide education on cardiovascular disease risk factors: The Five-City Project. *Journal of the American Medical Association, 264,* 359–365.

Fawcett, S., Lewis, R., Paine-Andrews, A., Francisco, V., Richer, K., Williams, E., & Copple, B. (1997). Evaluating community coalitions for prevention of substance abuse: The case of Project Freedom. *Health Education and Behavior, 24,* 812–828.

Fawcett. S., Paine, A., Francisco, V., & Vliet, M. (1993). Promoting health through community development. In D. Glenwick & L. A. Jason (Eds.), *Promoting health and mental health in children, youth and families* (pp. 233–255). New York: Springer.

Feighery, E., & Rogers, T. (1990). *Building and maintaining effective coalitions.* Palo Alto, CA: Health Promotion Resource Center, Stanford Center for Research in Disease Prevention.

Florin, P., Mitchell, R., & Stevenson, J. (1993). Identifying training and technical assistance needs in community coalitions: A developmental approach. *Health Education Research, 8,* 417–432.

Florin, P., & Wandersman A. (1990). An introduction to citizen participation, voluntary organizations, and community development: Insights for empowerment research. *American Journal of Community Psychology, 18,* 41–54.

Foster-Fishman, P., Berkowitz, S., Lounsbury, D., Jacobson, S., & Allen, N. (2001). Building collaborative capacity in community coalitions: A review and integrative framework. *American Journal of Community Psychology, 29,* 241–257.

Giamartino, G., & Wandersman, A. (1983). Organizational climate correlates of viable urban block organizations. *American Journal of Community Psychology, 11,* 529–541.

Glidewell, J., Kelly, J., Bagby, M., & Dickerson, A. (1998). Natural development of community leadership. In R. S. Tindale, Heath, L., Edwards, J., Posavac, E., Bryant, F., Suarez-Balcazar, Y., Henderson-King, E., & Myers, J. (Eds.), *Theory and research on small groups.* New York: Plenum Press.

Goodman, R. M,, Speers, M., McLeroy, K., Fawcett, S., Kegler, M., Parker, E., Smith, S., Sterling, T., & Wallerstein, N. (1998). Identifying and defining the dimensions of community capacity to provide a basis for measurement. *Health Education and Behavior, 25,* 258–278.

Goodman, R. M., & Steckler, A. (1989). A model for institutionalization of health promotion programs. *Family and Community Health, 11,* 63–78.

Goodman, R. M., & Wandersman, A. (1994). FORECAST: A formative approach to evaluating community coalitions and community-based initiatives. *Journal of Community Psychology* [Special issue], 6–25.

Goodman, R. M., Wandersman, A., Chinman, M., Imm, P., & Morrisey, E. (1996). An ecological assessment of community-based interventions for prevention and health promotion: Approaches to measuring community coalitions. *American Journal of Community Psychology, 24,* 33–61.

Gray, B. (1989). *Collaboration: Finding common ground for multiparty problems.* San Francisco: Jossey-Bass.

Gray, B., & Wood, D. (1991). Collaborative alliances: Moving from practice to theory. *Journal of Applied Behavioral Science, 27,* 3–22.

Green, L. (2000). Caveats on coalitions: In praise of partnerships. *Health Promotion Practice, 1,* 64–65.

Green, L. (2001). From research to "best practices" in other settings and populations. *American Journal of Health Behavior, 3,* 165–178.

Green, L., & Kreuter, M. (1992). CDC's planned approach to community health as an application of PRECEDE and an inspiration for PROCEED. *Journal of Health Education, 23,* 140–147.

Gulati, R. (1995). Social structure and alliance formation patterns: A longitudinal analysis. *Administrative Science Quarterly, 40,* 619–652.

Herman, K., Wolfson, M., & Forster J. (1993). The evolution, operation, and future of Minnesota SAFEPLAN: A coalition for family planning. *Health Education Research, 8,* 331–344.

Holden, D., Pendergast, K., & Austin, D. (2000). *Literature review for American Legacy Foundation's Statewide Youth Movement Against Tobacco Use—Draft report.* Research Triangle Park, NC: Research Triangle Institute.

Houseman, C., Butterfoss, F. D., Morrow, A. L., & Rosenthal, J. (1997). Focus groups among public, military and private sector mothers: Insights to improve the immunization process. *Journal of Public Health Nursing, 14,* 235–243.

Israel, B. A. (1982). Social networks and health status: Linking theory, research and practice. *Patient Counseling and Health Education, 4,* 65–79.

Israel, B. A., Checkoway, B., Schultz, A., & Zimmerman, M. (1994). Health education and community empowerment: Conceptualizing and measuring perceptions of individual, organizational and community control. *Health Education Quarterly, 21,* 149–170.

Kaye, G., & Wolff, T. (1995). *From the ground up: A workbook on coalition building and community development.* Amherst, MA: Area Health Education Center/Community Partners.

Kegler, M., Steckler, A., Malek, S., & McLeroy, K. (1998a). A multiple case study of implementation in ten local Project ASSIST coalitions in North Carolina. *Health Education Research, 13,* 225–238.

Kegler, M., Steckler, A., McLeroy, K., & Malek, S. (1998b). Factors that contribute to effective community health promotion coalitions: A study of ten Project ASSIST coalitions in North Carolina. *Health Education and Behavior, 25,* 338–353.

Kegler, M., Twiss, J., & Look, V. (2000). Assessing community change at multiple levels: The genesis of an evaluation framework for the California Healthy Cities and Communities Project. *Health Education and Behavior, 27,* 760–779.

Kreuter, M. (1992). PATCH: Its origins, basic concepts, and links to contemporary public health policy. *Journal of Health Education, 23,* 135–139.

Kreuter, M., Lezin, N., & Young, L. (2000). Evaluating community-based collaborative mechanisms: Implications for practitioners. *Health Promotion Practice, 1,* 49–63.

Kumpfer, K., Turner, C., Hopkins, R., & Librett, J. (1993). Leadership and team effectiveness in community coalitions for the prevention of alcohol and other drug abuse. *Health Education Research, 8,* 359–374.

Labonte, R. (1994). Health promotion and empowerment: Reflections on professional practice. *Health Education Quarterly, 21,* 253–268.

Lasker, R., Weiss, E., & Miller, R. (2000, April–May). *Promoting collaborations that improve health.* Paper commissioned for the Fourth Annual Community-Campus Partnerships for Health Conference, Arlington, VA.

Lasker, R., Weiss, E., & Miller, R. (2001). Partnership synergy: A practical framework for studying and strengthening the collaborative advantage. *Milbank Quarterly, 79*(2), 179–205.

Lefebvre, R., Lasater, T., Carleton, R., & Petersen, G. (1987). Theory and delivery of health programming in the community: The Pawtucket Heart Health Program. *Preventive Medicine, 16,* 80–95.

Mansergh, G., Rohrbach, L., Montgomery, S., Pentz, M., & Johnson, C. (1996). Process evaluation of community coalitions for alcohol and other drug abuse: A case study comparison of researcher- and community-initiated models. *Journal of Community Psychology, 24,* 118–135.

Mayer, J., Soweid, R., Dabney, S., Brownson, C., Goodman, R., & Brownson R. (1998). Practices of successful community coalitions: A multiple case study. *American Journal of Health Behavior, 22,* 368–377.

McLeroy, K., Bibeau, D., Steckler A., & Glanz, K. (1988). An ecological perspective on health promotion programs. *Health Education Quarterly, 15,* 351–377.

McLeroy, K., Kegler, M., Steckler, A., Burdine, J., & Wisotzky, M. (1994). Editorial: Community coalitions for health promotion: Summary and further reflections. *Health Education Research, 9,* 1–11.

McMillan, B., Florin, P., Stevenson, J., Kerman, B., & Mitchell, R. (1995). Empowerment praxis in community coalitions. *American Journal of Community Psychology, 23,* 699–727.

Milio, N. (1989). *Promoting health through public policy.* Ottawa: Canadian Public Health Association.

Minkler, M. (1994). Ten commitments for community health education. *Health Education Research, 9,* 527–534.

Mittelmark, M. (1999). Health promotion at the communitywide level: Lessons from diverse perspectives. In N. Bracht (Ed.), *Health promotion at the community level.* Thousand Oaks, CA: Sage.

Mittelmark, M., Luepker, R., Jacobs, D., Bracht, N., Carlaw, R., Crow, R., Finnegan, J., Grimm, R., Jeffery, R., Kline, F., Mullis, R., Murray, D., Pechacek, T., Perry, C., Pirie, P., & Blackburn H. (1986). Community-wide prevention of cardiovascular disease: Education strategies of the Minnesota Heart Health Program. *Preventive Medicine, 15,* 1–17.

Mizrahi, T., & Rosenthal, B. (1992). Managing dynamic tensions in social change coalitions. In T. Mizrahi & J. Morrison (Eds.), *Community organization and social administration.* New York: Haworth Press.

Mizruchi, M., & Galaskiewicz, J. (1994). Networks of interorganizational relations. In S. Wasserman & J. Galaskiewicz (Eds.), *Advances in social network analysis: Research in the social and behavioral sciences.* Thousand Oaks, CA: Sage.

Moos, R. (1986). *Group environment scale manual* (2nd ed.). Palo Alto, CA: Consulting Psychologists Press.

Morrow, A. L., Rosenthal, J., Lakkis, H., Bowers, J. C., Butterfoss, F. D., Crews, R. C., & Sirotkin, B. (1998). A population-based study of risk factors for under-immunization among urban Virginia children served by public, private and military health care systems. *Pediatrics, 101,* E5.

Nelson, G. (1994). The development of a mental health coalition: A case study. *American Journal of Community Psychology, 22,* 229–255.

Nezlek, J., & Galano, J. (1993). Developing and maintaining state-wide adolescent pregnancy prevention coalitions: A preliminary investigation. *Health Education Research, 8,* 433–447.

Norton, B., Kegler M., & Aronson, R. (May 2000). *Measuring community capacity in healthy cities initiatives.* Paper presented at the SOPHE 2000 Midyear Scientific Conference, Denver.

Penner, S. (1995). A study of coalitions among HIV/AIDS service organizations. *Sociological Perspectives, 38,* 217–239.

Perkins, D. (1995). Speaking truth to power: Empowerment ideology as social intervention and policy. *American Journal of Community Psychology, 23,* 765–794.

Perkins, D., Florin, P., Rich, R., Wandersman, A., & Chavis, D. (1990). Participation and the social and physical environment of residential blocks: Crime and community context. *American Journal of Community Psychology, 18,* 83–115.

Prestby, J., & Wandersman, A. (1985). An empirical exploration of a framework of organizational viability: Maintaining block organizations. *Journal of Applied Behavioral Science, 21,* 287–305.

Prestby, J., Wandersman, A., Florin, P., Rich, R., & Chavis, C. (1990). Benefits, costs, incentive management and participation in voluntary organizations: A means to understanding and promoting empowerment. *American Journal of Community Psychology, 18,* 117–149.

Provan, K., & Milward, H. (1995). A preliminary theory of interorganizational network effectiveness: A comparative study of four community mental health systems. *Administrative Science Quarterly, 40,* 1–33.

Putnam, R. (1993). *Making democracy work.* Princeton, NJ: Princeton University Press.

Rappaport, J. (1987). Terms of empowerment/exemplars of prevention: Toward a theory for community psychology. *American Journal of Community Psychology, 15,* 121–144.

Reininger, B., Dinh-Zarr, T., Sinicrope, P., & Martin, D. (1999). Dimensions of participation and leadership: Implications for community-based health promotion for youth. *Family and Community Health, 22,* 72–82.

Roberts-DeGennaro, M. (1986). Factors contributing to coalition maintenance. *Journal of Sociology and Social Welfare, 13*(2), 248–264.

Robertson, A., & Minkler, M. (1994). New health promotion movement: A critical examination. *Health Education Quarterly, 23,* 295–312.

Rogers, T., Howard-Pitney, B., Feighery, E., Altman, D., Endres, J., & Roeseler, A. (1993). Characteristics and participant perceptions of tobacco control coalitions in California. *Health Education Research, 8,* 345–357.

Roussos, S., & Fawcett, S. (2000). A review of collaborative partnerships as a strategy for improving community health. *Annual Review of Public Health, 21,* 369–402.

Sanchez, V. (2000). Reflections on community coalition staff: Research directions from practice. *Health Promotion Practice, 1,* 320–322.

Sharfman, M., Gray, B., & Yan, A. (1991). The context of interorganizational collaboration in the garment industry: An institutional perspective. *Journal of Applied Behavioral Science, 27,* 181–208.

Shea, S., & Basch, C. (1990). A review of five major community-based cardiovascular disease prevention programs. Part 1: Rationale, design and theoretical framework. *American Journal of Health Promotion, 4,* 203–213.

Stokols, D. (1992). Establishing and maintaining healthy environments: Toward a social ecology of health promotion. *American Psychologist, 47,* 6–22.

Tesh, S. (1988). *Hidden arguments: Political ideology and disease prevention policy.* New Brunswick, NJ: Rutgers University Press.

Thompson, B., & Kinne, S. (1990). Social change theory: Applications to community health. In N. Bracht (Ed.), *Health promotion at the community level.* Thousand Oaks, CA: Sage.

Wallerstein, N. (1992). Powerlessness, empowerment and health: Implications for health promotion programs. *American Journal of Health Promotion, 6,* 197–205.

Wandersman, A., & Alderman, J. (1993). Incentives, barriers and training of volunteers for the American Cancer Society: A staff perspective. *Review of Public Personnel Administration, 13,* 67–76.

Wandersman, A., Florin, P., Friedmann, R., & Meier, R. (1987). Who participates, who does not and why? An analysis of voluntary neighborhood associations in the United States and Israel. *Sociological Forum, 2,* 534–555.

Whetten, D. (1981). Interorganizational relations: A review of the field. *Journal of Higher Education, 52,* 1–28.

Whitt, M. (1993). *Fighting tobacco: A coalition approach to improving your community's health.* Lansing: Michigan Department of Public Health.

Wolff, T. (2001). Community coalition building—Contemporary practice and research. *American Journal of Community Psychology, 29,* 165–172.

Wood, D., & Gray, B. (1991). Toward a comprehensive theory of collaboration. *Journal of Applied Behavioral Science, 27,* 139–162.

Zapka, J., Marrocco, G., Lewis, B., McCusker, J., Sullivan, J., McCarthy, J., & Birth, F. (1992). Inter-organizational responses to AIDS: A case study of the Worcester AIDS consortium. *Health Education Research, 7,* 31–46.

Zimmerman, M. A., & Rappaport, J. (1988). Citizen participation, perceived control, and psychological empowerment. *American Journal of Community, 16,* 725–750.

CHAPTER EIGHT

COMMUNITY CAPACITY

Concept, Theory, and Methods

Barbara L. Norton
Kenneth R. McLeroy
James N. Burdine
Michael R. J. Felix
Alicia M. Dorsey

For the past two decades, there has been a dramatic increase in the interest of public health researchers and practitioners in community-based approaches to improving the health of the public, particularly in the areas of health promotion and disease prevention. This increased emphasis on community approaches is due to a variety of factors, including an understanding of the complex etiology of contemporary health problems (Florin & Chavis, 1990), an appreciation for the importance of the interplay between humans and their environments (Green, Richard, & Potvin, 1996; Heller, 1990), and a recognition among public health professionals of limits to fostering individually oriented strategies for behavior change (Steckler et al., 1995).

Despite this increased attention, there is considerable variation in the extent to which community is incorporated in interventions ranging from community as the setting or context of interventions to intensive community involvement in defining social problems, identifying solutions, and evaluating outcomes (Minkler & Wallerstein, 1997). Advocates for more intensive community involvement in public health programming suggest that the results of efforts to change individual health behaviors significantly within communities, when treated as settings, have been disappointing (Hawe, 1994; Florin & Chavis, 1990). Moreover, although characteristics of communities may inhibit action in addressing social problems, the nature of community relationships may also be part of the solution (Chavis, Speer, Resnick, & Zippay, 1993). For example, it has been noted that community has a powerful influence on individuals, symbolically and tangibly, by shaping identity and meaning, communicating norms, and offering and limiting opportunities for behavior (Thompson & Kinne, 1999). Communities offer a resource for change because they can be mobilized to identify, plan, channel resources, and undertake effective action for health promotion and health-enhancing social change.

A 1988 Institute of Medicine report, *The Future of Public Health,* issued a call for public health organizations to reorient their activities to ensure conditions for health and give prominence to the community as not only the logical setting but also the catalyst for health promotion. Building on the concept of community as problem and solution, a number of researchers have urged an ecological approach to public health interventions (McLeroy, Bibeau, Steckler, & Glanz, 1988; Stokols, 1992). An ecological framework uses a systemic perspective regarding the interdependence of people, institutions, services, and the broader social and political environment. When used to examine the nature and extent of social relationships that exist within communities and the presence of community factors that may affect the ability of communities to mobilize to address systemic problems, this approach is based on a theoretical concept known as *community capacity.*

Community capacity has recently fostered inquiry by foundations, government agencies, and a wide array of nonprofit organizations and academic institutions to identify and measure its associated factors. Funding organizations view building capacity, which has become an integral goal of numerous grant initiatives, as an untapped resource for improving health status. Grant-making institutions are keenly interested in improving their tools for identifying communities with the capacity to foster positive change, and community capacity may provide a useful criterion for the awarding of grants or tailoring of interventions (Easterling, Gallagher, Drisko, & Johnson, 1998a; Goodman et al., 1998). If community capacity is found lacking, it may be possible to adapt health-related interventions or develop antecedent capacity-building activities prior to implementing health promotion programs.

In addition to community capacity as a means for achieving community health improvement, it can also be viewed as an important outcome of public health interventions (Steckler, Dawson, Israel, & Eng, 1993). Many public health interventions have as desired outcomes strengthening the capacity of individuals, families, social networks, organizations, communities, public policy, and the broader social environment (McLeroy, Kegler, Steckler, Burdine, & Wisotsky, 1994). Foundations view capacity building as an essential strategy for sustaining programs and health improvements long after grant funding periods have ended because organizational infrastructure and the community commitment for continuation are created in the process.

Interest in community capacity touches many disciplines, including organizational development, community development, sociology and social work, criminal justice, political science, and public health. Some of this inquiry focuses on civic infrastructure, social service reform, and urban revitalization. Although the end goals of these various fields differ, they share a common interest in drawing on and building the capacity of communities to address their problems effectively. This has involved a fundamental shift away from a focus exclusively on deficit and scarcity to an assets perspective, embodying a dynamic and positive understanding of human, material, power, and social resources.

Interest in community capacity touches many disciplines, including organizational development, community development, sociology and social work, criminal justice, political science, and public health.

Despite the current interest, effective application is limited because measurement of community capacity is still in its infancy. Over the past five years, the U.S. Centers for Disease Control and Prevention and the Robert Wood Johnson Foundation have called on experts to develop a framework for understanding community capacity and developing useful and valid measures of capacity building (Goodman et al., 1998; Ricketts, 2001). We would like to believe that public health interventions always have positive and lasting outcomes. However, without a metric for measurement, it will remain a matter of conjecture whether community health interventions result in increased sustainability and capacity for future problem solving. Thus, the identification and assessment of community capacity, as both an input and an outcome, is important to those striving to develop healthy communities.

Our aim in this chapter is to provide a clearer conceptual understanding of community capacity, which will contribute to the development of measurable indexes and greater practical application of the construct of community capacity in the field of public health.

The Concept of Community

How we think about community will affect how we think about the concept of community capacity, including the resources that may exist within communities to address common problems. The concept of community has a history that places it squarely in opposition to the idea of individualism and traditional liberalism (Reynolds & Norman, 1988).

Beginning with Thomas Jefferson's vision of democratic ideals and notions about "public work" to Tocqueville's astute observations about America's vibrant associational life (Tocqueville, 2000), the importance of communal bonds in providing essential ballast for grounding the country's moral and social fabric was established. Yet a number of contemporary trends have confounded the practice of these American habits (Bellah, Madsen, Sullivan, Swidler, & Tipton, 1985; Elshtain, 1999), including massive demographic shifts, an explosion in the power and consumption of mass media and technology, and the erosion in the authority of moral institutions and organizational groups that were previously used as forums for community problem solving (Putnam, 2000).

Scholars within the fields of sociology, psychology, and political science have examined the community and constructs related to community dimensions (Bellah et al., 1985; Bellah, Madsen, Sullivan, Swidler, & Tipton, 1991; Iscoe, 1974; Sarason, 1974; Rappaport, 1981; Berger & Neuhaus, 1977; Putnam, 2000). These scholars see community not as simply a collection of individuals or the locus of a set of problems to be addressed but as an integrated ecosystem composed of assets and capabilities.

The term *community* carries a wide range of meanings, and although we assume a shared understanding of the term, its definition is problematic and multidimensional. In common usage, the term *community* represents something both real and ideal. Community is real in that it is considered concrete—for example, as a set of individuals delineated by physical, social, or jurisdictional boundaries. Yet it is also viewed as intangible—as a process of civil society and community development (Smith, 1996). Regardless of whether one views community as real or abstract, the term is replete with symbolic and pragmatic meaning, and it resonates with our ideals about the nature of human life.

How we think about community will affect how we think about the concept of community capacity, including the resources that may exist within communities to address common problems.

Community is most commonly described in geographically or relationally bounded terms (Hillery, 1955; McMillan & Chavis, 1986; Kumpfer, Turner, Hopkins, & Librett, 1993; Hawe, 1994). Usually communities share values and institutions (Thompson & Kinne, 1999). A shared identity and interdependency are extremely important, as highlighted in this definition: a sense of membership; common symbol systems; common values; reciprocal influence; common needs and a commitment to meeting them; and a shared history (Israel, Checkoway, Schulz, & Zimmerman, 1994).

Nature of Community Capacity

The concept of community capacity is consistent with Kretzmann and McKnight's conception (1993) of functional communities being defined by human and material resources that are the building blocks for assets; these assets can be identified, mobilized, and used to address issues of concern and bring about change. Although community capacity is not inherently a health construct in the narrow

Although community capacity is not inherently a health construct in the narrow or traditional sense, it is tightly bound to the World Health Organization's expanded definition of health.

or traditional sense, it is tightly bound to the World Health Organization's expanded definition of health (1984), which emphasizes the importance of control over health determinants and the inclusion of "social and personal resources, as well as physical capacities" (p. 73). This suggests that community capacity is linked to quality of life and public health's goal of fostering conditions conducive to health for all. However, there are real differences in conceptions of just how community capacity contributes to health.

Some have asserted that the purpose of community capacity is to strengthen the characteristics of communities that enable them to plan, develop, implement, and sustain effective community programs (Poole, 1997; Fawcett et al., 1996; Cottrell, 1976), that is, to serve as a mechanism for achieving a more coordinated and effective health and social service delivery system. Kingsley and colleagues (1997), referring to the new community-building movement to address poverty, identified its central theme as "rebuilding hope" (p. 13), in addition to building the ability of individuals, groups, and organizations to plan, implement, and manage community ventures. Others view community capacity as enhancing health outcomes directly, although the specific mechanisms are yet unclear (Freudenberg et al., 1995). One mechanism, for example, may be through an enhanced sense of community, social ties, and community cohesiveness (Israel, 1985).

Theoretical Perspective

Because it is an evolving construct, it is important to examine some of the fundamental assumptions and variations in assumptions about community capacity. These assumptions are portrayed in Figure 8.1. Each assumption stands on its own and is not necessarily vertically linked to others. Although each of these assumptions is described as a set of bipolar extremes, and examples or references are offered to illustrate these extremes, it is important to stress that no theory of community capacity is represented in such absolute terms. Rather, perspectives on community capacity are oriented, explicitly or implicitly, toward one side or the other of a continuum.

Value System. Community capacity has been presented by many as a value-free concept—something that assists communities in accomplishing their purposes as they choose (National Civic League, 1999; Mattessich & Monsey, 1997). One

FIGURE 8.1. CONTRASTING THEORETICAL PERSPECTIVES ON COMMUNITY CAPACITY.

Value-free ———————	**Value System**	——————— Value-based
Individual ———————	**Level of Analysis**	——————— Social organization
Harmonious and consensus-driven ———————	**Approach**	——————— Open to conflict and risk-driven
Homogeneous ———————	**Community Composition**	——————— Heterogenous
Locational ———————	**Definition of Boundaries**	——————— Relational
Fixed ———————	**Stability of Social System**	——————— Dynamic
Emic ———————	**Point of View**	——————— Etic
Specific ———————	**Issue Focus**	——————— Generalized

example from the community development literature is the definition of community capacity as "the abilities of residents to organize and mobilize their resources for the accomplishment of consensually defined goals" (Garkovich, 1989, p. 200). However, a value-free approach must allow for the possibility that a community may engage in capacity-building activities that enhance the well-being of one particular community or segments within it yet are harmful to those outside it. Carried to its logical end, rapacious communities can appropriate and dominate resources to the exclusion of others, such as weaker communities or disenfranchised groups.

The self-determined values of a community could run counter to the democratic values of free and open participation or could contradict the idea of community capacity as health enhancement. For example, as emphasized in the edited volume *Community in America* (Reynolds & Norman, 1988), communities are identified as much by whom they exclude as whom they include. A community could exclude minorities, rural residents, the young, the old, women, men, or other community members from their definition of the community. A number of writers are critical of value-free conceptualization (Fukuyama, 1995; Elshtain, 1999).

Level of Analysis. Community capacity may be described as an underlying framework for understanding human behavior, interaction, and organization (Turner, Beeghley, & Powers, 1998). The level of analysis may range from an individual orientation that emphasizes concepts from social psychology, such as trust, identity, self-efficacy, or the psychological sense of community, to those prominent in social organization theory, like ties that exist among community organizations and the extent to which individual social networks share members or network ties. When community capacity is examined through an individual or psychological lens, it is viewed primarily as a set of belief systems and resources that can be measured on an individual basis and then aggregated for approximation of a community-level phenomenon. An example would include measuring the self-efficacy or competence of members of a group and averaging the competence of the members as an indicator of group self-efficacy or competence. This aggregation may then be represented as the totality of sentiments and attitudes that bind people together for community problem solving and action (Hillery, 1955).

In contrast, social organization theorists highlight the importance of structural features and processes within the social environment as essential for community capacity. For example, a more structural view of capacity would focus on the availability and accessibility of mediating structures, interorganizational relationships, and distribution of power and authority.

Approach. Perspectives on community capacity are infused with the idea of seeking a common ground in developing community solutions. Processes that accommodate and integrate different perspectives through use of a consensus-based, collaborative process are highly valued. The heavy emphasis on consensual politics is aimed at keeping all parties at the table in the interests of developing comprehensive solutions that include everyone's interests, resources, and needs. The optimistic assumptions about human behavior and development that are inherent in collaborative models have been challenged from within the field of community development (Biddle & Biddle, 1965) and by those who broke off from it (Alinsky, 1971). Community organizing is premised on the belief that inequities and injustices are directly related to a lack of political power, that resources are finite, and that a shift in power relationships will lead to a redistribution of resources.

Conflict is inherent in the nature of community life and under some circumstances may play an important role in building capacity by serving as a catalyst for action (Labonte, 1997; Chaskin, Brown, Venkatesh, & Vidal, 2001). Clearly, conflict resolution skills are an important predictor of community coalition development (Butterfoss, Goodman, & Wandersman, 1996), one of the principal strategies currently employed in public health community development models. In communities with large disenfranchised populations and community norms that mitigate against political and social participation of significant minorities, consensus-based approaches may not be the only, or even the most appropriate, solution to building capacity. The heavy reliance on collaborative models may be related to the fact that the primary funding sources of public health are federal, state, and local governments. It may also be related to an idealized notion of community that many individuals hold. Regardless of its origins, mechanisms for building capacity, including conflict strategies and the circumstances under which these strategies are effective, are an important part of the research agenda for community capacity.

Definition of Boundaries. Definition of a community and its subsequent community capacity may be dramatically affected by the boundaries though which the community is defined. At one extreme, a locational perspective defines a community by geographical boundaries, such as streets, freeways, or other man-made or natural features. At the other extreme, a relational perspective defines a community by social networks or associational patterns.

The use of geographically defined communities is based, at least in part, on the assumption that people's lives are greatly influenced by their propinquity. There is considerable literature to support this assumption, and face-to-face interactions are an essential part of social capital, an element of community capacity. However, a locality-based definition—physical, political, or economic—may not correspond with the way people cultivate and exercise their personal relationships and group affiliations. Participation in planning, organizing, and implementing community development programs is unfamiliar to many individuals and communities, so social groups often serve as a starting point for engendering effective community involvement. Churches, voluntary associations, and neighborhood groups serve as mediating structures to encourage interactions among members and between members and the broader community (Berger & Neuhaus, 1977). Experiences with these groups serve as stepping-stones for further engagement in community affairs and decisions.

There is a wide variety of relational communities and criteria for defining boundaries, including those defined by network ties, common interest, or symbolic identity. Relational communities have membership, leadership, and social network structure. A relational community can be a geographical one, as long as the community's pattern of relationships corresponds to geographical boundaries. The importance of relational communities is that they are important pathways for social resources, such as information, assistance, and access to other people (Israel, 1985), and they are a part of our social identity and definition of personal community.

Bronfenbrenner (1986) indicated that boundaries established by social address (physical or demographic) are very different from perceptions of social network or community relationships. As a result, geographically defined communities, established to meet the needs of local, state, and federal institutions or those of grant-making entities, may not be adequate for addressing issues on a community-wide basis. In defining community capacity, it is important to focus not only on geographical or geopolitical boundaries, but also on the nature of ties or connections that exist within communities, including network connections among individuals and interorganizational relationships.

Community Composition. With relational communities defined, at least in part, by shared social norms, the extent of homogeneity in a community will have considerable influence on the ease or challenge of fostering greater connectedness among community members and on the strengthening of community capacity. More homogeneous communities may find it easier to build a sense of trust and sense of belonging. However, they may lack the variety of different perspectives inherent in more heterogeneous settings, hampering the long-term development of a civil society (O'Connell, 1999). Granovetter (1973) highlighted the importance of weak ties that bridge social distance between different sectors or social groupings. These bridging ties have value in diffusion of innovations, access to mobility opportunities for individuals, and enhancing cohesion for community building.

The increasing diversity of American society requires that communities adapt to the presence of different cultures, languages, and norms. At one extreme, community adaptations may take the form of multiple cultures independently coexisting, either peacefully or in conflict, within a particular locale. At the other extreme, there may be a merging or fusing of diverse cultures into a single, more coherent whole. How we manage our increasing diversity will have a dramatic effect on our ability to develop community capacity and sustain the ability of communities to address local, regional, and national problems.

Stability of Social Systems. A critical issue in using community capacity to strengthen community bonds is the extent to which interaction patterns, social norms, and organizational structures are malleable. We may regard community capacity as resulting from an evolutionary process that has historical foundations in the development of solidarity and social institutions over time. If we assume that it, like social capital (Putnam, 2000), is relatively immutable, we would restrict its application to readiness assessments for community-based interventions. However, if we assume that key aspects of capacity can be built and uncovered or animated for use in community problem solving, then application of the construct could encompass capacity building within an intervention design and might prescribe it as a desired outcome as well. Allen and Dillman (1994) found that even when communities face tremendous forces working against cohesion, they may still be effective in community problem solving by leveraging external resources, activating informal communication systems, and exercising horizontal leadership structures. So for certain outcomes and certain circumstances, different combinations of capacity can be effectively drawn on for community and health improvement. Although some aspects of capacity are more challenging to modify, others may be more sensitive to change. Yet even if this latter assumption is made, respect for the stability, longevity, and functional role of existing social systems is paramount. Dimensions of social systems are fragile and more vulnerable to erosion than to fortification.

Many of our community-based intervention strategies, such as community coalitions, are specifically designed to strengthen capacity through community participation in assessment, problem definition, and intervention development and to enhance interorganizational relationships (McLeroy et al., 1994). However, it may be argued that coalitions or related strategies simply impose a new set of organization on existing social structures, and it is not clear under what conditions these interventions have a lasting effect in modifying underlying community processes, such as social networks, sense of community, and interorganizational relationships. Moreover, we know relatively little about what happens to communities in the long term, once funding for infrastructure development is no longer available. As a result, interventions are constrained by deficits in community capacity even as they are directed at its amplification.

Insider Versus Outsider Point of View. Although used primarily within the field of anthropology to describe the two principal approaches to the study of native peoples (Lett, 1990), the constructs of emic and etic points of view are useful in the discussion of community capacity. An emic view represents concepts and categories that are meaningful and appropriate from the perspective of the people being studied; an etic view presents constructs that are meaningful and appropriate to those conducting the analysis. The importance of this distinction is more than simple semantics. A lack of sensitivity to native wisdom or view of community members about what constitutes community and capacity may threaten the validity of findings and conclusions, our ability to work productively with communities, and our capacity to inform broader audiences.

To date, much of the discussion of community capacity has been dominated by professionals and academic researchers attempting to understand and transform into generalizable models the complexity and subtlety of community change processes. The lens used for these discussions has largely been that of professional outsiders, despite the dominant rhetoric about community self-determination and use of local community assets. Uphoff (1992), aware of the risks of an etic approach, has made the following recommendations to the World Bank: (1) emphasize capacity over achieving targets, (2) weave participation into every aspect of a project from the start, (3) accommodate flexibility for learning, and (4) make an investment in building a locality's participatory capabilities.

Issue Focus. A very practical and theoretical issue with community capacity is whether it is a generalized state or condition in communities or a specific response to a given problem or concern. By looking at key community characteristics as indicators of capacity—social and interorganizational networks, leadership, psychological sense of community, skills and resources, citizen participation, mediating structures, reflective learning, leadership, and the exercise of power—it is tempting to conclude that community capacity is a generalized condition. However, the extent to which capacity is mobilized to address a specific problem may be contingent on the extent to which a social issue is on the public agenda and the extent to which individuals or organizations are available to serve a catalytic or leadership role.

Theoretically, community capacity consists of characteristics that affect a community's mobilization of resources, the extent to which communities are open to new problem definitions, and their ability to disseminate information and develop consensus. However, communities, like individuals, may have a limited span of attention. Too many items on the public agenda may lead to a less effective allocation of resources and reduced capacity around specific concerns.

Related to the issue of the public's span of attention is the amount of time that issues remain on the public agenda. Particularly for social problems, the attention span in communities may be limited. There are always new problems, issues, and concerns competing for attention and resources. Moreover, we tend to be a society enamored with quick fixes and expectations that problems are addressed, so that we can move on to the next problem. This raises a substantial issue about how we maintain public attention and how we can continue directing resources to high-priority concerns.

Definitions of Community Capacity

Chaskin and colleagues (2001), with the support of the Chapin Center for Children and Families at the University of Chicago, drew on their experiences with comprehensive community initiatives to develop a definition of community capacity that incorporates the influence of community context and desired outcomes and also addresses ways to build capacity:

> Community capacity is the interaction of human capital, organization
> resources, and social capital existing within a given community that can be
> leveraged to solve collective problems and improve or maintain the well being

of that community. It may operate through informal social processes and/or organized efforts by individuals, organizations, and social networks that exist among them and between them and the larger systems of which the community is a part [p. 7].

The Aspen Institute (1996) calls community capacity "the ability of individuals, organizations, businesses, and governments in their community to come together, learn, make well-reasoned decisions about the community's present and future, *and* to work together to carry out those decisions" (p. 1). The MacArthur Foundation (2001) expands on these expectations and defines its purpose when it describes community capacity as "the ability to mobilize the energy and talents of its members and to secure outside resources, such as capital investment and public services, to foster individual growth and improve quality of life." Within a public health context, McLeroy (1996) provides a definition of community capacity as "characteristics of communities that affect their ability to identify, mobilize, and address social and public health problems." Hancock (2001), one of the founders of the "healthy cities" movement, describes a similar construct, community capital, as the combination of social ecological, human, and economic capital. The healthy cities movement, fostered primarily through the efforts of the World Health Organization, represents an ecological approach to health promotion.

For the purposes of this chapter, community capacity is regarded as a set of dynamic community traits, resources, and associational patterns that can be brought to bear for community building and community health improvement. Captured within the definition are structural networks and the processes to cultivate and maintain them, as well as the perceptions, skills, and resources of individuals that are channeled through these social structures. This definition makes clear a theoretical position of community capacity as a value-laden concept focused on the attributes of both individuals and social structures.

> *Community capacity is regarded as a set of dynamic community traits, resources, and associational patterns that can be brought to bear for community building and community health improvement.*

Dimensions of Community Capacity

A number of researchers have sought to develop a set of dimensions or characteristics for the construct of community capacity. Table 8.1 provides a sense of the dimensions various researchers view as most important. Seven research models and their dimensions are presented in the order in which they were published.

TABLE 8.1. DIMENSIONS OF COMMUNITY CAPACITY AND COGNATE CONSTRUCTS.

	Cottrell, 1976 (Community Competence)	Harwood Group, 1996[a] (Public Capital)	Goodman et al., 1998 (Community Capacity)	Easterling et al., 1998a (Community Capacity)	National Civic League, 1992, 1999[b] (Civic Capital)	Chaskin et al., 2001 (Community Capacity)	Saguaro Seminar, 2001 (Social Capital)
Skills and resources	Articulateness		Skills	Skills and knowledge	Skills *in* inter-community cooperation	Access to resources	
	Management of relationships with the larger society		Resources (for example, financial, technological, other material)				
Nature of social relationships	Commitment		Sense of community	Trusting relationships and norms of reciprocity	Positive intergroup relationships	Commitment among community members	Social trust
	Conflict containment and accommodation		Social capital/trust (listed as type of "resource")	Sense of efficacy and confidence among residents		Sense of community	
Structures and mechanisms for community dialogue	Communication	Informal networks and links[2]	Social and inter-organizational networks		Community information sharing	Mechanisms of problem solving	Diversity of friendships
	Machinery for facilitating participant interaction and decision making	Abundance of social gatherings[1]	Mechanisms for communication across the community and for citizen input (listed as type of resource)		Capacity for cooperation and consensus building		Associational involvement
		Organized spaces for interaction[1]					Informal socializing
		Catalytic organizations[1]					
		Safe havens for decision makers[1]					

		Strong, diverse leadership [2]	Leadership	Leadership	Community leadership	Civic leadership (listed with "associational involvement")
Leadership						
Civic participation	Participation		Participation; Distribution of community power		Citizen participation	Political participation; Faith-based engagement; Equality of civic engagement across the community
Value system		Shared purpose for the community [3]; Community norms [3]	Community values		Community vision and pride; Volunteerism and philanthropy	Giving and volunteering
Learning culture	Self-other awareness and clarity of situational definitions	Conscious community discussion [2]	Understanding of community history; Critical reflection	Culture of learning	Civic education; Ongoing learning	

Note: Certain dimensions of the models, as originally developed by the researchers, have been split into more than one category to correspond to categories discussed in this chapter. For example, under the Goodman et al. (1998) model, participation and leadership is considered one dimension. If the way that researchers originally classified a dimension differs from our display, this is noted in parentheses. In some cases, italicized words clarifying the meaning of various dimensions have been added to the researchers' terminology.

[a] The Harwood Group's model of public capital defines categories of dimensions, indicated as 1 through 3: 1: tangible dimensions, 2: links between the tangible dimensions, 3: underlying values.

[b] The NCL model includes a dimension that is, in our opinion, an ecological or contextual factor: that of government performance. As a result, it is not reflected in this table of categories defining dimensions of community capacity.

Three models describe dimensions of what the researchers call community capacity: Goodman et al. (1998) from the field of public health; Easterling, Gallagher, Drisko, and Johnson (1998b) writing on behalf of a Colorado-based philanthropic organization; and Chaskin et al. (2001) from the field of social work and urban policy. The other four research models in the table and their dimensions are displayed to highlight the similarities and illustrate a few areas of departure from the construct of community capacity as we describe it. These cognate constructs are community competence (Cottrell, 1976); public capital (Harwood Group, 1996); civic capital, commonly referred to as the Civic Index (National Civic League, 1992, 1999); and social capital (Saguaro Seminar, 2001).

Cottrell (1976) described community competence as the ability of a community to draw together its parts to collaborate effectively in identifying its problems and needs, developing a consensus on solutions, and implementing their planned actions. He outlined eight dimensions that he saw as critical to community competence. A community psychologist by training, he placed his greatest emphasis on individual perceptions, skills, and consciousness. Among the elements, he included a mechanism for facilitating interaction but made no mention of social networks or leadership, two essential dimensions of community capacity.

Public capital and civic capital, highly similar constructs, emerge from the civic renewal field of inquiry, but they have been developed to emphasize slightly different components. Public capital (Harwood Group, 1996) is a model with nine dimensions that have been organized into three categories: tangible dimensions, links between the tangible dimensions, and underlying values. This categorical framework aids in clarifying our understanding of the construct, but at the same time it constrains the range of its application since it tends to bypass important human capital elements like skills, knowledge, and resources. The notion of civic capital, also known as the Civic Index, was developed more as a tool (National Civic League, 1992, 1999) than as a theoretical construct. As such, its dimensions have been defined first to make sense to civic and political leaders rather than be responsive to a researcher's need for conceptual clarity. Although the dimensions of civic capital appear to overlay well with the categories of community capacity, many important subdimensions are omitted. Like public capital, civic capital gives scant attention to human capital and resource availability; social trust and networks are similarly given only cursory mention. Despite this, through the National Civic League's Healthy Communities planning process, for example (Norris, 1993), the Civic Index is adapted to each local context, and many subdimensions, not elaborated on in their literature, are addressed within the day-to-day interactions of conducting a community project.

Social capital, a prominently used but variously defined construct, is the last of the four complementary models shown in Table 8.1. This construct originally emerged out of the education and sociology fields, but it has become a part of the popular vernacular with the writings of political scientist Robert Putnam (1993, 1995, 1996, 2000). Rather than a structure or an observable process, it is the value embedded within social networks and other associations that individuals draw on to achieve individual and collective goals (Putnam, 2000; Popapchuk, Crocker, Schechter, & Boogaard, 1998; Smedley & Syme, 2001). Because social networks are the foundation for collaboration and coalition building, they are an essential part of community capacity. But as the societal analogue to human and material capital, social capital represents a more enduring characteristic of communities and a more limiting construct than community capacity. It is interesting to note, however, that the way in which the Saguaro Seminar operationalized the construct for its Community Benchmark Survey (2001) involves a broad scope, touching on many more dimensions than has been the case with most other social capital research.

A set of seven dimensions defining the community capacity construct is distilled from this analysis (Table 8.1). These dimensions are constructed to represent the highest degree of consensus among researchers while preserving the particular character and emphasis of each model. The categories are labeled to avoid jargon and any explicit terms used for the various constructs themselves (for example, *social capital*). Because of the variability in the way that researchers characterize different dimensions of these models, the placement of any dimension within a given model is open to debate. However, this display represents one attempt at illustrating both the similarities and the differences among these cognate constructs and various interpretations of community capacity.

Level of Skills, Knowledge, and Resources

Skills and knowledge are identified as critical to community capacity by many researchers. This dimension includes skills for strategic planning and those related to interpersonal communication and group process. Chaskin et al. (2001) discussed this in terms of human capital and leadership. He linked human capital and leadership by explaining that the use of skills, knowledge, and resources by residents through participation in community improvement activities entails the exercise of leadership. This could involve a grassroots leader, who uses persuasive skills and his knowledge of community networks to mobilize neighbors, local churches, and store owners to become involved in cleaning up the area, or it could involve a local school principal who uses her school's resources and personal influence to garner community resources for an after-school and Saturday enrichment program for the neighborhood.

Although the most common emphasis is placed on internal community resources—a community's gifts and assets (Kretzmann & McKnight, 1993)—access to resources external to the community may be equally vital. An excessive or a deficient level of resources available to a community can impair the process of building capacity. External resources are not viewed as capacity enhancing unless they reduce dependency through the transfer of skills from external to internal sources. A reliance on externally imported skills and expertise is viewed as counter to capacity-building goals. Interventions typically stress the benefits of expanding a community's information base, that is, data and knowledge. Technical assistance has been the principal vehicle for achieving this purpose, but asset mapping and skill and resource inventories are increasingly used (Garkovich, 1989).

Nature of Social Relationships

The concept of social relationships builds on the idea of communities as social networks and social ties and is integral to the construct of social capital as defined in most of the scholarly literature. The notion of social connectedness highlights the quality of ties that exist among community members and the type and strength of sentiments embodied within those relationships. Included in this dimension is the belief that individuals matter to the community; that there is sufficient strength of social ties to work through serious differences; and that individual and collective actions will have desired results. For this reason it includes a sense of community, a sense of commitment and harmony, social trust, norms of reciprocity, and positive intergroup relations.

Structures, Mechanisms, and Spaces for Community Dialogue and Collective Action

This dimension represents a collection of tangible assets that provide the structural framework for community capacity. Included are social and interorganizational networks, especially voluntary associations; mechanisms for prompting and conducting community planning and action; community spaces for socializing and for problem solving; and systems for communitywide communication.

Social networks refer to the extent to which individuals are connected to each other through formal and informal networks of relationships and the extent to which social networks in the community share linkages or members. Because social resources—including instrumental assistance, emotional support, social identity, access to new social contacts, and information—flow across network ties, their distribution will be affected by the nature and extent of connectedness that exist in a community (Israel, 1985).

Social networks, such as friendship groups, are frequently developed within the context of the workplace, neighborhood, church, school, or other informal and formal organizations to which individuals belong. Thus, an important part of a community's capacity is its voluntary associational life. Many associations are formed for mutual aid, socialization, or social or political participation. More recently, associations have been formed as community planning and action groups or coalitions. These collaborative groups may be broad in scope or issue specific, ongoing entities or time limited, but they are often newly created in response to external funding opportunities. Unfortunately, many externally prompted efforts do not dedicate sufficient time or development resources to fostering local organizations or network building because of a need to demonstrate specific outcomes (Garkovich, 1989).

In addition to social networks and collaborative interorganizational structures, mechanisms for community dialogue may include catalytic organizations within communities and gathering spaces for interaction and public debate. Both are important to capacity because they help prompt community problem solving and reflection (Harwood Group, 1996; Chaskin et al., 2001). Catalytic organizations can provide the impetus for changing the status quo by making visible to leaders and community members the gap between what is and what could be. Examples of catalytic organizations within some communities are community foundations, community development corporations, chambers of commerce, citizen task forces or roundtables, and other community and voluntary organizations.

Quality of Leadership and Its Development

Leadership is critical in identifying problems, fostering community change activities, and providing opportunities for citizen participation. Given the increasing interdependence of individuals and groups within communities, it is essential that community leaders are knowledgeable about the broader community and its resources and have a sense of the common good (Esman & Uphoff, 1984). Effective leadership, then, requires qualities of communication, analysis and judgment, coaching, visioning, trust building, teamwork, reflection and learning, and partnering (Human Resources Development Canada, 2000).

Several issues are important for this dimension: the types of community leaders used, the development of leadership roles and new leaders, and the process for making the transition from old to new leadership. There are two ways of identifying leadership: positional and reputational. Communities with greater capacity not only draw on the skills of those in positions of office, supervision, or management but also tap the talents of those who are extensively connected within and across diverse community constituencies. In addition, new leaders are needed as new leadership positions develop and as older leaders retire, step down, or move on to other interests. Various studies show that the most effective community organizations are those that can successfully move new people into leadership positions over time (Presby & Wandersman, 1985).

With the rapid changes in the demographic composition of many communities—including the rapid growth in populations from other cultures and ethnic backgrounds, the aging of society, and changes in gender, age, and marital status roles—the development of new community leaders is critical. New leadership must represent the increasing diversity of groups, cultures, and orientations present in many of our communities.

Extent of Civic Participation

The importance of civic participation as an essential element in community capacity is inconsistently addressed by researchers who have defined community capacity and similar constructs (although it may be implied within other dimensions by those who fail to specify it explicitly). It is maintained here as an explicit and distinct dimension to emphasize its significance and because it serves as an important area of capacity-building leverage for health improvement interventions. This dimension describes the extent to which individuals within a community concern themselves with issues of broad public concern, including those relating to governance. It encompasses everything from parent-teacher association membership to voting behavior, from volunteering to participation in small social groups. These participatory mechanisms allow for specific constituencies to provide input to institutions at higher organizational or community levels.

Attributes of participation relate to breadth, depth, and intensity. A broad and representative base of citizen involvement is made possible when there is continuous conversation with all community segments. This requires constant outreach efforts and communication on the part of community leaders and members. It also requires vigilance in the cultivation of mutual trust and a vitality of neighborhood and social networks that link with each other, not simply within themselves. Achieving a depth of participation means that a community offers a multitude of creatively structured participation opportunities, making them widely and continually known, and that concerted efforts are undertaken to reduce individual and community-level barriers (Brown, 1991). Mediating structures play a critical role in defining the nature, extent, and intensity of civic participation because they provide the primary vehicle for its expression. Successful health improvement initiatives use existing institutions to organize and champion participation roles in their planning, implementing, and evaluating phases.

Another critical aspect of this dimension relates to community power structures and the distribution of power, which have been widely studied in the sociologic literature (Hunter, 1953). Power structures affect which problems are placed on the public agenda, the allocation of community resources, and the extent to which community participation in decision making is encouraged and facilitated. Although centralized power structures may facilitate decision making and allocation of resources, they may also limit participation and access to resources by relatively disenfranchised groups.

Value System

Community capacity is not value free and must encompass the norms, standards, expectations, and desires of particular communities. What is essential to capacity is not only that a community be able to articulate a clear and shared set of values, but that these values reflect a public moral philosophy (Elshtain, 1999). Warren (1980) defined a "good" community as one where people deal with each other on a personal basis; there is a broad distribution of power; a diversity of income, ethnic, and interest groups come together to work in common endeavors; there is a high degree of autonomy at the local level; and cooperation is highly valued. Many researchers agree that core values enhancing the capacity-building process include equity, democratic participation, collaboration, inclusion, and social responsibility (Goodman et al., 1998). Legal and procedural norms are secondary to these moral values in undergirding community capacity building.

Learning Culture

This dimension defines a community's ability to think critically and reflect on assumptions underlying one's ideas and actions, consider alternative ways of thinking and doing, and mine lessons from one's actions. This reflects a high degree of self-awareness about a community's values and interests and a strong institutional memory. The community culture must be one in which errors and failures are viewed as resources for learning instead of excuses for nonaction or instruments of blame. Management guru Peter Senge (1994) described learning as "the continuous testing of experience, and the transformation of that experience into knowledge—accessible to [all] . . ., and relevant to its core purpose" (p. 49). The concept of a learning culture has also been explored within the field of empowerment education and is defined by Paulo Freire (1970) as "critical consciousness." Communities that can reflect on the outcomes of their actions and on new options available to them may be more effective in maintaining change and improvements in social and health-related conditions. Chavis (1995) described capable communities as "learning communities."

Case Study: Applying the Concepts of Community Capacity to Health Development

This case study is a limited but illustrative example that employs the concept of community capacity to improve population health. This case, featuring a project conducted in Hartford, Connecticut, is not intended as a best practices model. Rather, its value may lie more in suggesting both the limitations and the potential of capacity approaches. A conceptual model for community capacity was developed and used in organizing this project by two of this chapter's authors, who served as outside facilitators for the process. In this example, the concept of building community capacity, as one of the goals of the project, was part of the original community dialogue and stated purposes of the community task force. The challenge of the project was to broaden the discussion from building the capacity of a single agency (the city's health department) to strengthening ties with the larger community and incorporating citizens in defining, implementing, and evaluating the overall program. Thus, the collaborative strategy used in Hartford stressed the building of community capacity as a central theme.

Development of the Project's Conceptual Model

Public health is predicated on the value of collective action and the belief that community is a significant unit of analysis and arena of practice (Rosen, 1958; Blum, 1974; Institute of Medicine, 1988; Amick, Levine, Tarlov, & Walsh, 1995). Numerous scholars have developed models of the factors that influence health and their interactions within communities (Rose, 1992; Tarlov, 1992; Evans & Stoddart, 1990; Patrick & Wickizer, 1995; McLeroy, et al., 1988). Documented success with the application of these models for improving overall community health, however, has been limited (Hancock et al., 1992; Israel, Schultz, Parker, & Becker, 1998). The value of a model is to focus the application of efforts and resources to improve health status more effectively. In these models, community capacity for health status improvement can be thought of as a tool and target for intervention, as well as a predictor of results.

The framework developed for this project contains four major elements: ecological factors, community capacity factors, health and human services system factors, and the outcome measure, population health status (Figure 8.2). Ecological factors include demographics, community history, organizational and public policies, participant expectations, and community resources. Community capacity includes two major elements: supporting or enabling functions and those related to a community's social capital. Supporting functions are skills or abilities within communities that allow them to accomplish tasks that enhance the likelihood of improving health status. These include exchange of information and resources, effective and accessible provision of services, training and technical assistance, monitoring and evaluation, and acquisition and management of resources. The second element of community capacity in this model, social capital, relates to "the features of social organization, such as networks, norms and social trust that facilitate coordination and cooperation for mutual benefit" (Putnam, 1995, p. 67). Numerous elements are posited to represent social capital, among them trust, goodwill, cooperation, civic engagement, reciprocity, collective efficacy, social networks, obligations, norms, and sense of community (Putnam, 1995; Kawachi, Kennedy, & Lochner, 1997b; Chavis & Wandersman, 1990; Sirianni & Friedland, 1995). Kawachi and colleagues (Kawachi, Kennedy, & Glass, 1999; Kawachi, Kennedy, Lochner, and Prothrow-Stith, 1997) established a linkage between social trust and health status; however, they depended exclusively on secondary data. The Hartford study was designed in part to advance research by developing valid indicators of social capital and by examining the association between these indicators and standardized measures of functional health status.

The last elements of the model, health and health system characteristics, are factors related to the accessibility of care, quality of care, financing of care, and adequacy of the service delivery system. This model acknowledges the practical reality that the health and human services system, with all of its limitations, is a fundamental tool used for health improvement. At the same time, it recognizes

FIGURE 8.2. A MODEL FOR COMMUNITY CAPACITY
FOR HEALTH STATUS IMPROVEMENT.

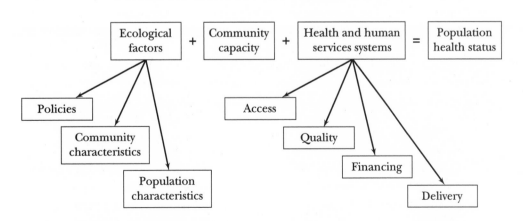

Source: Felix-Burdine & Associates (2000).

that the dynamic tension between solutions that focus on the financing and delivery of services and their quality and accessibility, and it also acknowledges the complex social determinants of health.

Background

In 1993, the mayor of Hartford, Connecticut responded to concerns about declining health status in the city and the inadequacy of the public health infrastructure. A Blue Ribbon Task Force was formed to coordinate a community health assessment and establish a system for monitoring health status, needs, and threats to public health. The task force incorporated the Institute of Medicine's recommendations from *The Future of Public Health* (1988), which emphasized the role of local public health in assessment, policy development, and assurance. As a result of its planning process, the task force recognized the need for a community vehicle in developing collaborative solutions to public health problems. Initially sponsored by local hospitals, the Community Health Partnership Committee (CHPC) became the vehicle through which an organized effort to build community capacity for health improvement was implemented.

From 1996 through 1998, the CHPC identified the individual, community, and broader social factors influencing health status and the local capacity and resources that could be used and enhanced in their strategy for improving community health. The assessment of local community capacity began with a series of interviews and community discussion groups with approximately 150 individuals, representing major sectors of the community, key decision makers, and groups not normally included in community decision making. Information was collected on issues of concern, resources available to address issues, the community's collaborative history, advice for the CHPC, and input regarding the role of the City of Hartford Health Department, including suggestions for developing its organizational effectiveness.

A number of major themes emerged from the community discussion groups, including several dimensions of organizational and community capacity:

- The presence of several sophisticated institutions and community-based research organizations, with competitive and uncoordinated organizational relationships
- Economic issues, including lack of coordination of block grant resources, and the organization of many city services along racial lines
- An abundance of health resources but problems of access for selected populations

- Opportunities for an expanded role for the city health department as a result of its recent restructuring and physical relocation
- A significant Hispanic population, largely Puerto Rican, characterized by a high degree of mobility between the mainland and the island, as well as fragmented political allegiances

The Community Health Improvement Strategy and Results

The CHPC used the information collected through the community discussion groups to create a community health improvement strategy. In addition, it created three subcommittees to engage other community stakeholders: public health strategic planning, public health assessment, and a steering committee. The assessment process continued with the planning and conduct of a general population survey ($n + 1,450$) and additional community discussion groups focusing on hard-to-reach audiences. The results of this assessment were presented in a community forum resulting in a "call to action" strategy: a commitment of community resources to address each priority issue and population within a limited time frame and with explicit outcomes.

This process had the following results:

- A community structure (the CHPC) through which efforts to improve access to care were, and continue to be, implemented
- A restructuring of local public health services, administration, roles, and resources
- A more integrated health services system, achieved through improved communication and coordination among local hospitals, public health, and individual providers
- Systemic use of consistent, high-quality health information across multiple organizations through coordinated collection, analysis, and applications
- The development of needed new community leadership and enhanced participation of existing leadership in health improvement efforts.
- Increased community participation in health improvement activities

When we examine the framework for building community capacity that appears in Figure 8.2, we can see that each element was identified and incorporated into the overall community health improvement strategy for this community. For example, ecological factors like local and state infrastructure issues, racial and ethnic factors, and community history were explored to determine how strengths and weaknesses could be addressed through a community health improvement strategy.

Community capacity building in this example was focused on the city health department at the request of the leaders initiating the process. As a result, primary attention was focused on improving access to care and the health status of the general population. To address this goal, changes were implemented in the organization of health services, and calls to action were issued for diabetes, hypertension, and other preventive-health topics. Among the by-products of the community development strategy were greater perceptions of trust, increased interorganizational information sharing, a positive experience with collaboration, and improved leveraging of external resources.

Future Directions

Contemporary emphasis on and interest in community capacity is intricately linked to the increased focus within public health and other disciplines on community-based, collaborative models to address social and health problems. Current interest is largely governed by instrumental motivations of funding agencies that seek to develop measures of capacity as both inputs and outcomes of community problem-solving interventions. High levels of community capacity may become an additional criterion for favorable funding decisions. Ratings of low capacity could lead to the development of antecedent interventions, so that lack of community capacity can be addressed before interventions are developed or as part of a health improvement intervention. Enhanced community capacity is also directly related to the sustainability of health improvement initiatives and is believed to possess inherent health benefits for individuals and communities.

A significant direction for future research entails refining the dimensions of community capacity, increasing our understanding of their interactions, and developing tools for measuring them. Without the ability to measure this construct, it will continue to remain uncertain whether or not public health and related interventions are effective in strengthening capacity. The difficulty in measuring community capacity is partly a function of the complexity of the construct even though each of the dimensions discussed in this chapter has existing methodologies for assessment. For example, the nature and extent of organizational cooperation within a community can be measured through network surveys of key respondents in community organizations. Civic participation may be assessed through population sample surveys designed to measure the extent of community

A significant direction for future research entails refining the dimensions of community capacity, increasing our understanding of their interactions, and developing tools for measuring them.

participation in voluntary groups. Connectedness of social networks may be measured through sample surveys of individuals using network sampling designs (Goodman et al., 1998; Ricketts, 2001).

However, it is important to recognize that we lack information on which dimensions of community capacity are important for what purpose. For example, is connectedness among informal social networks important for the purpose of strengthening referral patterns among community service organizations? We also do not know the extent to which the various dimensions of capacity tend to be interrelated. For example, are communities that are high in connectedness across social networks also high in interorganizational collaboration? Is the psychological sense of community linked to participation in voluntary groups and organizations? If the dimensions of capacity are strongly interrelated, then it will simplify our task of measuring overall capacity but confound our ability to sort out which dimensions may require augmentation.

Although measures for individual dimensions of capacity are available, assessment of multiple dimensions is a daunting, expensive, and time-consuming task. We also lack standards for making decisions about whether one or more of the dimensions constitutes sufficient capacity for undertaking effective interventions.

Given multiple measures and a lack of standards, one of the goals of assessment is to create an index of community capacity that is easily measured and useful for funding decisions and assessing outcomes across communities. For example, the Robert Wood Johnson Foundation has recently funded two studies (Ricketts, 2001; Felix-Burdine & Associates, 2000) to address the methodological, conceptual, and practical issues in the development of an index of capacity. Methodological issues include the unit of analysis, timing of measures, reliability and validity, the use of aggregate measures, and the availability of secondary measures or indicators.

Unit of Analysis

The unit of analysis or the definition of community that is the focus of data collection and analysis is critical to the utility of any measure of capacity. According to Ricketts (2001), if the definition of community for measurement purposes does not correspond to community as experienced by its members or community as the unit of solution (for example, states control the funds for a neighborhood program), looking at a neighborhood or census block or tract may not be useful. Conversely, if the unit of measurement is too large, then important differences across communities within the measurement definition may be overlooked, with community capacity representing nothing more than the average of capacity across units of solution.

Timing of Measurement

The frequency and timing of measurement can influence the utility of measures of community capacity. Single assessments may be most useful for funding decisions. However, if communities expect to be measured only once cross-sectionally, they may not invest in developing capacity. On the other hand, if the measurement of community capacity is designed for serial assessments that incorporate feedback toward the goal of improving capacity, then multiple measures across time are essential.

Reliability and Validity

Reliability and validity are issues with any measurement approach and are particularly critical when the consequences of measurement, such as funding decisions, are of such vital importance to individuals and communities. The development of appropriate measures of capacity requires that they be both reliable (that is, provide consistent results) and sensitive to change. Moreover, the predictive validity of measures of capacity is critical for establishing the importance of capacity as a predictor of community mobilization efforts.

Related to the issue of validity are the problems attendant on developing and using an index measure of capacity. Indexes may be useful in summarizing multiple measures and facilitating decision making. However, the benefits of indexes are also limitations. By creating indexes, we lose variability and obscure what may be important differences. Moreover, the weighting and inclusion of specific measures of capacity in an index score may have different meaning for different communities or stakeholders.

Primary and Secondary Measures

An important issue in measuring community capacity is the availability and utility of primary and secondary data. The principal challenge facing most states and communities interested in measures of community capacity is that useful data may not be available from existing sources. Data that are available are likely to be several years out-of-date or based on inappropriate units of analysis, such as a county or state. Primary data collection through surveys or other strategies is much more costly than reanalysis of existing data. However, the length of time required to gather, analyze, and report primary data may result in long delays and have a chilling effect on community participants. Thus, primary data collection may be cost prohibitive, particularly given the range and types of data that must now be collected to measure each of the dimensions of capacity.

Ethical Issues

In addition to measurement issues, there are important ethical issues in using community capacity as a criterion for funding or as an outcome of community interventions. One issue concerns the meaning of a high or low score on capacity. It may eventually be possible and desirable to compare ratings of communities and to establish standards for a high or low score on an index or the various dimensions of community capacity. But this raises the issue of what a high or low score means and the consequences of scoring high or low.

In diagnosing a community as low in community capacity, funding or sponsoring agencies may reduce the flow of financial support or other resources to it, although it is likely to be in great need of support. This may further increase health and other disparities between it and high-scoring communities. Low ratings may also demoralize community members and reduce the psychological sense of community (who would want to identify with a low-scoring community)? Labeling a community as high in capacity may strengthen access to resources and the psychological sense of community, even if a community lacks diversity and already has ready access to the services and resources it needs. Similarly, findings of minimal change or low-capacity outcomes resulting from a community intervention may inappropriately jeopardize its sustainability or its adoption by other communities.

Ranking communities on the basis of capacity alone presents inherent risks in interpretation and application. Any ranking system is based on an assumption of comparability across settings and requires simplification of complex and nuanced information about community characteristics. Ranking systems may lead to explicit or implicit labeling and often simplistic, value-laden categorization, such as high-low, strong-weak, or good-bad. Labeling communities may not only hamper access to resources, but can also have an adverse impact on community capacity itself, particularly in communities with the most need. Furthermore, ratings and labels tend to endure long after a rating is assigned and even when its accuracy or utility has changed. Thus, the concept of community capacity, if applied, must be used in conjunction with a host of other information about communities, including needs, resources, and diversity.

Conclusion

These measurement and ethical issues suggest that the idea of community capacity is in no small part a research and practice agenda. We are in the early stages of the development of appropriate measures, particularly index measures.

Furthermore, there are significant political and social issues in the construction and use of such indexes. So where do we go from here?

Two broad research frameworks may be of use in developing a community capacity research agenda. The first framework is a theory-driven model of measurement development in which we use the concept of community capacity dimensions to develop standardized measures that may be examined for internal consistency and associations among subscale scores. Thus, we may examine the relationships among standardized measures of interorganizational relationships, citizen participation, and the psychological sense of community across a number of communities. We could examine the extent to which measures of specific dimensions are predictive of community mobilization efforts and the extent to which a composite score or index is more or less predictive than the individual measures. We could compare different approaches to measuring individual dimensions, with particular attention to the availability and costs of data collection.

Such scale development would be an expensive task, but it is feasible. Once standardized measures were developed, they could be applied to comparison communities for purposes of funding decisions and for examining the effects of interventions on community capacity. Part of the difficulty with this theory-driven model of measurement is that we lack good theory about how the various dimensions of capacity affect community actions. It is not clear at this stage of our understanding whether we have adequately captured or understand the various ways in which community characteristics may affect community development and mobilization efforts. Without a shared understanding within communities of the importance and nature of community capacity, our efforts to develop and implement valid and reliable measures may be difficult.

An alternative approach to developing measures of community capacity focuses on strengthening our understanding of how communities develop and evolve through grounded theory or comparative case studies. Using the dimensions of capacity as a general framework for investigation, we can examine how the various components of capacity facilitate or inhibit the ability of individual communities to address health problems, particularly communities with different characteristics, developmental histories, agendas, and capacity. By using comparative case study approaches, we can compare findings across communities to draw broader conclusions, identify common themes, and develop a better understanding of the way community contextual factors affect the interplay of community characteristics and actions. A more ethnographic approach may help us to appreciate the different ways communities understand the concept of capacity and to translate our social science understandings into a shared language. Approaching community capacity through this research framework would also facilitate viewing communities as partners that may contribute to our common understanding of community development.

References

Alinsky, S. (1971). *Rules for radicals.* New York: Random House.

Allen, J. C., & Dillman, D. A. (1994). *Against all odds: Rural community in the information age.* Boulder, CO: Westview Press.

Amick, B. C., Levine, S., Tarlov, A. R., & Walsh, D. C. (Eds.). (1995). *Health and society.* New York: Oxford University Press.

Aspen Institute. (1996). *Measuring community capacity: A workbook-in-progress for rural communities.* Washington, DC: Aspen Institute Rural Economic Development Policy Program.

Bellah, R. N., Madsen, R., Sullivan, W. M., Swidler, A., & Tipton, S. M. (1985). *Habits of the heart.* Berkeley: University of California Press.

Bellah, R. N., Madsen, R., Sullivan, W. M., Swidler, A., & Tipton, S. M (1991). *The good society.* New York: Knopf.

Berger, P. L., & Neuhaus, R. J. (1977). *To empower people: The role of mediating structures in public policy.* Washington, DC: American Enterprise Institute for Public Policy Research.

Biddle, W. W., & Biddle, L. J. (1965). *The community development process: The rediscovery of local initiative.* New York: Holt, Rinehart & Winston.

Blum, H. L. (1974). *Planning for health.* New York: Human Science Press.

Bronfenbrenner, U. (1986). Ecology of the family as a context for human development: Research perspectives. *Developmental Psychology, 22,* 723–754.

Brown, E. R. (1991). Community action for health promotion: A strategy to empower individuals and communities. *International Journal of Health Services, 21,* 441–456.

Butterfoss, F., Goodman, R., & Wandersman, A. (1996). Community coalitions for prevention and health promotion: Factors predicting satisfaction, participation and planning. *Health Education Quarterly, 23,* 65–79.

Chaskin, R. J., Brown, P., Venkatesh, S., & Vidal, A. (2001). *Building community capacity.* New York: Aldine de Gruyter.

Chavis, D. M. (1995). Building community capacity to prevent violence through coalitions and partnerships. *Journal of Health Care for the Poor and the Underserved, 6,* 234–265.

Chavis, D. M., Speer, P. W., Resnick, I., & Zippay, A. (1993). Building community capacity to address alcohol and drug abuse: Getting to the heart of the problem. In R. C. Davis, A. J. Lurigio, & D. P. Rosenbaum (Eds.), *Drugs and the community* (pp. 251–284). Springfield, IL: Thomas.

Chavis, D. M., & Wandersman, A. (1990). Sense of community in the urban environment: A catalyst for participation and community development. *American Journal of Community Psychology, 18,* 55.

Cottrell, L. (1976). The competent community. In B. Kaplan, R. Wilson, & A. Leighton (Eds.), *Further explorations in social psychiatry.* New York: Basic Books.

Easterling, D., Gallagher, K., Drisko, J., & Johnson, T. (1998a). *Promoting health by building community capacity: Evidence and implications for grantmakers.* Denver: Colorado Trust.

Easterling, D., Gallagher, K., Drisko, J., & Johnson, T. (1998b). *Promoting health by building community capacity: Summary.* Denver: Colorado Trust.

Elshtain, J. B. (1999). Symposium: Civil society and the American family—A call to civil society. *Society, 36,* 11–19.

Esman, M. J., & Uphoff, N. T. (1984). *Local organizations: Intermediaries in rural development.* Ithaca, NY: Cornell University Press.

Evans, R. G., & Stoddart, G. L. (1990). Producing health, consumer care. *Social Science and Medicine, 31,* 347.

Fawcett, S. B., Paine-Andrews, A., Francisco, V. T., Schultz, J. A., Richter, K. P., Lewis, R. K., Harris, K. J., Williams, E. L., Berkley, J. Y., Lopez, C. M., & Fisher, J. L. (1996). Empowering community health initiatives through evaluation. In D. M. Fetterman, S. J. Kaftarian, & A. Wandersman (Eds.), *Empowerment evaluation: Knowledge and tools for self-assessment and accountability.* Thousand Oaks, CA: Sage.

Felix-Burdine & Associates (2000). *Model of community capacity for health improvement.* Report submitted to the Robert Wood Johnson Foundation, Allentown, PA.

Florin, P., & Chavis, D. (1990). Community development and substance abuse prevention. In *Community development, community participation and substance abuse prevention.* Santa Clara, CA: Prevention Office, Bureau of Drug Abuse Services.

Freire, P. (1970). *Pedagogy of the oppressed.* New York: Seabury Press.

Freudenberg, N., Eng, E., Flay, B., Parcel, G., Rogers, T., & Wallerstein, N. (1995). Strengthening individuals and community capacity to prevent disease and promote health. In search of relevant theories and principles. *Health Education Quarterly, 22,* 290–306.

Fukuyama, F. (1995). *Trust: The social values and the creation of prosperity.* New York: Free Press.

Garkovich, L. E. (1989). Local organizations and leadership in community development. In J. A. Christenson & J. W. Robinson (Eds.), *Community development in perspective.* Ames: Iowa State University Press.

Goodman, R. M., Speers, M. A., McLeroy, K. L., Fawcett, S., Kegler, M., Parker, E., Smith, S., Sterling, I. T., & Wallerstein, N. (1998). An attempt to identify and define the dimensions of community capacity to provide a basis for measurement. *Health Education and Behavior, 25,* 258–278.

Granovetter, M. (1973). The strength of weak ties. *American Journal of Sociology, 78,* 1360–1379.

Green, L. W., Richard, L., & Potvin, L. (1996). Ecological foundations of health promotion. *American Journal of Health Promotion, 10,* 270–281.

Hancock, L., Sanson-Fisher, R., Redman, S., Burton, R., Burton, L., Butler, J., Girgis, A., Gibberd, R., Hensley, M., McClintock, A., Reid, A., Schofield, M., Tripodi, T., & Walsh, R. (1992). Community action for health promotion: A review of methods and outcomes. *American Journal of Preventive Medicine, 13,* 229–239.

Hancock, T. (2001). People, partnerships and human progress: Building community capital. *Health Promotion International, 16,* 275–280.

Harwood Group. (1996). *Public capital: The dynamic system that makes public life work.* Bethesda, MD: Harwood Group.

Hawe, P. (1994). Capturing the meaning of "community" in community intervention evaluation: Some contributions from community psychology. *Health Promotion International, 9,* 199–210.

Heller, K. (1990). Social and community intervention. *Annual Review of Psychology, 41,* 141–168.

Hillery, G. A. (1955). Definitions of community: Areas of agreement. *Rural Sociology, 20,* 111–123.

Human Resources Development Canada. (2000). *Community capacity building toolkit.* Her Majesty the Queen in Right of Canada. Human Resources Development Canada, New Brunswick Region. Available: www.participation.net/english/ccbgoc.htm.

Hunter, F. (1953). *Community power structure: A study of decision makers.* Chapel Hill: University of North Carolina Press.

Institute of Medicine. (1988). *The future of public health.* Washington, DC: National Academy Press.

Iscoe, I. (1974). Community psychology and the competent community. *American Psychologist, 29,* 607–613.

Israel, B. A. (1985). Social networks and social support: Implications for natural helper and community level interventions. *Health Education Quarterly, 12,* 65–80.

Israel, B. A., Checkoway, B., Schulz, A., & Zimmerman, M. (1994). Health education and community empowerment: Conceptualizing and measuring perceptions of individual, organizational, and community control. *Health Education Quarterly, 21,* 149–170.

Israel, B. A., Schultz, A. J., Parker, E. L., & Becker, A. B. (1998). Review of community-based research: Assessing partnership approaches to improve public health. *Annual Review of Public Health, 19,* 173–202.

Kawachi, I., Kennedy, B. P., & Glass, R. (1999). Social capital and self-rated health: A contextual analysis. *American Journal of Public Health, 89,* 1187–1193.

Kawachi, I., Kennedy, B. P., & Lochner, K. (1997). Long live community: Social capital as public health. *American Prospect, 35,* 56–59.

Kawachi, I., Kennedy, B. P., Lochner, K., & Prothrow-Stith, D. (1997). Social capital, income inequality, and mortality. *American Journal of Public Health, 87,* 1491–1498.

Kingsley, G. T., McNeely, J. B., & Gibson, J. O. (1997). *Community building: Coming of age.* Washington, DC: Development Training Institute and the Urban Institute.

Kretzmann, J., & McKnight, J. (1993). *Building communities from the inside out.* Evanston, IL: Center for Urban Affairs, Northwestern University.

Kumpfer, K. L., Turner, C., Hopkins, R., & Librett, J., (1993). Leadership and team effectiveness in community coalitions for the prevention of alcohol and other drug abuse. *Health Education Research, 8,* 359–374.

Labonte, R. (1997). Community, community development, and the forming of authentic partnerships. In M. Minkler (Ed.), *Community organizing and community building for health.* New Brunswick, NJ: Rutgers University Press.

Lett, J. (1990). Emics and etics: Notes on epistemology of anthropology. In T. N. Headland, K. L. Pike, & M. Harris (Eds.), *Emics and etics: The insider/outsider debate.* Thousand Oaks, CA: Sage.

MacArthur Foundation. (July 15, 2001). Building community capacity. Available: www.macfound.org/research/hcd/bcc.htm.

Mattessich, P., & Monsey, B. (1997). *Community building: What makes it work, a review of factors influencing successful community building.* St. Paul, MN: Amherst H. Wilder Foundation, Wilder Research Center.

McLeroy, K. R. (February 1996). *Community capacity: What is it? How do we measure it? And what is the role of the prevention centers and the CDC?* Paper presented at the Sixth Annual Prevention Centers Conference, National Centers for Disease Control and Prevention, National Center for Chronic Disease Control and Prevention, Atlanta.

McLeroy, K. R., Bibeau, D., Steckler, A., & Glanz, K. (1988). An ecological perspective on health promotion programs. *Health Education Quarterly, 15,* 351–377.

McLeroy, K. R., Kegler, M., Steckler, A., Burdine, J., & Wisotsky, M. (1994). Editorial: Community coalitions for health promotion: Summary and further reflections. *Health Education Research, 9,* 1–11.

McMillan, D. W., & Chavis, D. M. (1986). Sense of community: A definition and theory. *Journal of Community Psychology, 14,* 6–23.

Minkler, M., & Wallerstein, N. (1997). Improving health through community organization and community building: A health education perspective. In M. Minkler (Ed.), *Community organizing and community building.* Princeton, NJ: Princeton University Press.

National Civic League. (1992.) *The Civic Index: A new approach to improving community life.* Denver, CO: National Civic League Press.

National Civic League. (1999). *The Civic Index: Measuring your community's civic health.* Denver, CO: National Civic League.

Norris, T. (1993). *The healthy communities handbook.* Denver, CO: National Civic League.

O'Connell, B. (1999). *Civil society.* Hanover, NH: University Press of New England.

Patrick, D. L., & Wickizer, T. M. (1995). Community and Health. In B. C. Amick, S. Levine, A. R. Tarlov, & D. C. Walsh (Eds.), *Society and health.* New York: Oxford University Press.

Poole, D. L. (1997). Building community capacity to promote social and public health. *Health and Social Work, 22,* 163–170.

Popapchuk, W. R., Crocker, J. P., Schechter, W. H., and Boogaard, D. (1998). *Building community: Exploring the role of social capital and local government.* Washington, DC: National Civic League.

Presby, J. E., & Wandersman, A. (1985). An empirical exploration of a framework of organizational viability: Maintaining block organizations. *Journal of Applied Behavioral Science, 21,* 287–305.

Putnam, R. D. (1993). *Making democracy work: Civic traditions in modern Italy.* Princeton, NJ: Princeton University Press.

Putnam, R. D. (1995). Bowling alone: America's declining social capital. *Journal of Democracy, 6,* 65–78.

Putnam, R. D. (1996). The strange disappearance of civic America. *American Prospect, 24,* 34–48.

Putnam, R. D. (2000). *Bowling alone.* New York: Simon & Schuster.

Rappaport, J. (1981). In praise of paradox: A social policy of empowerment over prevention. *American Journal of Community Psychology, 9,* 1–25.

Reynolds, C. H., & Norman, R. V. (Eds.). (1988). *Community in America: The challenge of habits of the heart.* Berkeley: University of California Press.

Ricketts, T. (2001). *Community capacity for health: How can we measure it?* (Tech. Rep.). Research Triangle Park, NC: Research Triangle Institute.

Rose, G. (1992). *The strategy of preventive medicine.* New York: Oxford University Press.

Rosen, G. (1958). *A history of public health.* New York: MD Publications.

Saguaro Seminar. (2001). *The social capital community benchmark survey: Executive summary.* Cambridge, MA: John F. Kennedy School of Government, Harvard University. Available: www.cfsv.org/communitysurvey.

Sarason, S. B. (1974). *The psychological sense of community: Prospects for a community psychology.* San Francisco: Jossey-Bass.

Senge, P. (1994). *The fifth discipline fieldbook: Strategies and tools for building a learning organization.* New York: Doubleday.

Sirianni, C., & Friedland, L. (1995). Social capital and civic innovation: Learning and capacity building from the 1960s to the 1990s. *Civic Practices Network.* University of Wisconsin and Brandeis University. Available: http://cpn.journalism.wisc.edu/cpn.

Smedley, B. D., & Syme, S. L. (2001). Promoting health: Intervention strategies from social and behavioral research. *American Journal of Health Promotion, 15,* 149–166.

Smith, G. (1996). *Community-arianism.* London: UK Communities. Available: www.communities.org.uk/greg/gsum.html.

Steckler, A., Allegrante, J. P., Altman, D., Brown, R., Burdine, J. N., Goodman, R. M., & Jorgensen, C. (1995). Health education intervention strategies: Recommendations for future research. *Health Education Quarterly, 22,* 207–239.

Steckler, A. B., Dawson, L., Israel, B. A., & Eng, E. (1993). Community health development: An overview of the works of Guy W. Steuart. *Health Education Quarterly* (Suppl. 1), S3-S20.

Stokols, D. (1992). Establishing and maintaining healthy environments: Toward a social ecology of health promotion. *American Psychologist, 47,* 6–22.

Tarlov, A. (1992). The coming influence of a social sciences perspective on medical education. *Academic Medicine, 67,* 722.

Thompson, B., & Kinne, S. (1999). Social change theory: Applications to community health. In N. Bracht (Ed.), *Health promotion at the community level.* Thousand Oaks, CA: Sage.

Tocqueville, A. (2000). *Democracy in America.* (Harvey Mansfield, Trans.) Chicago: University of Chicago Press.

Turner, J. H., Beeghley, L., & Powers, C. H. (1998). *The emergence of sociological thought.* Belmont, CA: Wadsworth.

Uphoff, N. T. (1992). *Local institutions and participation for sustainable development.* London: International Institute for Environment and Development, Sustainable Agriculture Programme.

Warren, R. (1980). The good community revisited. *Social Development Issues, 4,* 18–40.

World Health Organization. (1984). *Health promotion: A discussion document on the concepts and principles.* Copenhagen, Denmark: WHO Regional Office for Europe.

CHAPTER NINE

SOCIAL CAPITAL THEORY

Implications for Community-Based Health Promotion

Marshall W. Kreuter
Nicole Lezin

Social capital is a term that is almost self-explanatory. People easily grasp its meaning and, more often than not, interpret it with a positive sentiment. It is closely linked to other social processes; some scholars consider it a subset of the theory of social cohesion (Berkman & Glass, 2000). At the same time, however, it is a complex concept that is difficult to pin down, much less measure with precision. Is social capital a sentimental extension of Alexis de Tocqueville's perception of American democracy, or might it represent a piece of a complex puzzle that, if seriously examined and prudently applied, would add to our understanding of community-based strategies? This chapter addresses that question by trying to unpack the complexities of social capital through a review of the knowledge that we have in hand, fully acknowledging that our current knowledge is partial. The discussion of social capital in this chapter is, for the most part, delimited by the connections between the notion of social capital and the process of community-based health promotion. Especially relevant is the distinction between bonding social capital and bridging social capital, because the latter is so closely tied to the interorganizational collaboration so essential to the basic tenets of "community-based" health promotion programs.

Community-Based Health Promotion: Key Principles

A number of aphorisms—for example, "Rich together, poor if separated" (from Laos), "One finger cannot lift a pebble" (from Iran), and "United we stand, divided we fall" (from the United States)—suggest that the idea of people and groups forming alliances and coalitions and the inherent value of such action is universal. In democratic societies, the notion of local community and local control offers a potent political and social symbol. It is this general sentiment that is at the heart of what Morone (1990) has termed the *democratic wish:* "the image of a single, united people, bound together by a consensus over the public good, which is discerned through direct citizen participation in community settings" (p. 7).

The principles of collaboration and participation are cornerstones for community health promotion strategies (Evans, Barer, & Marmor, 1994). The terms *community* and *community based* have particular appeal in public health, where they are virtual shorthand for a number of basic tenets. First, they highlight public health's emphasis on populations, as opposed to the medical care system's focus on individual health. Second, a community focus acknowledges that individual health behaviors are strongly influenced by the infrastructure, policies, and social norms that can affect health actions positively or negatively. More specifically, even a casual examination of the health issues addressed by the community-based approach (such as diabetes, breast cancer, violence, infant mortality, human immunodeficiency virus infection, teen smoking, and unplanned pregnancies) will reveal the connections between health problems and their social, economic, and historical determinants—employment, housing, culture, and education. The fact that these complex determinants tend to cluster by neighborhoods and communities is perhaps the strongest single justification for community-based public health strategies (Gerstein, Labelle, MacLeod et al., 1991; Green & Kreuter, 1999).

Programs That Work

In the literature, there is good news and not-so-good news about the effectiveness of community-based approaches. The good news is that in addition to its compelling philosophical and intuitive appeal, there are numerous published studies indicating that well-planned community-based programs do yield positive effects (Kreuter, 1993; Kotchen et al., 1986; Centers for Disease Control and Prevention, 1991; Puska et al., 1985; Vartiainen et al., 1986; Lando, Loken, Howard-Pitney, & Pechacek, 1990; Pierce, Macaskill, & Hill, 1990). Accounts of intervention strategies applied in these and other studies have strengthened our understanding of the theories, processes, and methods required to implement community-based health promotion programs that work. In this context, the phrase *programs that work* is preferable to the term *efficacy* because, as Fishbein (1996) points out, the latter implies a precise level of outcome that is often unrealistic for community-based interventions.

The not-so-good news is that the ratio of successful to not-so-successful programs is disappointing. For example, in their assessment of the effectiveness of community-based health promotion, Hancock et al. (1997) reported mixed and somewhat equivocal results. This was true even for some programs where it seemed apparent that appropriate standards for planning and implementation had been applied and funding was allotted for the intervention.

These findings were similar to those based on our analysis of approximately one hundred published articles describing the use of coalitions or collaborative approaches to attain either health or system change effects. Although there were clear examples that some programs did yield strong, positive outcomes, the ratio of those programs that achieved their target goals compared to those that did not was disappointing. This analysis led to three general conclusions: (1) planners, stakeholders, and funders tend to grossly underestimate the complexity, resources, and time required to carry out an effective community-based collaborative initiative; (2) stakeholders hold unrealistic expectations about what a collaboration can do; and (3) in the absence of a sound theoretical framework and logic model for evaluating community-based health promotion, program effects may be going undetected (Kreuter, Lezin, & Young, 2000).

One possible explanation for the third point most certainly lies in the complexity of measuring community-level effects. Academicians, grant makers, and practitioners have yet to reach consensus on what constitutes an appropriate and coherent methodology for assessing the impact and effectiveness of community-based health promotion strategies (Schwab & Syme, 1997). Unlike assessing the impact of specific vaccines, which are created in controlled, laboratory settings to act on predictable biological properties, community-based health promotion interventions strive to have an effect in a dynamic context where social, cultural, and political factors are controlled for or factored out. As Rootman, Goodstadt, Potvin, and Springett (1996) have said more directly, failure to take social and political context into account is a major barrier to the effective evaluation of community-based health promotion.

It seems reasonable to assume that at least some portion of what we interpret to be social and political context will be reflected by the extent to which a community's institutions get along with one another on matters of common interest to that community. The idea that the willingness and capacity to collaborate may mediate the effectiveness of a health promotion program is inherent in studies and commentaries on community competence (Clark & McLeroy, 1995), community readiness (Bowen, Kinne, & Urban, 1997; Eng & Parker 1994), empowerment (Wallerstein & Bernstein, 1994), and participatory research (Green et al., 1995). In reviewing two decades of their pioneering community-based cardiovascular disease prevention experience in Finland, Puska and his colleagues (1995) concluded that even programs employing the best methods and practices face substantial resistance in the absence of community participation and collaboration.

Cooperation and the factors that make it possible are key aspects, if not essential ingredients of, community health promotion. The concept of social capital suggests that collective actions requiring collaborative efforts are mediated by the presence or absence of trust, reciprocity, and cooperation. Might a better understanding of these factors and how to measure and influence them help public health researchers and practitioners enhance the effectiveness of community-based health promotion?

The Concept of Social Capital

James Coleman, Pierre Bourdieu, Alejandro Portes, Robert Putnam, and Francis Fukuyama are among the scholars most often cited as the principal theorists of social capital. A sampling of the definitions of social capital they have offered is presented in Table 9.1. Although the definitions differ in length and wording, the central themes that emerge from them are conceptually consistent and reveal the following dimensions of social capital:

It is defined by its function.

It is lodged neither in individuals nor in physical implements of production but instead is a property of the individual's set of relationships with others.

It facilitates certain actions of the individuals who are within the structure to pursue shared objectives.

It is expressed by networks, norms, and trust that enable participants to act together more effectively.

It is able to command scarce resources by virtue of membership in networks or broader social structures.

In summarizing their analysis of the definitions of social capital, Hawe and Shiell (2000) conclude that "social capital is not 'one thing.' It has relational, material, and political aspects and it may have positive or negative effects. It can refer to both dense and loose networks and it takes on the different form depending upon whether one is concerned with the individual and his or her immediate group membership or the interaction between social institutions" (p. 873).

In virtually all conceptualizations of social capital, trust and reciprocity emerge as especially salient components, or constructs. Coleman and Hoffer (1987) described the logic of social capital in terms of its potential to produce a

TABLE 9.1. DEFINITIONS OF SOCIAL CAPITAL.

Author	Definition
Bourdieu (1985)	"The aggregate of the actual or potential resources which are linked to possession of a durable network of more or less institutionalized relationships of mutual acquaintance or recognition."
Coleman (1990)	"Social capital is defined by its function. It is not a single entity, but a variety of different entities having two characteristics in common: They all consist of some aspect of social structure and they facilitate certain actions of the individuals who are within the structure. Like all forms of capital, social capital is productive, making possible the attainment of certain ends that would not be possible in its absence. Like physical and human capital, social capital is not completely fungible with respect to certain activities. A given form of social capital that is valuable in facilitating actions may be useless or even harmful for others. Unlike other forms of capital, social capital inheres in the structure of relations between persons and among persons. It is lodged neither in individuals nor in physical implements of production."
Portes (1995)	"The capacity of individuals to command scarce resources by virtue of their membership in networks, or broader social structures. . . . The ability to obtain [social capital] does not inhere in the individual . . . but instead is a property of the individual's set of relationships with others."
Putnam (1996)	"The features of social life—networks, norms, and trust—that enable participants to act together more effectively to pursue shared objectives. (Whether or not their shared objectives are praiseworthy is, of course, another matter.)"
Fukuyama (1999)	"A set of informal values or norms shared among members of a group that permits cooperation among them. If members of the group come to expect that others will behave reliably and honestly, then they will come to trust one another. Trust is like the lubricant that makes the running of any group more efficient."

stronger social fabric because it builds bonds based on trust. Trust nurtures solidarity between people, often as by-products of other activities. That logic is clearly reflected in Fukuyama's definition.

Reciprocity refers to the expectation of a return on one's investment—the faith that an action or good deed will be returned in some form in the future. According to Taylor (1982), reciprocity is "made up of a series of acts, each of which is short-run altruistic (benefitting others at a cost to the altruist), but which together typically make every participant better off" (pp. 28–29). Reciprocity has special relevance when it comes to the interactions and exchanges that must occur when multiple organizations are called on to collaborate and cooperate with one another around a common cause.

To illustrate how our understanding of an academic construct like trust has relevance to public health, consider a common situation. The selection and purchase of food is made easier when people trust the private and public institutions responsible for food safety. That trust will certainly influence opinions about and support for those institutions. However, that trust can be put into jeopardy as a result of outbreaks in foodborne diseases or when confidence in government erodes due to communication that is not timely or appears to be less than forthright, or both.

The Popularization of Social Capital

In the past decade, the concept of social capital has undergone a most interesting transition. In that time, it has emerged from occasional references in the academic literatures of the social and political sciences and economics to everyday language in the popular media; this has been a global phenomenon. In a view shared by several other scholars, Portes (1998) has expressed concern that this popularization has led some to assume that social capital is a cure-all for the problems of society and warns that we may be "approaching the point at which social capital comes to be applied to so many events and in so many different contexts as to lose any distinct meaning" (p. 2). We shall return to this cautionary note later in this section.

In the past decade, the concept of social capital has undergone a most interesting transition. In that time, it has emerged from occasional references in the academic literatures of the social and political sciences and economics to everyday language in the popular media; this has been a global phenomenon.

The catapulting of social capital from its somewhat obscure academic origins to much broader discussion was in large part triggered by the widespread interpretation of Putnam's research on the evolutionary patterns of local government in Italy (1993) and his related inquiry in the United States popularized by his book *Bowling Alone: The Collapse and Revival of the American Community* (2000). Both triggered considerable discussion and debate in the mainstream media.

Over two decades, Putnam studied the performance of regional governments in Italy and concluded that those regions demonstrating superior governance had more social capital (manifested by a public spiritedness among citizens), higher levels of civic participation, and the tendency to form collaborative, often nonpolitical associations. The phrase "bowling alone" was derived from Putnam's observation that although the number of individual bowlers in the United States rose by 10 percent between 1980 and 1993, league bowling ("bowling in groups") declined by 40 percent. The implication was that this trend in team bowling reflects a decline in the social camaraderie and civic conversations that were an inherent part of the bowling league experience. Putnam also offered a number of other measures to bolster his argument that the American public was losing the social bonds that fueled American civil society and its participatory democratic traditions. These include declines in voter turnout, church attendance, and membership in everything from unions to volunteer organizations, as well as declines in overall trust in government.

Putnam has suggested that the core elements of social capital—trust and cooperation—could be developed over time by repeated interaction of people involved in long-term relationships that are supported by community institutions. As such, those core elements are learned behaviors. Putnam's assertion that key elements of social capital are learned behaviors probably inspired hope that social capital could be created. According to Coleman, however, increases in social capital will not come easily. He pointed out that the property that distinguishes social capital from other forms of capital—a commitment to public good—may act as a barrier to its investment. Coleman reminds us that many individual actors (as either individuals or members of organizations) who make an investment in the betterment of the whole community capture personally only a small portion of the benefits. For some, the realization that benefits accrue to others in the community and not to them can lead to an *underinvestment* in social capital (Coleman, 1988). This kind of attitude might explain why taxes earmarked for school improvement may get voted down by those with little or no affiliation with children. In the parlance of social capital, paraphrasing Portes's definition, the investment (vote of support) is withheld because the voter in question is not part of the broader network. Because the voter is, in effect, an outsider, one cannot expect him or her either to trust or act on behalf of that broader network.

Scholars who study social capital generally agree that social capital increases when it is spent: the more one uses, the more one produces (Cox, 1995). In theory, social capital metaphorically functions much as wisely invested financial capital does: by generating further production.

Debates and Controversy

Putnam's principal thesis—that civic participation in America (based on macrolevel indicators) is in decline, and, as a result, its civic and political fabric is at risk—has triggered controversy and debate. Several critics have asserted that the macrolevel measures that Putnam used to illustrate his point, while symbolic, do not reflect a true picture of civic connections among Americans. Bowling alone instead of in a league, for example, does not necessarily imply that solitary bowlers are filling the bowling alleys. Instead, bowling continues to be a more informal social event—still in groups, but with bowling itself perhaps taking a backseat to general camaraderie.

Some critics have pointed out that most of the membership decline in organizations that Putnam cited were fixtures of an earlier time: 4-H Clubs, Knights of Columbus, American Legion, Shriners, and others. New civic activities have filled that void, including youth soccer and environmental groups like Adopt-a-Highway. Similarly, while participation in the Episcopal church declined by 26 percent between 1980 and 1995, the number of Pentecostals grew by 469 percent and Jehovah's Witnesses by 286 percent (Putnam, 2000b; Lemann, 1996).

Others have also protested that all memberships should not be counted equally. For example, trust and collaboration related to governance may be more likely (or more profound) by-products for organizations devoted to some type of community problem solving, such as substance abuse coalitions, rather than more social or recreational groups (Verba, Schlozman, & Brady, 1995). Furthermore, membership alone may not reflect the intensity of civic activity. For example, some individuals' church memberships may in fact reflect a high degree and variety of volunteerism through a variety of church-sponsored events, such as building houses through Habitat for Humanity, which are not reflected accurately in the single count of one individual's church affiliation.

These represent legitimate questions and concerns. Social capital theory remains in its formative stages. Researchers and practitioners interested in studying and applying social capital theory should keep these concerns in mind and maintain the perspective that although social capital is quite likely an important determinant of community group process, it is no panacea.

An Early Definition and a Caveat

Because it is easy to grasp the meaning of the words *social* and *capital,* together they create a concept that is intuitive. It is understandable that the origins of the term *social capital* have been difficult to pin down. One of the earliest documented applications of the term was found in *Community Center,* by L. J. Hanifan, published in 1920:

> In the use of the phrase "social capital" no reference here is made to the usual acceptation of the term "capital," except in a figurative sense. We refer not to real estate or to personal property or to cash, but rather to that in life which tends to make those tangible substances count for most in the lives of people: namely good will, fellowship, sympathy, and social intercourse among the individuals and family that make up a social unit. . . . The community as a whole will benefit by the cooperation of all of its parts, while the individual will find

in his [her] associations the advantages of help, the sympathy, and fellowship of his neighbors. First then, there must be an accumulation of community social capital [p. 130].

Although this early conceptualization is remarkably consistent with the definitions previously cited, elements of it enable us to explore an important conceptual caveat. Hanifan's use of phrases like "good will . . . fellowship . . . sympathy. . . community as a whole will benefit" implies that the effects of social capital are inherently good. Recall in Putnam's definition the parenthetical statement, "Whether or not their shared objectives are praise worthy is, of course, another matter." This caveat is universally shared by all contemporary scholars on the subject because it is evident that norms of trust and strong associational ties do not inherently produce social good. The antisocial consequences of terrorist groups are grounded in trust and networking. Fukuyama (1999) has pointed out that one may characterize the norms of the mafiosi as "take advantage of people outside of your immediate family at every occasion because otherwise they will take advantage of you first" (p. 17). Paradoxically, the reality that social capital can propel action for social good or social disruption adds validity to the assumption that it is a powerful social force. As such, public health researchers, planners, practitioners, and policy makers must ensure that its application is framed in the context of social benefit.

Researchers and practitioners interested in studying and applying social capital theory should keep these concerns in mind and maintain the perspective that although social capital is quite likely an important determinant of community group process, it is no panacea.

Simply stated, the constructs of social capital, depending on the context and intent, have the power to facilitate social benefits or wreak havoc. Recognizing the potential power of social capital, a reluctance to try to harness it for health improvement or other social good seems like an opportunity lost.

We have already highlighted Portes's concern that the popularization of social capital may lead to its becoming diluted by its application in different contexts. However, especially given the importance that context plays in the interpretation of social capital, we argue that its popularization and the attendant efforts to broaden its application are likely to have the opposite effect implied by Portes. Purposeful efforts to seek citizen participation can lead to a sharper delineation of the theory and provide a rich context for more robust tests of its practical application.

Elsewhere, using the principles and constructs of social capital prominently described in the literature, we crafted an operational definition that would be compatible with the goals of health promotion and the context of community: "Those specific processes among people and organizations, working collaboratively in an atmosphere of trust, that lead to accomplishing a goal of mutual social benefit" (Kreuter, Lezin, Koplan, & Young, 2001)

By specifying that the processes of social capital are intended to lead to a goal of mutual social benefit, the ambiguity of its intent is removed. Community-based health promotion has an unambiguous goal: health improvement. This gives rise to important empirical questions: Can social capital, at the community level, be measured? If it is measurable, is there any evidence that it mediates health conditions or health status? If it mediates health conditions or health status, is it amenable to change? The following literature review provides some basis for framing preliminary responses to those questions.

Health-Related Research Applications

Social support networks form the initial informal links among individuals that are a key ingredient of social capital. House et al. (1988) discussed powerful findings from prospective studies conducted during the 1980s indicating that measures of social support networks could predict mortality. Globally, studies indicate that social support networks, including marriage, family contacts, and group affiliations, can be linked to mortality after controlling for baseline differences in health status. Later studies refined the association between mortality and social support networks and have also explored its relationship to disease incidence. A 1996 study of more than thirty-two thousand men indicated that there is a strong association between social isolation and increased risk of certain types of mortality, specifically cardiovascular disease, unintentional injuries, and suicides. This study also linked social support networks to disease incidence, specifically stroke (Kawachi et al., 1996).

Kawachi and his colleagues conducted a nationwide study of social capital and state-level health outcomes using data on trust and group membership from the General Social Survey to assess levels of social capital in thirty-nine states (Kawachi, Kennedy, Lochner, & Prothrow-Smith, 1997). Findings revealed that levels of social trust and group membership were significantly associated with overall mortality, specifically, with deaths from coronary heart disease and malignant neoplasms, and with infant mortality. Regression analysis indicated that for a single standard deviation increase in trust, overall age-adjusted mortality would decrease by 67.1 individuals per 100,000, and for each incremental increase in group membership, mortality would decrease by 83.2 individuals per 100,000. These associations remained significant after controlling for state differences in income and poverty levels.

In a case control study of 667 at-risk children in four communities across the country, Runyan et al. (1998) measured social capital as an index of five factors:

presence of two parents or parent figures in the household, maternal caregiver's perception of social support, number of children in the household, neighborhood support, and regular church attendance by the family. When foster care placement, maternal depression, family income, maternal education, and site differences were controlled, data showed that adding a single social capital indicator to a child's situation increased the odds of "doing well" by 29 percent. Adding two indicators increased a child's odds of doing well by 66 percent.

In 343 Chicago neighborhoods, Sampson, Raudenbush, and Earls (1997) studied the relationship between collective efficacy, defined as "social cohesion among neighbors combined with their willingness to intervene on behalf of the common good," (p. 919) and levels of violent crime among juveniles. The study controlled for three variables generally assumed to be associated with high levels of violent crime: concentrated disadvantage (a composite variable that included age composition, income, and employment indicators, as well as a measure of single female–headed households), immigrant concentration, and residential stability. Results showed that high levels of "collective efficacy" were a significant predictor of lower levels of juvenile delinquency, crime victimization, and homicide rates (Sampson et al., 1997).

Higgins (1997) conducted a study to determine how individual perceptions of social capital were associated with selected actions taken by low-income, volunteer peer educators working in human immunodeficiency virus (HIV) prevention projects in Denver, Colorado, and New York City. She found that those with high social capital scores also had higher involvement in the community, were more likely to seek screening themselves, and had enlarged their social networks through participation in the project. The study findings also provided modest evidence that participation in a community-based intervention may itself have furthered or fostered social capital.

Project Northland was a communitywide demonstration research project designed to be conducted in multiple school districts in Minnesota. Perry et al. (1996) designed the project to determine whether active coordination of a theoretically sound school curriculum, parental involvement, and community task force support could have an impact on youth alcohol consumption. Differences between intervention and control districts after three years revealed that Project Northland was effective in reducing alcohol use. In an editorial independently critiquing Project Northland, Wechsler and Weitzman (1996) called specific attention to the role that social capital, manifested by patterns of trust, mutual obligation, and supportive informal and formal social networks, may have had on the project. They hypothesized

that it is the accrual and expenditure of social capital through sharing responsibility, resources, and roles to achieve reductions in youth substance use that will, in the end, achieve sustained reductions in the extent of use and the progression to abuse [p. 925].

This sampling of research studies reveals a rather consistent pattern in which the presence of high levels of social capital is associated with desirable public health objectives and outcomes.

Social Capital at Two Levels: Bonds and Bridges

Focusing on the role that social capital plays in influencing community change, Tempkin and Rohe (1998) found that it was a major predictor of neighborhood stability. Their study employed a model of neighborhood change that conceptualized two operational levels of social capital: sociocultural milieu and institutional infrastructure. They defined sociocultural milieu as the manifestation of residents' identity with the neighborhood and the degree of social interaction that neighbors have with one another. *Institutional infrastructure* refers primarily to the presence of neighborhood organizations (community-based organizations, CBOs) and the actual ability of those CBOs to act on behalf of the residents. Rohe and Tempkin also indicated that an essential ingredient of the institutional infrastructure concept was a strong commitment by those organizations to form alliances with influential sources outside the neighborhood: "The neighborhood must be able to leverage a strong sense of place into a collective movement that is able to form alliances with actors outside the community and influence decisions that affect the neighborhood's character over time" (p. 70).

These two operational levels of social capital cited are consistent with the distinction between bonding social capital and bridging social capital that Putnam (2000) described. Bonding social capital, similar to sociocultural milieu, is assumed to be a critical factor in creating and nurturing the kind of group solidarity that one sees in close neighborhoods and within ethnic enclaves. Bridging social capital, analogous to institutional infrastructure, is detected at the organizational level where norms, values, and social structures facilitate more macroconnections: the linking together of different organizational entities within a community around a common purpose and access to resources and assets outside the community. Putnam has observed that exhaustive descriptions of social networks in the United States do not yet exist, even at a single point in time, and he has found no reliable measures of social capital that neatly distinguish bridgingness and bondingness. He adds that these distinctions are relevant because they clearly imply that bridging and bonding social capital are *not* interchangeable concepts.

Two Midwestern Communities

Findings from a study by Kreuter et al. (1998) support Putnam's conclusion. The study was designed to determine the validity of different measures of social capital at the community level. The study sites were two small (population twenty thousand), demographically matched midwestern towns. The towns, referred to as Town A and Town B, differed in their levels of what the authors termed *prima facie social capital*. Prima facie social capital was established through a consensus process undertaken by state health department officials. The process involved a review of multiple communities within the state; judgments about levels of social capital were based on the past record of interorganizational collaboration and performance on health initiatives manifested over time in various communities. A summary consensus process yielded two pools of five communities each. One pool was judged to have high levels of social capital and the other low levels. Town A was selected from the pool judged to have high levels of social capital; Town B was selected from the other pool.

Social capital was independently assessed in the two communities using two complementary measurement strategies. One was a qualitative approach that employed the triangulation of structured interviews with thirty community leaders and stakeholders from each community, newspaper content analysis, and interviews with county extension agents. The other was a quantitative measure obtained from telephone surveys of a random sample of community residents from each of the two sites.

Results from the qualitative assessment revealed marked differences between the two communities in the same direction as the prima facie estimate. Town A was high in social capital, and Town B was low. Themes that emerged from the structured interviews revealed that organizational leaders in Town A described their town and the activities of their various organizations using collaborative examples and language much more so than their counterparts in Town B did.

An interesting manifestation of this pattern was found in the actions of churches. Churches and religious groups were referenced with positive regard in both towns. However, in Town A, there were repeated references and examples of interfaith collaboration through ministerial alliances—different denominations coming together to address a common community need or problem. Mentions of such collaboration in Town B's faith community were noticeably absent. Following are examples of comments from leaders in Town A:

"There isn't a church in town that would turn its back on those not in its congregation."

"We have twenty-four churches that support our program. We get about a thousand hours of volunteer work each month, and we get them from the Catholics, Baptists, and Methodists. They all work together very well."

And here are comments from leaders in Town B:

"Churches are mediocre to the general public, but okay to their parishioners."

"I think a lot of churches have strong youth programs, but churches don't work very well together."

"There is no central body that we can go to and say among the clergy, 'Here is something we can do together.' There has been a long history here of mistrust among the churches; I think that no one wants to resurrect that history of mistrust. This in not an indictment of history; it is an indictment of mistrust."

This pattern was consistent across all three dimensions of the qualitative measures of social capital. These parallel patterns, evident in Town A but not Town B, seemed to be associated with positive references to trust, the broad perception that collaboration was an expected mode of operation, and that service to everyone in the town was a community value.

In spite of this consistent pattern, the authors found that the estimated perceptions of social capital, based on the random telephone surveys, did not confirm the prima facie judgment. In fact, the survey results indicated that both Town A and Town B were relatively high in social capital.

Why the Difference?

The towns selected for this study were demographically matched, stable communities with rich cultural histories. Visitors to the two towns, frequenting local shops and restaurants, would discover the residents to be friendly, pleasant, and engaging; they would probably notice nothing unusual about either community. The telephone survey revealed that the residents of the two towns appeared to hold generally positive perceptions about their relationships and connections with one another as neighbors and acquaintances: bonding social capital was relatively high in both places.

One explanation for the stark difference between this finding and those expressed by the organizational leaders in the respective communities may lie in the contextual differences between the qualitative and quantitative methods used. Observations by Tourangeau and Rasinski (1988) provide added perspective on this issue. They note that when individuals are asked to respond to attitude questions using an attitude framework that they rarely access or that is not strongly formed, strong context effects and measurement error are introduced. Recall also that in the Sampson et al. (1997) study revealing the positive effects of high levels of collective efficacy, the measure of collective efficacy (social capital) was framed within the context of a specific dependent variable: youth violence.

Thus, it could be that the residents of the two towns responded to general questions about the constructs of social capital (trust, reciprocity, civic engagement) with little frame of reference to make decisions about the constructs being assessed. On the other hand, all three dimensions of the qualitative measures were in large part framed around the interactions of community organizations and their leaders in the context of their day-to-day operation and politics of the community.

A second possible explanation for the lack of association between the results of structured interviews with community leaders and those from the telephone survey is that organizational-level social capital and population social capital may be interdependent parts of a larger model of social capital. The differences that Kreuter et al. found led them to a model that offers a conceptualization of the role that bonding social capital may play in mediating the effects of community-based programs. That conceptualization is depicted in Figure 9.1. Several assumptions were made in constructing that model:

- The ultimate outcome (indicator of success) of community-based health promotion programs is health improvement: evidence of enhancements in health and quality of life.
- The presence of high levels of interorganizational trust and cooperation (bridging social capital) will enhance the probability that a community-based health promotion program will be successful.
- Bridging social capital between and among organizations will vary across communities.
- Although levels of bonding social capital will vary across communities, levels in this instance were high, consistent with the findings from the Kreuter et al. study.

The flow of the model follows the above assumptions in reverse. It begins with the notion that the level of a community's bonding social capital is positive, as was the case with Towns A and B. On the left side of the figure, the level of organizational trust and cooperation (bridging social capital) is high. Because the combination of positive bonding and bridging social capital nurtures community

FIGURE 9.1. BRIDGING SOCIAL CAPITAL: A MEDIATING FACTOR IN COMMUNITY PROGRAMS.

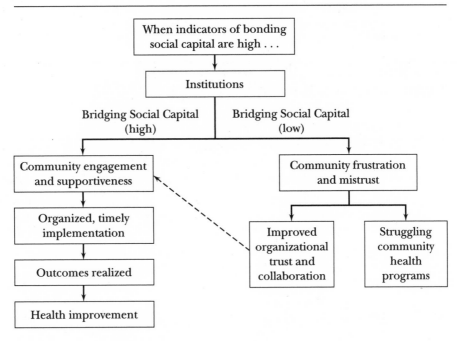

support and participation, timely implementation, achievement program objectives, and outcomes, the probability for program success is substantially increased.

The right side of the figure implies that where bridging social capital is weak; dissonance is created and is manifested by community frustration or mistrust. Communities capable of acknowledging the extent to which their bridging social capital reserves are low can undertake strategies to build or rebuild the trust needed to undertake cooperative efforts toward the goal of community health improvement. If successful, such communities would move to the left side of the model. If it remains unaddressed, this frustration can lead to programs that struggle, do not realize their hoped-for goals, and consequently do little to enhance quality of life in the community.

The dissonance just cited may be put into perspective by these observations by Tempkin and Rohe (1996) about the determinants of neighborhood stability in the face of potential negative external forces:

> A strong social fabric is a necessary, but not sufficient, condition for successful neighborhood defense. To successfully resist the forces of change, neighborhood

residents must be able to influence larger political, financial and other institutional actors whose decisions affect neighborhood stability or change. . . . Neighborhoods can collectively shape their futures, but they must do so in a complex social and uncertain political and economic environment [p. 166].

Bridging Social Capital: Implications for Community-Based Health Promotion

Globally, the majority of funding to support the application of community-based health promotion strategies continues to be tied to specific health problems: heart disease, asthma, tobacco, HIV and acquired immunodeficiency syndrome (AIDS), domestic violence, and so on. In virtually all instances, the funding protocols typically indicate that resources will be awarded for activities that are directly linked to the resolution of the health problem in question. However, those protocols frequently require some evidence that the intervention strategy includes the formation of a coalition or organizational partnership.

Paradoxically, however, the investment in the science and art of building community capacity remains a low priority for funding agencies. On the surface, it appears that the reluctance to invest in these more generic areas is tied to one or more of the following reasons: funding agencies either (1) believe that such allocations are inappropriate for categorical "health" funding, (2) are not aware of the existing evidence, or (3) are aware of the existing evidence but consider it weak. Hawe and Shiell (2000) reinforce the last point in this passage:

> The science of social capital is weak, by which we mean its empirical capacity to explain health patterning is relatively weak at present. The concept is too broad relative to more precise, alternative constructs. The distinctions between micro and macro levels of social capital are qualitatively different things. . . . Empirically, however, the distinction between the levels of social capital has not been adequately captured [p. 880].

To better understand both the potential benefits and limits of social capital as it relates to community-based health promotion, the most immediate challenge is one of measurement. Valid measurement of relevant levels or dimensions of social capital, clearly linked to the effective application of community-based public health programs, would give public, private, and philanthropic organizations the information they need to make more informed decisions about the most productive ways to contribute infusions of health-related funding to a given community—either to bolster the capacity that is requisite for successful interventions or to move directly to the interventions themselves.

Where Are We?

The following assumptions profile the current status of social capital in the context of community health promotion:

- Principles and theories, supported by evidence, suggest that collaboration and participation are essential and fundamental ingredients of community-based health promotion initiatives that seek to improve health.
- Although there is research evidence demonstrating that community-based health promotion initiatives yield positive benefits, the ratio of effective to not-so-effective examples is low.
- The low ratio of success is in part due to the fact that researchers, practitioners, and funding agencies have underestimated the complexity, time, and cost of activating collaborative networks.
- Theory, combined with growing empirical evidence, indicates that key constructs of social capital are likely to have a major influence on the way collaborative networks function.
- There appear to be valid macrolevel (national, state, provincial) measures of the principal constructs of social capital, and there is evidence that progress is being made on assessing those constructs at the community level.
- The ability to assess validly bridging (organizational) social capital at the community level could improve our understanding of the way community health promotion coalitions or networks function. Furthermore, the capacity to do such assessment may help explain some portion of the discrepancy between effective and not-so-effective community-based health promotion initiatives.

Bridging Social Capital: Recommended Next Steps

The first step in developing a valid assessment of bridging social capital is to stay focused. Recognizing that social capital is a large, complex theory, we believe that attention should be directed to that dimension of the theory that will enhance our knowledge of how social structures and connections: (1) facilitate the linking together of different organizational entities within a community around a common purpose and (2) access assets outside the community. We encourage delimiting the development of bridging social measures to the specific context of community health promotion strategies because (1) the goal of such strategies is to achieve a social benefit: health improvement, (2) the actions necessary for effective community-based health promotion parallel the constructs and conditions that foster bridging social capital, and (3) globally, community-based health promotion programs constitute a large cross-cultural reservoir of sites to examine the question at hand.

The second step would begin by reaching consensus on an operational definition of bridging social capital that clearly delineates its constructs. We offered a definition earlier in this chapter that could serve as a possible point of departure for this step. This would serve as the basis for the development of a conceptual logic model illustrating how the principal constructs of bridging social capital (for example, social structures and networks, history, norms and trust) interact to influence health improvement.

We encourage delimiting the development of bridging social measures to the specific context of community health promotion strategies.

A bridging social capital logic model will provide a basic frame of reference not only for the development and testing of tools and methods to measure the concept, but also for the eventual conceptualization and testing of strategies to develop and nurture it. This task will not require starting from scratch. An excellent point of departure would be to examine existing logic models for social capital, social networks, and community capacity. How might these models help advance our current thinking? Goodman (1996), in exploring ways to assess the capacity of communities to implement complex community-based programs, found it useful to identity different general domains for assessing community capacity. One of those domains, "rich social networks," was characterized by the following indicators:

- Reciprocal links throughout the community network
- Frequent supportive interactions
- The ability to form new associations
- Trust and cooperation
- More horizontal than vertical ties and relationships
- Cooperative decision-making processes
- The existence of similar network properties within and between organizations and groups

Berkman and Glass (2000) have created a multilevel conceptual model of social networks. The model is framed as a causal chain that starts with social-cultural conditions at the macrolevel, moves to social networks at the mezzolevel, and then moves on to social and interpersonal behaviors. As is the case with Goodman's conceptualization, operational constructs at the mezzolevel, and some at the macrolevel, seem to be in alignment with the notion of bonding social capital.

We strongly urge practitioners and policymakers not to view logic model conceptualizations like these as merely academic exercises. Not only do they help us see the salient parts of a complex system, but they also point out how these are connected to one another by time or space, or both. And by acknowledging that the parts are linked within a system, we are more likely to study and interpret each part in the context of that system. For the assessment of community coalitions, such a contextual or ecological analysis will be more appropriate and robust than the examination of the parts as independent or isolated variables. All of these concepts warrant serious consideration and bring us to yet another critical challenge: investing in the measurement of bridging social capital.

Measurement Resources

The references to the assessment of social capital, primarily through the specific measurement of its theoretical constructs, have been cited throughout this chapter. However, these references represent a very small sampling of social capital study and research. Globally, published descriptions of efforts to develop, revise, and apply various measures of social capital continue to grow exponentially. Thanks to computer and communications technology, most of that new knowledge is accessible on-line.

For example, through the support of the Danish Government and World Bank, Krishna and Shrader have published the Social Capital Assessment Tool (SCAT), which includes a set of tools and multiple methodologies intended to contribute to a uniform measurement methodology (www.worldbank.org/poverty/scapital/index.htm). The Social Capital Community Benchmark Survey describes the rationale and methods of a national survey of different dimensions of social capital of three thousand respondents in forty communities in the United States. The survey questionnaire is available in its entirety and asks questions about dimensions of social capital, including trust in government, political engagement, diversity of social networks, and religious participation (www.cfsv.org/communitysurvey). Under the leadership of Richard Rose, the Center for the Study of Public Policy at the University of Strathclyde in Glasgow, Scotland, has undertaken major projects to measure social capital in Russia and in Africa. Among numerous categories of survey items available through this resource are those that explicitly assess connections with, and perceptions of, community associations (www.socialcaptial.strath.ac.uk/).

Anne Spellerberg leads a team that has developed the Framework for the Measurement of Social Capital in New Zealand, with special emphasis on the inclusion of the Maori culture. Four well-defined structural components of social capital measurement are presented, with specific indicators spelled out for each. (To review this framework, see Paper 14 at the project's Web site: www.stats. govt.nz/domino/external/web/aboutsnz.nsf/htmldocs).

Finally, practitioners and researchers alike will find Wendy Stone's *Measuring Social Capital: Towards a Theoretically Informed Measurement Framework of Researching Social Capital in Family and Community Life* a thorough and readable treatment of the subject. It includes a well-documented measurement framework and a comprehensive sampling of measurement strategies, including sample questions (www.aifs. org.au/institute/pubs/stone.html).

The Inevitable Question: Can Social Capital Be Changed?

If valid measurement can show that social capital or some other aspect of community capacity is clearly linked to the effective application of community-based public health programs, those who provide funding would have valuable information to justify a reexamination of current policies. Specifically, public, private, and philanthropic funders would be able to make more informed decisions about the most productive ways to contribute infusions of health-related funding to a given community—either to bolster the capacity that is requisite for successful interventions or to move directly to the interventions themselves. Such progress would give rise to yet another challenge. Virtually all social capital research has examined the concept as an independent variable—that is, exploring the extent to which levels of social capital influence an outcome, as Kawachi and colleagues (1997) found with premature mortality, Sampson et al. (1997) found with youth-related violence, Perry et al. (1996) found with a school-based program, and Tempkin and Rohe (1998) found with community stability. However, improved measurements of social capital (including bridging social capital) would clear the way to a serious investigation of social capital as a dependent variable—that is, examining the extent to which specific actions themselves promote, enhance, or create social capital.

In the study of two midwestern communities cited earlier, Town A was assessed to have much higher levels of bridging social capital than its counterpart, Town B. Anticipating that leaders in Town B would want some recommendation as to how they might develop social capital in their community, we envisioned a strategy based on Stages of Change theory, sometimes referred to as the Transtheoretical Model (Prochaska & DiClemente, 1992).

In brief, the model suggests an alternative to psychological models that urge or expect dramatic behavior change in one fell swoop. Instead, it theorizes that individuals move through stages of behavior change in incremental steps, punctuated by relapse and struggle. Each stage is characterized by a distinctive cluster of features and tasks; once these are addressed and conquered, the individual proceeds to the next stage.

Movement through each stage is not a smooth, linear progression. Rather, it is characterized as a spiral, with significant false starts and relapse before a new plateau is achieved. Indeed, the anticipation of relapse and the view of relapse as an opportunity to learn how to sustain change in future attempts are distinctive features of the Stages of Change model.

When the model is applied to individuals—for example, to individuals who smoke—the stages are defined as follows:

• *Precontemplation.* This first stage is akin to a form of denial; the individual genuinely does not perceive a problem or has established significant defense mechanisms to convince himself or herself that any problems associated with the behavior do not apply to his or her situation—for example, "I don't really smoke or drink that much, so I'm not going to experience those adverse health effects later in life."

• *Contemplation.* The individual is more open to discussion and a more realistic assessment, yet still feels unable to confront the problem or seriously consider changing the behavior—for example, "I know I really should think about quitting smoking, but I can't deal with it right now."

• *Preparation.* The individual moves away from contemplation and toward the next stage, action. During the preparation stage, the individual is actively gathering information and support for a near-term change in the behavior, recognizing that more than one attempt may be required. For example, a smoker might enlist a doctor's help, inform friends and family members of the intent to quit smoking, or even try to cut back on daily cigarette consumption.

• *Action.* This stage marks a clear change in behavior—again, an attempt that may have to be repeated, but one that clearly represents a break from the past. For a smoker, this would be akin to setting a quit date, wearing a nicotine patch, or making the decision to stop smoking cigarettes from that point forward.

• *Maintenance.* As the name implies, this is a stage of constant vigilance to avoid relapse. If relapse occurs, the model suggests that individuals learn from their relapse and repeat the preparation and action stages until they achieve longer and longer maintenance stages.

In this model, success is never fully ensured, because ingrained behaviors are so difficult to change. However, throughout the process, the pros or benefits of behavior changes gradually tip the scales, outweighing the cons or negative effects that loomed large earlier in the change process.

Social capital theory and constructs, especially as they were applied in the study of Town A and Town B, seemed to suggest that a process not unlike stages of change might serve as a framework to pursue actions intended to enhance levels of social capital. For example, Town A could be described accurately as a place that has, through a combination of good fortune and conscious choice, arrived at a maintenance stage that many other towns across the country would envy. Levels of trust, collaboration, voluntary activity, and civic engagement are high. Residents are proud of their town and of the collaborative spirit that is represented in various centers, buildings, and projects that benefit the town as a whole. People miss Town A when they leave it, and they often return.

Town B, on the other hand, is characterized by mistrust, cynicism, and a sense that opportunities have been lost. Some residents want things to be different and believe there is some hope for change, but the sentiment is one of cautious hope or wariness. Few residents or leaders are willing to risk new types of collaboration, for fear of being taken advantage of or of being tainted by a failed effort.

In terms of the Stages of Change model, if Town B wanted to become more like Town A, the following stages might apply:

- *Precontemplation.* With some exceptions, many residents of Town B could be described as precontemplators. They believe that Town B has always had strife and conflict and probably always will. Previous attempts to change the town's economic profile have failed or led to divisiveness among residents.

- *Contemplation.* A first step out of precontemplation would involve open discussion of problems, perhaps led by local news organizations, that sought to define reality in a balanced way, avoiding the blame and recrimination that seem to characterize many accounts of past events in Town B. It would be very important to highlight the town's many assets in such a discussion and not to dwell on only the negative legacy. In short, the leadership task would be to define and address the realities of Town B.

- *Preparation.* To prepare for future action and sustained change, key groups within the town should be identified to help find middle ground and move toward greater inclusiveness. Community forums could be convened in which information from the previous stage is discussed and used to create a positive, meaningful vision of Town B's future. Specific tasks might include learning how to agree to disagree in communitywide forums and keeping each other mindful of avoiding personal attacks and blame for things that go wrong. The goal of this stage would be to agree to try new collaborative efforts, realizing that they may be difficult and painful at first.

- *Action.* Collaborative efforts, however flawed or hesitant, are launched. The goals would be to create stronger norms for valuing collaboration. Individuals and organizations would specifically be asked (and be willing) to give up turf and act in good faith regarding the motives of others. As a result, social capital markers such as volunteerism, levels of trust, and civic engagement would increase over time.

• *Maintenance.* Town B's residents would now acknowledge the benefits of a more collaborative, trusting approach. Over time, peer pressure to maintain collaborative approaches would emerge as a reinforcement of collaborative behavior and as a disincentive for those who relapse into negative, personal attacks. As collaboration becomes the norm, there will be more and more examples of success, leading to more individuals and organizations willing to take the risk of collaborating with others for the collective good of the town.

As Figure 9.1 indicates, the route to a better quality of life will be most direct when perceptions of social capital at the population level are positive and community infrastructure is collaborative. Also, the model implies that when such enhancement occurs, it is a manifestation of what Putnam refers to as the civil society. However, the model also indicates that when population perceptions of social capital are less positive or community infrastructure is less collaborative, positive outcomes are still possible—through strategies designed to correct shortcomings in institutional infrastructure or to directly address and resolve community frustration.

Conclusion

The call for measuring social capital must not be mistaken for the siren of scientific reductionism. Attempts to reduce human behavior, individual or collective, are inherently futile. There are many ways to gain meaningful and valid insight into social actions that we do or do not choose to take. Although a commitment to valid, precise measurement should be paramount, care must be taken not to lose sight of the reality that there are many ways to study the meaning and influence of social capital. Philosopher Ken Wilber (1998) and health educator Lawrence Green (Green & Kreuter, 1999) both confirm what common sense tells us: that there are different ways of knowing and different interpretations of reality. Participatory research in public health has taught us that an epidemiologist, an anthropologist, a health educator, and a layperson are likely to view the same problem through different lenses. More important, each is quite likely to detect a glimpse of reality that the others may miss. All who have a stake in uncovering insights about social capital (practitioners; epidemiologists; social, behavioral, economic, and political scientists; and certainly those they seek to serve) need to explore seriously how their various views of reality can be combined to give us new knowledge.

References

Berkman, L. F., & Glass, T. (2000). Social integration, social networks, social support and health. In L. F. Berkman & I. Kawachi (Eds.), *Social epidemiology.* New York: Oxford University Press.

Bourdieu, P. (1985). The forms of capital. In J. G. Richardson (Ed.), *Handbook of theory and research for the sociology of education* (pp. 241–250). Westport, CT: Greenwood Press.

Bowen, D. J., Kinne, S., & Urban, N. (1997). Analyzing communities for readiness to change. *American Journal of Health Behavior, 21,* 289–298.

Centers for Disease Control and Prevention. (1991). Increasing breast cancer screening among the medically underserved, Dade County, FL. *MMWR, 40,* 261–263.

Coleman, J. S., & Hoffer, T. (1987). *Public and private high schools: The impact of communities.* New York: Basic Books.

Coleman, J. S. (1988). Social capital in the creation of human capital. *American Journal of Sociology, 94* (Suppl.), 95–120.

Coleman, J. S. (1990). *Foundations of social theory.* Cambridge, MA: Harvard University Press.

Cox, E. (1995). *A truly civil society.* Sydney, Australia: Australian Broadcasting Company Books.

Clark, N., & McLeroy, R. (Eds.). (1995). Creating capacity: A research agenda for public education. (1995, August). *Health Education Quarterly, 22.*

Eng, E., & Parker, E. (1994). Measuring community competence in the Mississippi Delta: The interface between program evaluation and empowerment. *Health Education Quarterly, 21,* 199–220.

Evans, R. G., Barer, M. L., & Marmor, T. R. (1994). *Why are some people healthy and others, not? The determinants of health in populations.* Hawthorne, NY: Aldine de Gruyter.

Fishbein, M. (1996). Great expectations, or do we ask too much from community-level interventions? *American Journal of Public Health, 86,* 1075- 1076.

Fukuyama, F. (1999). *The great disruption: Human nature and the reconstruction of social order.* New York: Free Press.

Gerstein, R., Labelle, J., MacLeod, S., Mustard, F., Spasoff, T., & Watson, J. (May 1991). *Nurturing health: A framework on the determinants of health.* Toronto, ON: Premier's Council on Health Strategy.

Goodman, R. (1996). *Measuring and nurturing community capacity in health promotion programs,* Paper presented at the 1996 Mid-Year Society for Public Health Education (SOPHE) Meeting, Westchester, PA.

Green, L. W., George, M. A., Daniel, M., Frankish, C. J., Herbert, C. U., Bowre, W. R., & O'Neil, M. (1995). *Study of participatory research in health promotion: Review and recommendations for the development of participatory research in health promotion in Canada.* British Columbia: Institute of Health Promotion Research–University of British Columbia and the British Columbia Consortium for Health Promotion Research, Royal Society of Canada.

Green, L. W., & Kreuter, M. W. (1999). *Health promotion planning: An educational and ecological approach* (3rd ed.). Mountain View, CA: Mayfield.

Hancock, L., Sanson-Fisher, R., Redman, S., Burton, R., Burton, L., Butler, J., Girgis, A., Gibberd, R., Hensley, M., McClintock, A., Reid, A., Schofield, M., Tripod, T., & Walsh, R. (1997). Community action for health promotion: A review of methods and outcomes. *American Journal of Preventive Medicine, 13,* 229–239; and the COMMIT Research

Group. Community Intervention Trial for Smoking Cessation (COMMIT): II Changes in Adult Cigarette Smoking prevalence. *American Journal of Public Health, 85,* 183–192.

Hanifan, L. J. (1916). The Rural School Center. *Annals of the American Academy of Political and Social Science, 67,* 130–138..

Hanifan, L. J. (1920). *The community center.* Boston: Silver, Burdett.

Hawe, P., & Shiell A. (2000). Social capital and health promotion: A review. *Social Science and Medicine, 51,* 871–885)

Higgins, D. L. (1997). *Social capital and HIV intervention.* Unpublished Doctor of Philosophy thesis, University of Nottingham.

House, J. S., Landis, K. R., & Umberson, D. (1988). Social relationships and health. *Science, 241,* 540–545.

Kawachi, I., Colditz, G., Ascherio, A., Rimm, E., & Giovannucci, E. (1996). A prospective study of social networks in relation to total mortality and cardiovascular disease in men in the USA. *Journal of Epidemiology and Community Health, 50,* 245–251.

Kawachi, I., Kennedy, B. P., Lochner, K., & Prothrow-Smith, D. (1997). Income inequality, social capital and mortality. *American Journal of Public Health, 87,* 1491–1498.

Kotchen, J. M., McKean, H. E., Jackson-Thayer, S., Moore, R. W., Straus, R., Kotchen, T. (1986). The impact of a rural high blood pressure control program on hypertension control and CVD mortality. *JAMA, 255*(16), 2177–2182.

Kreuter, M. W. (1993). Human behavior and cancer: Forget the magic bullet! *Cancer, 72,* 996–1001.

Kreuter, M. W., Lezin, N. A., Koplan, A. N., & Young, L. A. (2001). Social capital: Evaluation implications for community health promotion. In I. Rootman, M. Goodstadt, D. McQueen, L. Potvin, J. Springett, & Ziglio (Eds.), *Evaluation in health promotion: Principles and perspectives.* Copenhagen: European Regional Office of the World Health Organization.

Kreuter, M., Lezin, N. L., & Young, L. (2000, January). Evaluating community-based mechanisms: Implications for practitioners. *Health Promotion Practice, 1,* 49–63.

Lando, H. A., Loken, B., Howard-Pitney, B., & Pechacek, T. (1990). Community impact of a localized smoking cessation contest. *American Journal of Public Health, 80,* 601–603.

Lemann, N. (1996). Kicking in groups. *Atlantic Monthly, 27,* 22–26.

Morone, J. A. (1990). *The democratic wish: Popular participation and the limits of American government.* New York: Basic Books.

Perry, C. L., Williams, C. L., Veblen-Mortenson, S., Toomey, T. L., Komro, K. A., Anstine, P. S., McGovern, P. G., Finnegan, J. R., Forster, J. L., Wagenaar, A. C., & Wolfson, M. (1996). Project Northland: Outcomes of a community-wide alcohol use prevention program during early adolescence. *American Journal of Public Health, 86,* 956–965.

Pierce, J. P., Macaskill, P., & Hill, A. (1990). Long-term effectiveness of mass media led antismoking campaigns in Australia. *American Journal of Public Health, 80,* 565–569.

Portes, A. (1995). Economic sociology and the sociology of immigration: A conceptual overview. In A. Portes (Ed.), *Economic sociology of immigration: Essays on networks, ethnicity, and entrepreneurship.* New York: Russell Sage Foundation.

Portes, A. (1998). Social capital: Its origins and applications in modern sociology, *Annual Review of Sociology, 24,* 1–24.

Prochaska, J., & DiClemente, C. (1992). Stages of change in the modification of problem behaviors. *Progress in Behavior Modification, 28,* 183–218.

Puska, P., Nissinen, A., Tuomilehto, J., Salonen, J., Koskela, K., McAlister, A.., Koltke, T., Maccoby, N., & Farquhar, J. (1985). The community-based strategy to prevent coronary heart disease: Conclusions from the Ten Years of the North Karelia Project. *Annual Review of Public Health, 6,* 147–193.

Puska, P., Tuomilehto, J., Nissinen, A., & Vartianen, E. (1995). *The North Karelia Project: Twenty years results and experiences.* Helsinki, Finland: National Public Health Institute (KTL) Finland and WHO Regional Office for Europe and the North Karelia Project Research Foundation.

Putnam, R. D. (1993). *Making democracy work: Civic traditions in modern Italy.* Princeton, NJ: Princeton University Press.

Putnam, R. D. (1996, Winter). The strange disappearance of civic America. *American Prospect, 7*(24).

Putnam, R. D. (2000a). *Bowling alone: The collapse and revival of American community.* New York: Simon & Schuster.

Putnam, W. G. (2000b, July 17). *American Prospect,* 34–37.

Rootman, I., Goodstadt, M., Potvin, L., & Springett, J. (1996). A framework for health promotion evaluation. In I. Rootman, M. Goodstadt, D. McQueen, L. Potvin, J. Springett, & Ziglio, E. (Eds.), *Evaluation in health promotion: Principles and perspectives.* Copenhagen: European Regional Office of the World Health Organization.

Runyan, D. K., Hunter, W., Socolar, R., Amaya-Jackson, L., English, D., Landsverk, J., Dubowitzit, Browne, D., Bangdiwala, S., & Mathew, R. (1998). Children who prosper in unfavorable environments: The relationship to social capital. *Pediatrics, 101,* 12–18.

Sampson, R. J., Raudenbush, S. W., & Earls, F. (1997). Neighborhoods and violent crime: A multilevel study of collective efficacy. *Science, 277,* 918–924.

Schwab, M., & Syme, S. L. (1997). On paradigms, community participation, and the future of public health. *American Journal of Public Health, 87,* 2050.

Taylor, M. (1982). *Community, anarchy, and community.* Cambridge: Cambridge University Press.

Tempkin, K., & Rohe, W. (1996). Neighborhood change and urban policy. *Journal of Planning Education and Research, 15,* 159–170.

Tempkin, K., & Rohe, W. (1998). Social capital and neighborhood stability: An empirical investigation. *Housing Policy Debate, 9,* 61–68.

Tourangeau, R., & Raisinski, K. A. (1988). Cognitive processes underlying context effects in attitude measurement. *Psychological Bulletin, 103,* 299–314.

Vartiainen, E., Puska, P., Tossavainen, K., Viri, L., Niskanen, E., Moisio, S., McAlishr, A., & Pallonen, U. (1986). Prevention of non-communicable diseases: Risk Factors in Youth— the North Karelia youth project (1984–1988). *Health Promotion, 1,* 269–283.

Verba, S., Schlozman, K. L., & Brady, H. (1995). *Voice and equality: Civic voluntarism in American politics.* Cambridge, MA: Harvard University Press.

Wallerstein, N., & Berstein, E. (1994). Introduction to community empowerment, participatory education and health. *Health Education Quarterly, 21,* 141–148.

Wechsler, H., & Weitzman, E. R. (1996). Editorial: Community solutions to community problems: Preventing adolescent alcohol abuse. *American Journal of Public Health, 86,* 923–925.

Wilber, K. (1998). *Marriage of sense and soul: Integrating science and religion.* New York: Random House.

Winkelstein, W. (1996). Editorial: Eras, paradigms and the future of epidemiology. *American Journal of Public Health, 86,* 621–622.

CHAPTER TEN

PREVENTION MARKETING

An Emerging Integrated Framework

May G. Kennedy
Richard A. Crosby

H ealth behavior is subject to numerous influences, which can be organized conceptually into a multilevel system. The system would include health influences at the individual and interpersonal levels, as well as higher-order influences such as those at the organizational, community, and cultural levels. Limiting a theoretical framework to one level of influence may be convenient from a research perspective, but several emerging theoretical frameworks suggest that health behavior intervention programs should integrate multiple levels of influence (McLeroy, Bibeau, Steckler, & Glanz, 1988; Sallis & Owen, 1997). The research challenges inherent in the use of an integrated multilevel framework are offset by its potential to provide an adequate conceptual map of a complicated health problem (Reppucci, Mulvey, & Kastner, 1983). Using such a map to design a preventive intervention makes it more likely that the intervention will result in widespread and long-lasting health behavior change.

Prevention marketing is one example of an integrated multilevel approach to achieving communitywide change in health-relevant behavior. This approach employs principles from three disciplines that focus on various levels of the system of health influences: behavioral science, social marketing, and community development. Developed in the mid-1990s, prevention marketing guided several

We gratefully acknowledge the comments of Yuko Mizuno, Lydia Ogden, and Ann O'Leary on previous drafts of this chapter.

federal human immunodeficiency virus (HIV) prevention activities that targeted American youth (Ogden, Shepherd, & Smith, 1996).

This chapter examines prevention marketing in depth, beginning with a presentation of the key elements of the framework and some thoughts about its development. Throughout this chapter, we use three similar terms: prevention marketing, a theoretical framework; the Prevention Marketing Initiative, a national HIV prevention campaign; and the Prevention Marketing Initiative (PMI) Demonstration Project, a five-site project.

Key Elements of Prevention Marketing

Prevention marketing was conceived as the integration of three distinct fields (behavioral science, social marketing, and community development) that have been applied to public health problems in the past. As Figure 10.1 shows, each of these three fields has the ability to reach an audience and, perhaps, to have a somewhat independent and additive impact on the audience.

Prevention marketing was conceived as the integration of three distinct fields (behavioral science, social marketing, and community development) that have been applied to public health problems in the past.

The central premise of prevention marketing is that widespread behavior change can result from a particular strategic program planning and implementation process undertaken by (or in concert with) community representatives. The steps in the planning process, shown in Figure 10.2,

FIGURE 10.1. COMPONENTS OF THE PREVENTION MARKETING FRAMEWORK.

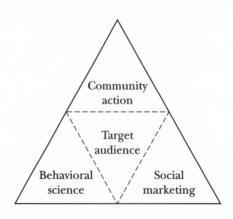

encompass social marketing and behavioral science practices that will be described in greater detail later in this chapter. In brief, these practices are defining the problem, conducting a needs assessment and audience research, segmenting audiences and tailoring activities on the basis of the audience research, and refining activities over time on the basis of additional feedback from the target audience.

Behavioral Science

Behavioral science is a term used in medicine and public health to describe methods of inquiry within several scientific disciplines (for example, psychology, sociology, and anthropology). Behavioral scientists ask questions about who is doing what, with whom, where, when, how, and how often. Why people behave as they do and how that behavior can be modified are central questions of behavioral science. Behavioral science theories try to explain what makes a particular behavior more or less likely. These theories maintain that behavior is determined largely by what people know; their skills, beliefs, and attitudes; and their social, cultural, and environmental circumstances. The Theory of Reasoned Action (TRA; Ajzen & Fishbein, 1980), the Health Belief Model (Becker, 1974), the Acquired Immuno-deficiency Syndrome (AIDS) Risk-Reduction Model (Catania, Coates, & Kegeles, 1994), Social Cognitive Theory (Bandura, 1986), Diffusion Theory (Rogers, 1995), the Transtheoretical Model (Prochaska & DiClemente, 1992), and Social Influence Theory (see Fisher, 1988) have been particularly influential in HIV prevention. Increasingly, HIV prevention efforts are being informed by behavioral and social science theories that go beyond analyzing the behavior of individuals to

FIGURE 10.2. STEPS IN THE
PREVENTION MARKETING PLANNING PROCESS.

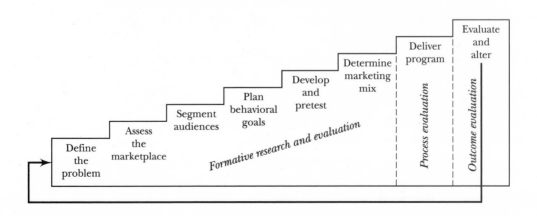

examine cultural and social factors that affect health behaviors (Lewis, 1993; Minkler & Wallerstein, 1997; Pasik, 1997; Roter & Hall, 1997; Wingood & DiClemente, 2000).

Studies have validated explanations of health behavior offered by behavioral science theories. For example, variables that are considered behavioral predictors in the Theory of Reasoned Action have been shown to predict a diverse group of health-relevant behaviors—for example, marijuana smoking, cigarette smoking, mammography, vaccination, oral contraceptive use, and condom use (Ajzen & Fishbein, 1980; Ajzen, 1988; Brown, DiClemente, & Park, 1992; Montano, Kasprzyk, & Taplin, 1997; Montano & Taplin, 1991; Montano, 1986; Weinstein, Lyon, Sandman, & Cuite, 1998). Similarly, the Health Belief Model has been successful in predicting behavior (Armstrong, Berlin, Schwartz, Propert, & Ubel, 2001; Liau & Zimet, 2000; Strecher & Rosenstock, 1997), as have Social Cognitive Theory (Baranowski, Perry, & Parcel, 1997; St. Lawrence et al., 1995), Diffusion Theory (Oldenburg, Hardcastle, & Kok, 1997), and other models.

Theoretical constructs from behavioral science have also been useful as outcome variables in intervention research. Theoretical intermediate outcome variables can be particularly valuable when behavior is constrained by external circumstances. For example, adolescents tend to have sporadic opportunities to have sex (Hofferth & Hayes, 1987). Their behavioral intentions are not constrained in the same way, and a postintervention change in intentions can be used to show that a preventive intervention had a positive effect.

Programs that have been shown to be effective in preventing HIV risk behavior (Centers for Disease Control and Prevention, 1999a) are usually based in (or are at least consistent with) behavioral science theory. Furthermore, the documentation of the success of these interventions has relied on the arsenal of behavioral science research methods. Research designs, measurement tools, strategies for collecting and summarizing data, analytic and modeling procedures, and other research methods from the behavioral and social sciences have been applied to HIV prevention (Kalichman, 1998), as well as to other public health problems.

Social Marketing

Social marketing is the application of commercial marketing principles and techniques to the achievement of socially beneficial goals (Kotler & Zaltman, 1971). Not a theory per se, social marketing is consistent with Economic Exchange Theory (Lefebre & Rochlin, 1997). Social marketing techniques have been used to persuade people to adopt effective family planning methods, employ sound nutritional practices, become literate, immunize infants, and educate daughters, among other worthy ends (Andreasen, 1995). Detailed definitions of social marketing generally describe either the components of social marketing programs or the stages or strategic decision points in the social marketing process. Integrating these two types of descriptions, social marketing can be thought of as a multistage strategic planning and implementation process that typically has five steps:

1. Conducting formative audience research
2. Using the research results to divide the target audience into segments with similar characteristics and tailoring messages to appeal to each segment
3. Identifying the costs and benefits of the product or behavior from the consumer's point of view and then designing messages that minimize the costs and promote the benefits to create the perception of a beneficial exchange
4. Employing a 4 P's analysis of campaign plans by considering the attractiveness of the offering or *product,* the affordability and perceived reasonableness of its *price* or nonmonetary costs, the convenience with which it can be accessed or its *placement,* and the best channels and messages to use in its *promotion* to the target audience
5. Revising campaign offerings based on ongoing consumer feedback

Social marketing "products" may be behaviors, such as condom use, or determinants of behaviors, such as more favorable attitudes toward condom use. Both kinds of products can be promoted at different points in the life span of a single social marketing project. Initial campaigns might promote an antecedent to a behavior—something that is logically or theoretically required before the ultimate project goal can be addressed successfully. Subsequent campaigns would promote action made possible by the success of the first campaign. For example, in some traditional societies, convincing husbands to allow their wives to visit a health clinic may be necessary before a campaign promoting the adoption of family planning methods could persuade the wives to seek reproductive health care.

Social marketing relies on feedback from members of the target audience, or "consumers," to guide product development and promotion, but in the past, the mechanics of campaign planning have remained largely in the hands of experts (Smith, 2000). For example, Project Action, a condom social marketing campaign in Portland, Oregon, that emphasized community support (Blair, 1995), was essentially an expert-driven endeavor that called on the community for background information, endorsement, or cooperation. Prevention marketing is a departure from this top-down process.

Community Development

The prevention marketing framework stipulates community action, which often requires community organization (Minkler & Wallerstein, 1997). Community organization involves conflictual or consensual interventions at the community level that influence community institutions and solve community problems (Alinsky, 1971; Braithwaite, Bianchi, & Taylor, 1994; Cox, Erlich, Rothman, & Tropman, 1970). One form of community organization, community development, is a consensus-building strategy that has been mandated by numerous federal agencies and several foundations since the end of World War II (Wandersman, 1984).

Clinard (1970, p. 126) identified the components of community development:

- Creation of a sense of social cohesion and strengthening of group interrelationships
- Encouragement and stimulation of self-help
- Reliance on persuasion rather than compulsion to produce change through the efforts of local people
- Identification and development of local leadership
- Development of civic consciousness and acceptance of civic responsibility
- Use of professional and technical assistance to support local efforts
- Coordination of local services to meet local needs and problems
- Provision of training in democratic procedures that may result in decentralization of some government functions

In public health areas ranging from drug abuse to cardiovascular disease, community development has often meant organizing local coalitions or collaborative bodies to identify and clarify problems and make plans to ameliorate them (Kaftarian & Hansen, 1994; Fawcett et al., 1995). This approach is resonant with democratic ideals, but it has generated few documented cases of success in changing health systems or health status (Kreuter & Lezin, 1998). Collaboration has been hampered by such factors as a legacy of mistrust, poor leadership, and conflicts of interest. Even when the collaborative process has run smoothly, events beyond the control of the coalition (for example, an economic recession) have blocked success. Furthermore, it is possible that some of the coalition-based, community-level interventions were successful but their success could not be detected. Confounding events that occur in the comparison or control areas, small sample sizes at the community level of analysis, and small effect sizes at the individual level of analysis make measuring the effects of community-level interventions highly problematic (Fishbein, 1996) but not impossible (Centers for Disease Control, 1999b).

A coalition-based prevention effort is more likely to succeed if members have realistic expectations. Part of what they should expect is that building a coalition takes a substantial amount of time and proceeds through stages. Researchers have pointed out that members of new coalitions (and new members of established coalitions) must learn about each other and build trust before joint strategic planning can begin (Sofaer & Myrtle, 1991).

It is also important to clarify tasks, roles, and procedures early in the process of community development (Bracht & Kingsbury, 1990) and for coalition members to know that their roles may change over time (Hare et al., 2000). For example, an informal coalition may become a formal organization that hires staff, and the staff may gradually assume decision-making roles in day-to-day matters. The power structures and decision-making processes within local communities should be understood as well, because new community mobilization efforts will build on existing structures (Sofaer, 1993). Some coalition members may play more central or more visible roles than others; making this clear at the outset may help avoid resentment later. Finally, as coalition tasks change, it may become necessary to recruit new coalition members who have specific technical skills or social network connections (Hare et al., 2000). If the original coalition members are aware of this possibility, they may feel more comfortable with changes in the groups' composition. Finally, coalition members should be aware that making a significant difference in a health or social problem requires sustaining an extremely high level of coalition functioning for several years.

Coalition members should be aware that making a significant difference in a health or social problem requires sustaining an extremely high level of coalition functioning for several years.

Origins of Prevention Marketing

Prevention marketing was developed in response to the epidemic of HIV infection among America's youth. As many as half of all new HIV infections in the United States occur among people under twenty-five years of age (Liao & Brookmeyer, 1995). The annual number of new HIV infections may be going down among some groups, but it does not appear to be dropping among young people (Rosenberg & Biggar, 1998), a group in which most diagnosed cases of HIV are the result of unprotected sexual activity (Centers for Disease Control and Prevention, 2001a). These trends were becoming apparent in 1993 when prevention marketing was conceived by the Centers for Disease Control (CDC), the federal agency responsible for disease prevention and health promotion in the United States.

Since the mid-1980s, CDC had been responding to the HIV threat to the nation's youth on two fronts: school systems and youth-serving organizations.

Unfortunately, despite receiving relevant training and technical assistance from CDC, most school districts were not offering HIV prevention programs that had scientifically credible evidence of effectiveness, and some were unwilling to allow an instructor to say that condoms are effective in preventing HIV infection (CDC, 2001b). Even where school policies were consistent with HIV prevention education guidelines (CDC, 1988), many adolescents at highest risk of HIV infection did not receive prevention education because they did not attend school regularly. CDC had been able to allocate some resources to national and community-based organizations to address HIV prevention, but high-risk and out-of-school youth remained underserved (National Research Council, 1995). Overall, there was a pressing need for a supplemental HIV prevention approach that could reach broad segments of the youth audience with messages that were effective in reducing sexual risk taking.

The Search for Relevant Theory

The attempt to find a formal theory comprehensive enough to guide this new endeavor was unsuccessful. Rogers's work on the diffusion of innovations (1995) seemed to come closest and did provide some guidance. For example, according to Diffusion Theory, innovators or early adopters of a new behavior such as condom use can be spurred to action by hearing about the need to act in school or through the mass media. However, to motivate behavior change in the majority of adolescents, Diffusion Theory posits that it is necessary to reinforce school and media messages with interpersonal influence. Unfortunately, Diffusion Theory offers little guidance for sparking influential interpersonal interactions on a communitywide scale. In fact, Rogers noted that communitywide health communication campaigns have had to seek direction not only from theory but also from lessons learned in the field (Rogers, 1996).

In lieu of a suitable comprehensive theory, CDC and other national prevention partners constructed the general conceptual framework they called prevention marketing. It set the broad content parameters for national prevention communication activities and a local demonstration project (Ogden et al., 1996).

Rationale for Selecting Behavioral Science, Social Marketing, and Community Action

Behavioral science was included in the prevention marketing framework because interventions grounded in behavioral and social science theory had already been shown to prompt adolescent HIV risk behavior change in small-group settings

(Jemmott, Jemmott, & Fong, 1992; Kirby, Barth, Leland, & Fetro, 1991). Moreover, behavioral science could contribute sound program evaluation methods. The relatively new field of social marketing was added because it had the potential for broad reach into the target audience and because its ability to promote widespread condom use had been demonstrated in other countries (Dubois-Arber, Keannin, Konings, & Paccaud, 1997). Community action, which generally followed community organization and development, was included because CDC believed that community involvement and support would legitimize speaking to young people about sex, make it possible to frame and target messages more efficiently and effectively, create the best chances for sustaining an intervention program, and thus foster long-term behavior change.

Previous work of the Academy for Educational Development (AED) was a central influence in limiting the number of disciplines in the prevention marketing framework to three. AED was the major technical assistance provider for PMI and had already developed a three-part model for progressive social change: technology, individual behavior, and participatory policymaking components (Booth, 1996). Using this scheme, this U.S.-based nonprofit consulting firm had amassed an impressive international track record in pollution prevention and other health and development areas. The mix of the three disciplines in prevention marketing disciplines also may have some intrinsic logical appeal; one scholar whose writing suggests that he was working wholly independently from AED (McKenzie-Mohr, 2000) has promoted the integration of social marketing with behavioral science and community action.

Political science, a discipline that covers a broad range of topics (for example, information relevant to structural interventions; see Sumartojo & Laga, 2000), could have filled the third slot in the prevention marketing framework that was ultimately filled by community action. Perhaps the major factor in choosing community action was that at the time prevention marketing was being conceptualized, CDC was establishing HIV Prevention Community Planning throughout the United States. This was a new system for allocating federal funding for local HIV prevention activities. It required that community volunteers who were infected or affected by HIV join local health department officials in a collaborative priority-setting process. Community members were being included to help HIV prevention respond more sensitively to cultural and epidemiological variations in the epidemic across the country, promote local ownership and support for HIV prevention, and build local community capacity for science-based decision making. In brief, prevention marketing included community action because it was the emerging standard in HIV prevention and because community planning groups were moving into position to be able to apply lessons learned by PMI.

The PMI Local Demonstration Project

Funded in 1993, the PMI local demonstration project was a five-year, five-site project with a primary goal of reducing sexual risk behavior among young people under twenty-five years of age. It served as a laboratory for learning how to integrate the three disciplines comprising prevention marketing at the local level.

The PMI local demonstration sites were Nashville, Tennessee; Newark, New Jersey; northern Virginia; Phoenix, Arizona; and Sacramento, California. Sites were selected to represent a range of geographical locations and AIDS incidence rates, in the hope that lessons learned eventually could be applied across the country. In addition, each site had an established agency with human service planning experience that was willing to serve as lead agency, providing space and administrative support for a small paid PMI staff.

During the first two years of the project, AED and other national partners gave formal training and a substantial amount of technical assistance to the PMI sites as they organized coalitions of community volunteers and trained them to think like marketers. The coalitions included young people and parents, as well as representatives from health departments, youth-serving and AIDS organizations, religious groups, and schools. During the third and fourth years of PMI, multimodal HIV prevention campaigns (see Table 10.1) were designed by each of the coalitions and implemented under their supervision.

Each PMI site targeted a carefully chosen subgroup of adolescents (and their parents, in some cases). Some campaign components (for example, thirty-second radio spots) had the potential for broad reach into a target audience, but they would expose adolescents to prevention messages only briefly and were not expected to elicit much behavior change on their own. Conversely, other components (such as multisession skills-building workshops) had the potential to change behavior because they were more intensive and included repeated exposure to prevention messages, but they could reach relatively few adolescents. The last group of campaign components (telephone information lines, logos, and slogans) was included to tie together the components of broad reach and intensive exposure into an integrated system with mutually reinforcing elements.

In the final year of PMI, evaluation activities were emphasized. These last months were also the time when site coalitions decided whether to sustain PMI after federal funding ended and tried to find ongoing financial support if they wanted to continue their activities.

Behavioral Science in the Demonstration Project

Behavioral science concepts, techniques, and findings were incorporated at every phase of PMI. Before the five PMI sites were chosen, an initial survey of young people in four cities was conducted to investigate underlying determinants of consistent condom use in this population (Middlestadt, Bhattacharyya, Rosenbaum, Fishbein, & Shepherd, 1996). After sites had been selected and coalitions organized, behavioral science was used to (1) define target audiences and behavioral objectives, (2) obtain local information about barriers to and facilitators of delaying sexual activity and condom use, (3) develop and test the programs on the list of effective intervention models, and (4) design and conduct the PMI program evaluation.

The initial four-city determinant survey used a qualitative elicitation technique to fill in information that program planners need when theoretical constructs have content that can vary. For example, the opinions of important others are a key predictor of behavior according to the Theory of Reasoned Action (Ajzen & Fishbein, 1980), but the membership of this group of influential people varies with the behavior in question. It is necessary to ask members of each target audience which reference groups are most important to them regarding a given behavior. When adolescents in the elicitation survey were asked whose opinions concerning condom use mattered to them, they surprised researchers by responding that the opinions of their parents were almost as salient as the opinions of sex partners. On the whole, most of the survey findings were consistent across the four cities, suggesting that they would be informative to the PMI sites that were eventually chosen.

Findings from the previously published behavioral science literature were also offered to PMI sites to inform their planning decisions, and some of this information was incorporated in campaign plans. For example, the consistent finding that condom use with a main or steady partner is less likely than with a casual partner (Carol, 1991; Magura, Shapiro, & Kang, 1994) was reflected in target audience definitions in two PMI sites.

When local data were available in time for use in planning, PMI coalition members preferred them over findings from the published scientific literature (Kennedy et al., 1997). Focus group data were some of the earliest local data collected, and focus group themes were used in a variety of ways. For example, the PMI program in Phoenix was called YouthCare because focus group participants said using a condom shows you care about your future and your partner's future. Focus group themes were also used in the development of slogans, public service announcements, and tailored skills-building workshop curricula.

TABLE 10.1. OVERVIEW OF PMI SITE PREVENTION PLANS.

Site	Target Audience	Behavioral Objective	Behavioral Determinants and Objectives	Intervention Components
Nashville, Tennessee	Sexually active twelve- to fifteen-year-old African Americans living in low-cost housing who want to avoid pregnancy and sexually transmitted diseases	Use condoms consistently and correctly	Increase knowledge and salience of STDs, including HIV Increase prevention intentions and perceptions of condom efficacy Improve communication, refusal, negotiation, and condom use skills Encourage handy plans Increase peer support for delay or condom use Increase perception that controlling your body is controlling your life Change norm of exchanging sex for gifts	Skills-building workshops Media (soap opera, posters) Promotional materials (T-shirts, key chains)
	Nonsexually active twelve- to fifteen-year-old African Americans living in low-income housing	Delay intercourse until after high school and graduation		
Newark, New Jersey	Sexually active thirteen- to sixteen-year-olds who want to avoid pregnancy and HIV	Use a condom the next time they have sex	Improve skills (see above) Improve parent-child communication Increase safer-sex self-efficacy Promote condom carrying and use norms Increase STDs/HIV salience	Skills-building workshops Parent network (workshops and meetings) Outreach at large public events
	Nonactive thirteen- to sixteen-year-olds	Continue to delay sex or use a condom the first time they have sex	For nonactive youth, increase delay self-efficacy and promote delay norm	

Location	Target population	Behavioral goal	Objectives	Activities
Northern Virginia	Sexually active fifteen- to nineteen-year-old African Americans	Use latex condoms correctly and consistently with all partners	Improve skills (see above) Increase perceived risk of HIV Improve access to condom distribution channels Promote teen and adult norms of consistent condom use for teens Encourage condom handy plans	Skills-building workshops Outreach to influential adults Media (cable TV public service announcements, posters, remote radio events, radio spots) Poster contest for scholarships
	Nonactive fifteen- to nineteen-year-old African Americans	Delay onset of penetrative sex	Improve skills (see above) Promote benefits of avoiding penetrative sex Promote norms of delaying penetrative sex among peers and influential adults	
Phoenix, Arizona	Sexually active sixteen- to nineteen-year-olds who have used a condom at least once and intend to use condoms	Use condoms consistently with steady or "familiar" partners	Reinforce positive beliefs and attitudes about using condoms with familiar partners Improve skills (see above) Encourage condom carrying and handy plans	Skills-building workshops Peer outreach Media (radio spots, billboards, zines) Web site Promotional materials (T-shirts, key chains)
Sacramento, California	Sexually active fourteen- to eighteen-year-olds in high-risk areas	Use condoms correctly and consistently with all partners in all situations	Reinforce community norms about using condoms all the time and carrying condoms Improve skills (see above) Encourage handy plans	Skills-building workshops Media (radio, print) Peer outreach Phone information line Promotional materials (palmcards, temporary tattoos, mugs, T-shirts)

Prior to program launch, baseline telephone survey evaluation data were collected in three PMI sites and tabulated quickly. An analysis of these data by Mizuno, Kennedy, Seals, and Myllyluoma at CDC (2000) assisted program planners. The analysis indicated that perceived norms were an important predictor of attitudes toward condom use for the target audience as a whole, but that girls and boys had slightly different patterns. For girls, there was an association between positive condom attitudes and the awareness that condoms were in widespread use among their peers. For boys, a passive awareness of peer practices was not enough; to have positive attitudes toward condom use, boys had to know that their "important others" (especially their girlfriends) really wanted them to use condoms. The Sacramento PMI site used these findings to develop separate radio spots for boys and girls. In the "girl" spot, several girls find a condom in another girl's backpack, the condom-carrying girl advises her friends to carry their own condoms, and the other girls giggle while they heed her advice by raiding her condom stash. The "boy" spot is a conversation in which, before they decide to have sex, a girl brings up the topic of condom use with her boyfriend. He assures her that condom use is very important to him too.

Overall, the PMI sites made limited use of the behavioral science literature until it was distilled into lists of specific options (Strand, Rosenbaum, Hanlon, & Jimerson, 2000; Hare et al., 2000). An acute need for this distillation was perceived after all five sites decided to mount skills-building workshops for small groups as part of their campaigns. The decision to offer workshops created a need for workshop curricula, and the planning process bogged down as the coalitions confronted the prospect of developing their own curricula or reviewing the extensive HIV prevention literature for suitable models. There was general relief at the news that the Division of Adolescent School Health at CDC had already reviewed the intervention literature and had identified three published curricula with credible evidence of adolescent behavior change (see www.cdc.gov/nccdphp/dash/rtc/index.htm for a regularly updated list, "Programs That Work," in reducing adolescent sexual risk behavior). Choosing among these three options and then tailoring the chosen curriculum to fit local circumstances nevertheless were considered demanding tasks in themselves. The committee members later remarked that after starting with model programs and then tailoring them exhaustively, they were proud of the quality of their final products.

Finally, well-established behavioral science techniques were used in CDC's evaluation of the PMI demonstration project. However, whether the results would meet the scientific standard of effectiveness is a question that reflects a larger debate currently under way in public health. The gold standard against which HIV prevention program evaluation designs have been judged to date is the randomized experimental design (or randomized controlled trial). In this design, there is a condition in which participants receive the intervention of interest and another, the control condition, in which participants do not receive the intervention. For reasons including cost, lack of control over potentially confounding conditions in the control community, ethical concerns about getting data from a community that receives no direct benefit in return, and community relations, many community-level health programs do not include control or comparison areas in their evaluation designs. There have been reviews of the literature in several areas of applied research, including smoking prevention, that used an alternative set of scientific criteria that are less stringent with regard to the comparison or control group issue but impose requirements for greater scientific rigor on other aspects of the research (Zaza & Pickett, 2001). (A discussion of these criteria is available in Zaza, 2000.) The PMI workshops were evaluated using control or comparison groups, but the overall multimodal campaign was not. If and when the standards for evidence-based HIV prevention programs adopt alternative evaluation criteria, the evaluated PMI campaign in Sacramento should have good prospects for inclusion in the list of CDC's "Programs That Work."

Social Marketing in the Demonstration Project

After the coalitions were organized, the PMI sites went through a complex strategic planning process that paralleled the five steps of social marketing listed earlier in this chapter:

1. AED gave the sites a review of the scientific literature on the determinants of condom use among adolescents, and each site conducted supplementary audience research. Local audience research included focus groups with adolescents (and parents, in some cases), an audit of the HIV-related health and prevention services that were already available to young people in each geographical area, and a teen HIV risk profile that compiled local epidemiological data (see CDC, 1999c, for a risk profile development guide based on PMI site experiences).

2. The results of the audience research informed the selection of the local target audiences, leading to definitions of the target audiences not only in terms of demographic variables like age, race, and residence in geographical areas with low-income housing or high rates of STDs or pregnancy among adolescents, but also in terms of psychological factors (referred to as psychographics in social marketing) and behavior.

3. Audience research also informed the development of specific prevention messages and the selection of the channels through which they would be sent. The focus groups captured adolescents' perspectives on the benefits of and barriers to avoiding sexual risk behavior. Their perceived benefits were promoted in

the PMI campaigns, and real and perceived barriers were addressed by a proactive issues management effort and other strategies.

4. A 4 P's (product, price, placement, and promotion) analysis was conducted to make sure that a planned mix of interventions and campaign activities would be accessible and appealing.

5. All materials and procedures were consumer tested until they were understood and liked by members of the adolescent target audiences and until audience members said the materials were "speaking to them."

At the end of the project, a social marketing perspective was helpful in identifying funding for long-term PMI site sustainability after conclusion of the federal demonstration period (Kennedy, Stover, & Tormala, 2000). Viewing potential donors as the target audience and giving as the goal behavior allowed the PMI staff and coalitions to employ the social marketing steps: conducting research on donors, segmenting this audience, and framing and conveying messages in ways that were likely to elicit donor support. Fundraising was hampered by a short time frame and an unfinished program evaluation, but two of the four PMI sites that attempted to find support were able to do so.

Community Action in the Demonstration Project

The protagonists of the PMI story were the coalition members. In the words of one member, being asked to join a new PMI coalition was like being told to climb a mountain that had no paths to the top. A student of previous federally mandated health service planning coalitions, Shoshana Sofaer, was brought in as an expert adviser early in the PMI process. Nonetheless, many lessons were learned by trial and error (Strand et al., 2000; Hare et al., 2000).

Himmelman's theoretical work (1996) on the stagelike evolution of intergroup collaboration was used mainly to justify to concerned CDC policymakers the amount of time that coalitions consumed prior to actually designing and launching programs for young people. Wandersman (1984) provided some direction, but the available literature contained no ready answers to questions like who should be at the table, how to ensure that PMI programs stayed on task in the face of shifting community concerns, how to overcome historical animosities between community factions, and how to accommodate federal funding timelines without stifling local debate.

Evidence for the Effectiveness of Prevention Marketing from PMI

Thus far, the major evidence supporting prevention marketing as a useful conceptual framework comes from the evaluation of the PMI local demonstration project. The two major goals of the evaluation were to document reductions in HIV risk behavior among adolescents in the target audiences and to provide qualitative information about the PMI process and how various stakeholders viewed it. Because evaluation resources were limited, these goals were not fully met in all five PMI sites.

There were a number of strategies for evaluating PMI. As part of process evaluation, exposure to PMI messages through the broad-reach media campaign components was estimated by the media outlets themselves, sometimes on the basis of tracking information commercially available from ARBITRON. The outcomes of the workshops held in each site were evaluated in an experimental study conducted collaboratively by CDC, AED, and the five sites. The cumulative exposure to and effect of an entire PMI campaign was evaluated in one site by means of a multiround random sample survey. Finally, two interview-based case studies chronicled the experiences of a large sample of PMI coalition members, site staff, and national partners. This qualitative study provided insight into stakeholders' views of PMI. The various components of the overall evaluation effort generated converging lines of evidence that the program had a positive outcome.

Evidence from Workshop Evaluations. Four of the five PMI sites adopted the Be Proud! Be Responsible! curriculum (Jemmott, Jemmott, & McCaffree, 1996) as the basis for their workshops and then adapted the curriculum to fit local circumstances. One site adopted the curriculum and implemented it as originally written. Although CDC scientists cautioned the PMI coalitions against making major revisions in this evidence-based curriculum, major alterations nevertheless were made; for example, the curriculum's videotape was replaced by another copyrighted videotape, which may or may not have had the same effect on viewers.

The effectiveness of the tailored workshops was tested in an experimental study in which participants were to be randomly assigned to either an immediate intervention group or a wait-list control group that would receive an unevaluated version of the study after all the follow-up data had been collected. Paper-and-pencil questionnaires were to be administered three times to the intervention group (before, just after, and one month after the intervention) and twice to the control group (once on the workshop day and again one month later).

Not all PMI sites were able to complete the full design. Studies in Nashville and Sacramento where the full design was implemented showed that the revised curricula had a measurable protective effect at one-month follow-up on some combination of determinants of safer-sex behavior (including HIV knowledge, communication skills, and talking to friends about HIV) and behavioral outcomes (carrying condoms and condom use at last sex; the difference in frequency of unprotected sex in the past thirty days was marginally significant). Findings in studies in the other three sites where partial designs were implemented were consistent with findings in Sacramento and Nashville (Kennedy, Mizuno, Hoffman, Baume, & Strand, 2000).

Evidence from Communitywide Surveys. Communitywide surveys of adolescents were initiated in the three PMI sites that targeted older adolescents, but it was not possible to attain the necessary sample sizes in two sites with small geographical target areas. The effect of a full PMI campaign was measured by means of a five-time-point random sample telephone survey of Sacramento adolescents between the ages of fifteen and eighteen who lived in a fifteen-postal-code target area. The total number of survey respondents was 1,402.

Over the year that the PMI program was in the field, there was a statistically significant, and increasing, trend in the direction of exposure to PMI, culminating in a 70 percent exposure rate. Exposure was beneficial; the more channels through which an adolescent was exposed to PMI messages, the more likely he or she was to have used a condom at last sex with a main partner. The odds that condom use at last sex would be reported increased 26 percent for each additional channel of exposure reported by the participants (odds ratio = 1.26, $p < .01$). Increased exposure to communication channels also increased the odds that adolescents carried condoms (odds ratio = 1.27, $p < .01$) and levels of psychosocial determinants of condom use, including intentions, subjective norms, and self-efficacy. After statistical adjustments for sex, age, and race and ethnicity to make survey rounds comparable, the subsample of sexually active adolescents who reported condom use at last sex increased 4.3 percentage points over the course of the study (this increase represented a 13.7 percent decrease in the proportion of adolescents who engaged in sexual risk behavior). By comparison, over a two-year period, there had been a nationally reported increase of 2.4 percentage points (Kennedy, Mizuno, Seals, Myllyluoma, & Weeks-Norton, 2000).

Information from the Case Studies. Interview-based case studies were conducted at two points during the project in all five PMI sites; the case studies put the quantitative findings into context and captured the participants' observations. The first set of case studies was done just after the planning phase of the PMI project, and the second was completed after the campaign plans had been implemented. Among numerous case study findings were the observations that (1) PMI increased the capacity of local participants to make data-based program decisions, (2) there was no organized resistance to or negative publicity about any of the PMI programs during the project, and (3) no other events occurred in Sacramento during the survey period that could account for the change in behavior reported in the communitywide survey. Additional lessons learned by participants at various levels of the project are reported in a special issue of the *Social Marketing Quarterly* that was devoted to PMI and in a series of technical assistance documents listed on the PMI Web site (www.cdc.gov/hiv/projects/pmi/index.htm).

Other Evidence Supporting Prevention Marketing. A recent statewide smoking prevention program in Florida called the "Truth" Campaign incorporated many of the same procedures and some of the technical assistance providers that PMI used. One year after the campaign started, there was a 19.4 percent decline in smoking among Florida middle school students (Zucker et al., 2000). The project did not organize community coalitions, but it did have heavy youth involvement. The state government obtained the resources for the multimedia campaign by winning court cases against tobacco companies and using the settlements to hire and manage the social marketing consultants that designed and implemented the campaign. This state government involvement could be considered analogous to the CDC role in the national media campaign that was part of the PMI, so this evidence pertains to a case that is within the range of permissible variations on the prevention marketing theme.

Strengths and Limitations of Prevention Marketing

Prevention marketing has proven to have many of the strengths it was expected to have. Nonprofessionals can employ aspects of behavioral science ranging from theoretical models to program evaluation techniques. Social marketing can bring potential recipients of health behavior messages into the process of developing and refining prevention campaign plans and content, and there is evidence that the resulting prevention messages can have broad reach and widespread effects on behavior. Sustainability—an increasingly important consideration in the allocation of federal funds for behavioral interventions designed to achieve public health objectives—may be fostered by community coalitions. Applications of behavioral science, social marketing, and community action to public health are not new, but prevention marketing is the first empirically validated approach to integrating these three disciplines into an effective framework of health promotion.

Applications of behavioral science, social marketing, and community action to public health are not new, but prevention marketing is the first empirically validated approach to integrating these three disciplines into an effective framework of health promotion.

The original architects of prevention marketing considered the scope of the framework broad enough to allow for innovation and creativity but focused enough to provide direction. However, a conceptual framework this general has a number of inherent limitations:

- *Unspecified technical requirements.* The PMI demonstration project was very ambitious and required some technical inputs that went beyond initial expectations based on the definition of prevention marketing. Two needs that PMI sites were unprepared to meet were developing their own local adolescent HIV risk profiles and managing what became very complex enterprises. It could be argued that the epidemiological risk profile was only one of several kinds of audience research and did not need to be mentioned specifically. It could also be argued that competence in the organizational functions (for example, personnel recruitment and training, budgeting, writing subcontracts, and project monitoring) that were essential to successful site operations was a given. The danger, however, is that implicit requirements in a very general framework may leave a prevention effort unprepared to meet inevitable challenges.
- *Unspecified sequence.* Project managers found the prevention marketing framework quite general, with no clear point of entry. The steps in social marketing (Ogden et al., 1996) provided some direction, and, to assist program managers, evaluation experts recommended the development of a supplementary logic model (Yin, 1989). A logic model is an articulation of the goals of a program and the specific means by which their achievement is expected.

Early attempts to develop a projectwide logic model were complicated by the different disciplinary perspectives of PMI participants. A further complication was that stakeholders held various opinions about the criteria that should be used to judge project success; some felt that it was enough to show that coalitions had been able to design and implement social marketing campaigns, and others were unsatisfied with anything short of demonstrated behavior change in the target audiences. A number of revisions were made to an initial draft of a projectwide logic model. Figure 10.3 displays two of the revisions. Unfortunately, even the most refined versions of the model failed to do justice to the complexity of project.

Eventually, the AED, the primary technical assistance provider for the PMI project, reduced some essential elements covered in "Applying Prevention Marketing" (Ogden et al., 1996) into a simple four-part, fill-in-the-blanks logic model that individual sites completed for themselves. There were blanks for target audience, behavioral objective, key determinants of the behavior, and feasible interventions likely to impact those determinants. Called the BEHAVE model, this tool helped sites clarify the logic inherent in their activities and also has been useful to other community practitioners (Strand et al., 2000).

FIGURE 10.3. EARLY PMI DEMONSTRATION PROJECT LOGIC MODELS.

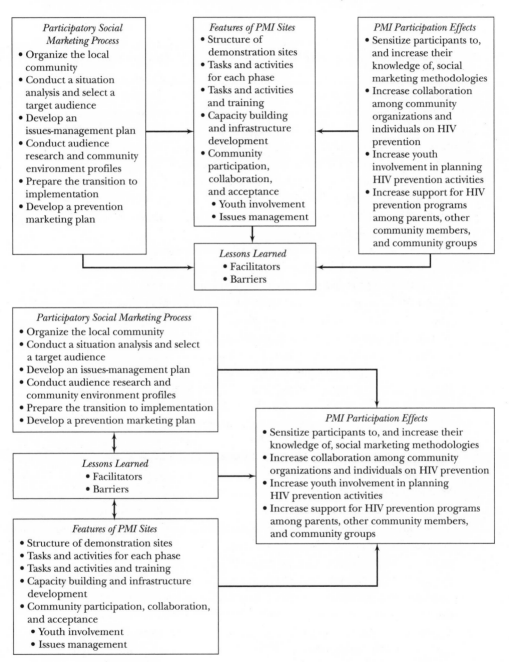

- *Unspecified discipline mix.* The specific contributions that social marketing, behavioral science, and community organizing should make are not explicitly outlined in the prevention marketing framework. Conversely, the framework fails to narrow the universe of possible contributions that each of the three disciplines might make to PMI. This lack of specificity often confused participants and sometimes created contention. For example, when a behavioral science design for program evaluation was being heavily emphasized at the end of the project, coalition members complained that they "thought PMI was a social marketing project"!

Sometimes behavioral science and social marketing techniques were similar or complementary, but the integration of these disciplines was not always smooth. For example, evaluation requirements conflicted with the social marketing admonition to revise a campaign constantly on the basis of consumer feedback. CDC evaluators had to insist that the PMI sites freeze the content of their skills-building workshops until enough participants had completed evaluation questionnaires to make statistical analysis possible.

Flexibility about the mix of disciplines has advantages, such as making it possible to subsume widely disparate but potentially complementary national communication activities under one rubric. Linking the three prongs of the PMI (the local demonstration projects, a youth-targeted national media campaign with the slogan "Respect Yourself! Protect Yourself!" and a national HIV prevention collaborative) facilitated the dissemination of breaking HIV prevention news and technical information. The inputs from and relative emphases on the three prevention marketing disciplines varied across the three communication activities. For example, community development was not heavily weighted in the national media campaign but was central to the development of the collaborative network, which used a very different organizing strategy than the local demonstration sites did. Still, the basic touchstones of broad reach and appeal, scientific rigor, and community involvement helped the three activities stay on track.

Although flexibility can be an advantage to seasoned professionals with a well-practiced repertoire of strategies, a lack of structure can be paralyzing for inexperienced community volunteers. If the contributions that the three prevention marketing disciplines should make to certain kinds of activities are not specified in much greater detail, the application of prevention marketing will continue to require a great deal of expert guidance (Smith, 2000).

Social marketing is a rapidly evolving field that incorporates constructs, theories, research methods, and findings from the behavioral sciences, economics, and other academic and applied disciplines. This diversity breeds overlap between disciplines and can obscure the theoretical origins and context of constructs. PMI coalition members often could not say where a key concept had come from, making it difficult to access relevant scholarly or professional literature. Failing to draw distinctions between superficially similar concepts and techniques can also create practical problems. For example, focus groups are conducted by social marketers and by behavioral scientists, but they often have very different purposes. Simply stated, the goal of the focus groups conducted by social marketers is to provide information that will lead to the design of campaign elements or offerings that are seen as fun, easy, and popular (AED, 1996). On the other hand, when focus groups are conducted as part of formative research by behavioral scientists, they can address other goals, including adapting theory-based research procedures to specific settings or populations. PMI sites muddied the distinction between the sets of goals, tried to accomplish too much with a single focus group procedure, and failed to get satisfying answers to some of their planning questions from focus group themes.

Future Research and Model Development

Many questions about local applications of prevention marketing remain unanswered, and their number and generality attest to the fact that this framework is truly at an emerging stage. There is even less information in the published scientific literature about national applications of the prevention marketing framework. Specifying the elements and procedures that are necessary and sufficient to define a prevention marketing program would probably speed progress in answering questions about local and national applications of the prevention marketing framework.

Many questions about local applications of prevention marketing remain unanswered, and their number and generality attest to the fact that this framework is truly at an emerging stage.

The most important outstanding question about local applications of prevention marketing may be whether this framework can be applied successfully in projects that are less expensive and take less time. Evidence suggests that the PMI demonstration project worked, but it was an extremely resource-intensive effort. Without substantial streamlining, this HIV prevention approach would not be feasible for most local areas. A prevention marketing intervention might be made more efficient in the following ways:

- Working with already organized community groups
- Using recorded or long-distance training modalities
- Preparing in advance short lists of options from which coalitions would choose at various program design decision points (Strand et al., 2000)

- Substituting program fidelity monitoring data for program outcome data when an evidence-based intervention is adopted as part of a campaign
- Using behavioral and disease surveillance data that are already routinely collected for other purposes to evaluate communitywide programs

These streamlining strategies should be employed and tested empirically.

Another broad question about local prevention marketing concerns the ability of a local campaign (with and without the support of national activities) to have a real impact on the health status of a target audience. Although factors such as prohibitive sample size requirements and incomplete HIV surveillance may preclude using HIV incidence rates as a measure of the success of an HIV prevention program, the effect of a prevention marketing approach on proxy measures of HIV incidence could be observed. For example, rates of common sexually transmitted diseases and adolescent pregnancy could be tracked; although their correlations with HIV incidence are far from perfect, their higher incidence would make program effects easier to detect, and they are themselves important targets of an intervention designed to reduce sexual risk behavior.

If using HIV proxies to assess the impact of the prevention marketing approach is not possible, then, at minimum, the long-term behavioral impact of this kind of program should be evaluated. Communities in which initial decreases in risk behavior or increases in protective behavior are reported should be studied for at least one year to examine the duration of these changes.

Evaluation resources in the PMI project were limited; consequently, several evaluation opportunities were missed. Among the unexamined program elements were a very popular radio soap opera broadcast by the Nashville PMI site and views of the program held by community members who had been outside the PMI process but were aware of it. Future research on local applications of prevention marketing should attempt to fill these information gaps.

Coalitions represent more to a community than just a means to a single public health end, and they are worthy subjects of study in themselves. Research on organizational climate (Moos, 1994; Goodman, Wandersman, Chinman, Imm, & Morrissey, 1996; Butterfoss, Goodman, & Wandersman, 1996) has already advanced our understanding of coalition-level outcomes such as member satisfaction, continued participation, and the quality of coalition plans. Evaluators of local prevention marketing campaigns should make every effort to further the investigation of coalition dynamics.

Based on observations of local PMI site decision making (Kennedy et al., 1997), CDC officials concluded that focus group data were easier for coalitions to use than findings from the national behavioral science literature. Observations also indicated that although trained coalition members could identify components of a multimodal intervention that were likely to be effective, they had difficulty tying these components together into integrated campaigns in which various pieces reinforced each other. Finding ways to ease the more difficult integration and planning tasks would be a valuable contribution.

There was no budget in PMI for tracking site activities after the conclusion of the demonstration project; in the sites that chose to sustain PMI activities after federal funding ended, there is no systematically preserved record of the programmatic activities that endured and how they changed over time. It would have been interesting, for example, to examine the ramifications of choosing to maintain a PMI coalition as an autonomous entity, as opposed to choosing to fold some or all of the PMI activities into a previously existing organization. This decision about organizational structure could affect a program's integrity, name recognition, growth, popularity, and longevity.

In a similar vein, there has been no systematic investigation of the dissemination of the prevention marketing model from program planners in PMI to nonparticipants, inside or outside the original PMI sites. PMI site coalition members reported using what they learned in PMI in their home agencies. It has also come to the attention of CDC officials that some of the PMI program components (for example, the radio soap opera) have been replicated in other cities and that the entire prevention marketing framework is being used in a communitywide antismoking project with adolescents; it is also under consideration for use in an HIV prevention project with adults (personal communications from Carol Bryant, December 1999 and William Darrow, February 2001). However, additional dissemination may have resulted from word of mouth, the dozens of conference presentations made by PMI participants and evaluators, and the publication of the program evaluation findings in scientific and professional journals. Without documenting this dissemination history, it will not be possible to learn lessons about which dissemination mechanisms are most useful with various audiences.

What other health and social problems could prevention marketing address domestically and overseas? In the case of a health area with no preexisting list of scripted "programs that work," would coalitions of community volunteers be able to apply prevention marketing? What other preconditions are necessary for the success of this approach? Answering questions about the generalizability of a model that takes years to apply will demand new techniques for assessing and synthesizing the results of prevention efforts.

In the long run, prevention marketing may make its greatest contribution by motivating joint action on the parts of individuals with marketing, behavioral science, and community organizing perspectives and experience. Program guidelines and other precedent-preserving mechanisms may enhance the positive synergy inherent in this kind of collaboration, but there should also be room for creative, unpredictable applications and syntheses of the three disciplines. A prevention marketing team has a collective understanding of what a community needs and will accept, which strategies researchers have shown to be promising, and how to make programs and products appealing to a target audience. This combination of insights can be a formidable force in the advancement of public health, and its potential should be explored more fully.

References

Academy for Educational Development. (July 1996). *Using the power of prevention science.* Poster distributed at the International AIDS Conference, Vancouver. Available: www.aed.org.

Ajzen, I. (1988). *Attitudes, personality, and behavior.* Chicago: Dorsey Press.

Ajzen, I., & Fishbein, M. (1980). *Understanding attitudes and predicting social behavior.* Upper Saddle River, NJ: Prentice Hall.

Alinsky, S. D. (1971). *Rules for radicals.* New York: Random House.

Andreasen, A. (1995). *Marketing social change.* San Francisco: Jossey-Bass.

Armstrong, K., Berlin, M., Schwartz, J., Propert, K., & Ubel, P. A. (2001). Barriers to influenza immunization in a low-income urban population. *American Journal of Preventive Medicine, 20,* 21-25.

Bandura, A. (1986). *Social foundations of thought and action: A social cognitive theory.* Upper Saddle River, NJ: Prentice Hall.

Baranowski, T., Perry, C. L., & Parcel, G. S. (1997). How individuals, environments, and health behavior interact: Social cognitive theory. In K. Glanz, F. M. Lewis, & B. K. Rimer (Eds.), *Health behavior and health education: Theory, research, and practice* (2nd ed., pp. 153–178). San Francisco: Jossey-Bass.

Becker, M. (1974). The health belief model and sick role behavior. *Health Education Monographs, 2,* 409–419.

Blair, J. (1995). *PSI/Project Action: Impact on teen risk reduction.* Washington, DC: Population Services International.

Booth, E. M. (1996). *Starting with behavior: A participatory process for selecting target behaviors in environmental programs.* Washington, DC: Academy for Educational Development.

Bracht, N., & Kingsbury, L. (1990). Community organization principles in health promotion: A five-stage model. In N. Bracht (Ed.), *Health promotion at the community level.* Thousand Oaks, CA: Sage.

Braithwaite, R. L., Bianchi, C., & Taylor, S. E. (1994). Ethnographic approach to community organization and health empowerment. *Health Education Quarterly, 21,* 407–419.

Brown, L. K., DiClemente, R. J., & Park, B. A. (1992). Predictors of condom use in sexually active adolescents. *Journal of Adolescent Health, 12,* 651–657.

Butterfoss, F., Goodman, R. M., & Wandersman, A. (1996). Community coalitions for prevention and health promotion: Factors predicting satisfaction, participation, and planning. *Health Education Quarterly, 23,* 65–79.

Carol, L. (1991). Gender, knowledge about AIDS, reported behavioral change, and the sexual behavior of college students. *Journal of American College Health, 40,* 5–12.

Catania, J. A., Coates, T. J., & Kegeles, S. (1994). A test of the AIDS risk reduction model: Psychosocial correlates of condom use in the AMEN cohort survey. *Health Psychology, 13,* 548–555.

Centers for Disease Control and Prevention. (1988). Guidelines for effective school health education to prevent the spread of HIV. *MMWR, 37*(S-2), 1–14.

Centers for Disease Control and Prevention (1999a). Compendium of HIV prevention interventions with evidence of effectiveness. National Center for HIV, STD, and TB Prevention: Atlanta, GA.

Centers for Disease Control and Prevention. (1999b). The CDC AIDS Community Demonstration Projects: A multi-site community-level intervention to promote HIV risk reduction. *American Journal of Public Health, 89,* 336–345.

Centers for Disease Control and Prevention. (1999c). *The Prevention Marketing Initiative: Constructing teen HIV risk profiles.* Atlanta, GA: Author.

Centers for Disease Control and Prevention. (2001a). *HIV/AIDS surveillance report.* Atlanta, GA: Author.

Centers for Disease Control and Prevention. (Updated September 19, 2001b). *CDC fact sheet: HIV-prevention education, from CDC's 1994 School Health Policies and Programs Study (SHPPS).* Atlanta, GA: Author. Available: www.cdc.gov/ncchphp/dcsh/shpps/factsheets/fs_hiv.htm.

Clinard, M. B. (1970). *Slums and community development: Experiments in self-help.* New York: Free Press.

Cox, F. M., Erlich, J. R., Rothman, J., & Tropman, J. E. (1970). *Strategies of community organization: A book of readings.* Itasca, IL: Peacock.

Dubois-Arber, G., Keannin, A., Konings, E., & Paccaud, F. (1997). Increased condom use without other major changes in sexual behavior among the general population in Switzerland. *American Journal of Public Health, 97,* 558–566.

Fawcett, S. B., Sterling, T. D., Paine-Andrews, A., Harris, K. J., Francisco, V. T., Richter, K. P., Lewis, R. K., & Schmid, T. L. (1995). *Evaluating community efforts to prevent cardiovascular diseases.* Atlanta, GA: CDC/National Center for Chronic Disease Prevention and Health Promotion.

Fishbein, M. (1996). Great expectations, or do we ask too much from community-level interventions? *American Journal of Public Health, 86,* 1075–1076.

Fisher, J. (1988). Possible effects of reference group–based social influence on AIDS-risk behavior and AIDS prevention. *American Psychologist, 43,* 914–920.

Goodman, R. M., Wandersman, A., Chinman, M., Imm, P., & Morrissey, E. (1996). An ecological assessment of community-based interventions for prevention and health promotion: Approaches to measuring community coalitions. *American Journal of Community Psychology, 24,* 33–61.

Hare, M. L., Orians, C. E., Kennedy, M. G., Goodman, K. J., Wijesinha, S., & Seals, B. F. (2000). Lessons learned from the PMI case study: The community perspective. *Social Marketing Quarterly, 6,* 54–65.

Himmelman, A. T. (1996). On the theory and practice of transformational collaboration: From social service to social justice. In Huxham, C. (Ed.), *Creating collaborative advantage* (pp. 19–43). Thousand Oaks, CA: Sage.

Hofferth, S. L., & Hayes, C. D. (Eds.). (1987). *Risking the future: Adolescent sexuality, pregnancy and childbearing.* Washington, DC: National Academy Press.

Jemmott, J., Jemmott, L. S., & Fong, G. (1992). Reductions in HIV risk-associated sexual behaviors among black male adolescents: Effects of an AIDS prevention. *American Journal of Public Health, 82,* 372–377.

Jemmott, J., Jemmott, L. S., & McCaffree, K. A. (1996). *Be Proud! Be Responsible! Strategies to empower youth to reduce their risk of AIDS.* New York: Select Media.

Kaftarian, S. J., & Hansen, W. B. (1994). Improving methodologies for the evaluation of community-based substance abuse prevention programs. *Journal of Community Psychology* (Special Issue), 3–5.

Kalichman, S. C. (1998). *Preventing AIDS: A sourcebook for behavioral intervention.* Hillside, NJ: Erlbaum.

Kennedy, M. G. (Guest Ed.). (2000). Special issue: CDC's Prevention Marketing Initiative Project. *Social Marketing Quarterly, 6*(1), 2–72.

Kennedy, M. G., Mizuno, Y., Hoffman, R., Baume, C., & Strand, J. (2000). The effect of tailoring a model HIV prevention program for local adolescent target audiences. *AIDS Education and Prevention, 12,* 225–238.

Kennedy, M. G., Mizuno, Y., Seals, B. F., Myllyluoma, J., & Weeks-Norton, K. (2000). Increasing condom use among adolescents with coalition-based social marketing. *AIDS, 14,* 1809–1818.

Kennedy, M. G., Seals, B., Nowak, G., Hare, M. L., Schechter, C., & Strand, J. (1997). The PMI demonstration project: Program evaluation, social marketing, and community coalitions. Presented at the Third Annual Social Marketing Conference, May 1997, Boston.

Kennedy, M. G., Stover, D. L., & Tormala, Z. L. (2000). Using social marketing to raise funds for prevention programs. *Social Marketing Quarterly, 4,* 44–53.

Kirby, D., Barth, R. P., Leland, N., & Fetro, J. V. (1991). Reducing the risk: Impact of a new curriculum on sexual risk-taking. *Family Planning Perspectives, 23,* 253–263.

Kotler, P., & Zaltman, Z. (1971). Social marketing: An approach to planned social change. *Journal of Marketing, 35,* 3–12.

Kreuter, M., & Lezin, N. (1998). *Are consortia/collaboratives effective in changing health status and health systems?* Atlanta: Health 2000.

Lefebre, C., & Rochlin, L. (1997). Social marketing. In K. Glanz, F. M. Lewis, & B. K. Rimer (Eds.), *Health behavior and health education: Theory, research and practice.* San Francisco: Jossey-Bass.

Lewis, A. M. (Ed.). (1993). *Behavioral and social sciences and the HIV/AIDS epidemic.* Washington, DC: National Commission on AIDS.

Liao, J., & Brookmeyer, R. (1995). An empirical Bayes approach to smoothing in back-calculation of HIV infection rates. *Biometrics, 51,* 579–588.

Liau, A., & Zimet, G. D. (2000). Undergraduates' perception of HIV immunization: Attitudes and behaviours as determining factors. *International Journal of STD and AIDS, 11,* 445–450.

Magura, S., Shapiro, J. L., & Kang, S. Y. (1994). Condom use among criminally involved adolescents. *AIDS Care, 6,* 595–603.

McKenzie-Mohr, D. (2000). Fostering sustainable behavior through community-based social marketing. *American Psychologist, 55,* 531–537.

McLeroy, K. R., Bibeau, D., Steckler, A., & Glanz, K. (1988). An ecological perspective on health promotion programs. *Health Education Quarterly, 15,* 351–378.

Middlestadt, S. E., Bhattacharyya, K., Rosenbaum, J., Fishbein, M., & Shepherd, M. (1996). The use of theory based semistructured elicitation questionnaires: Formative research for CDC's Prevention Marketing Initiative. *Public Health Reports, 111* (Suppl. 1), 18–27.

Minkler, M., & Wallerstein, N. (1997). Improving health through community organization and community building. In K. Glanz, F. M. Lewis, & B. K. Rimer (Eds.), *Health behavior and health education: Theory, research, and practice* (2nd ed., pp. 241–269). San Francisco: Jossey-Bass.

Mizuno, Y., Kennedy, M., Seals, B., & Myllyluoma, J. (2000). Predictors of teens' attitudes toward condoms: Gender differences in the effects of norms. *Journal of Applied Social Psychology, 2000, 30,* 1381–1395.

Montano, D. E. (1986). Predicting and understanding influenza vaccination behavior: Alternatives to the health belief model. *Medical Care, 24,* 438–453.

Montano, D. E., Kasprzyk, & Taplin, S. H. (1997). The theory of reasoned action and the theory of planned behavior. In K. Glanz, F. M. Lewis, & B. K. Rimer (Eds.), *Health behavior and health education: Theory, research, and practice* (2nd ed., pp. 85–112). San Francisco: Jossey-Bass.

Montano, D. E., & Taplin, S. H. (1991). A test of the expanded theory of reasoned action to predict mammography participation. *Social Science and Medicine, 32,* 733–741.

Moos, R. H. (1994). *A Social Climate Scale, Group Environment Scale Manual: Development, applications, research* (3rd ed.) Palo Alto, CA: Consulting Psychologists Press.

National Research Council. (1995). *Losing generations: Adolescents in high-risk settings.* Washington, DC: National Academy Press

Ogden, L., Shepherd, M., & Smith, W. A. (1996). *The Prevention Marketing Initiative: Applying prevention marketing.* Department of Health and Human Services. Atlanta, GA. Available: www.cdcnpin.org.

Oldenburg, B., Hardcastle, D. M., & Kok, G. (1997). Diffusion of innovations. In K. Glanz, F. M. Lewis, & B. K. Rimer (Eds.), *Health behavior and health education: Theory, research, and practice* (2nd ed., pp. 270–286). San Francisco: Jossey-Bass.

Pasik, R. J. (1997). Socioeconomic and cultural factors in the development and use of theory. In K. Glanz, F. M. Lewis, & B. K. Rimer (Eds.), *Health behavior and health education: Theory, research, and practice* (2nd ed., pp. 425–440). San Francisco: Jossey-Bass.

Prochaska, J. O., & DiClemente, C. C. (1992). The transtheoretical approach. In J. C. Norcross & M. R. Goldfried (Eds.), *Handbook of psychotherapy integration.* New York: Basic Books.

Reppucci, N. D., Mulvey, E. P., & Kastner, L. (1983). Prevention and interdisciplinary perspectives: A framework and case analysis. In R. D. Felner, L. A. Jason, J. N. Moritsugu, & S. S. Farber (Eds.), *Preventive psychology: Theory, research, and practice.* New York: Pergamon Press.

Rogers, E. M. (1995). *Diffusion of innovations* (4th ed.). New York: Free Press.

Rogers, E. M. (1996). The field of health communication today: An up-to-date report. *Journal of Health Communication, 1,* 15–23.

Rosenberg, P. S., & Biggar, R. J. (1998). Trend in HIV incidence among young adults in the United States. *Journal of the American Medical Association, 279,* 1894–1899.

Roter, D. L., & Hall, J. A. (1997). Patient-provider communication. In K. Glanz, F. M. Lewis, & B. K. Rimer (Eds.), *Health behavior and health education: Theory, research, and practice* (2nd ed., pp. 206–226). San Francisco: Jossey-Bass.

Sallis, J. F., & Owen, N. (1997). Ecological models. In K. Glanz, F. M. Lewis, & B. K. Rimer (Eds.), *Health behavior and health education: Theory, research, and practice* (2nd ed., pp. 403–424). San Francisco: Jossey-Bass.

Smith, B. (2000). Home grown social marketing—what next? *Social Marketing Quarterly, 6,* 66–68.

Sofaer, S. (1993). *The Prevention Marketing Initiative: Coalitions and public health.* CDC/AED technical assistance document. Available: www.cdcnpin.org (inventory number D398).

Sofaer, S., & Myrtle, R.C. (1991). Interorganizational theory and research: Implications for health care management, policy, and research. *Medical Care Review, 48,* 371–409.

St. Lawrence, J. S., Brasfield, T. L., Jefferson, K. W., Alleyne, E., O'Bennon, R. E., & Shirley, A. (1995). Cognitive-behavioral intervention to reduce African American adolescents' risk for HIV infection. *Journal of Consulting and Clinical Psychology, 63,* 221–237.

Strand, J., Rosenbaum, J., Hanlon, E., & Jimerson, A. (2000). The PMI local site demonstration project: Lessons in technical assistance. *Social Marketing Quarterly, 6,* 12–22.

Strecher, V. J., & Rosenstock, I. M. (1997). The health belief model. In K. Glanz, F. M. Lewis, & B. K. Rimer (Eds.), *Health behavior and health education: Theory, research, and practice* (2nd ed., pp. 41–59). San Francisco: Jossey-Bass.

Sumartojo, E., & Laga, M. (Eds.). (2000). Structural factors in HIV prevention. *AIDS, 14,* S1–S73.

Wandersman, A. (1984). Citizen participation. In K. Heller, R. H. Price, S. Reinharz, S. Riger, & A. Wandersman. *Psychology and community change.* Homewood, IL: Dorsey.

Weinstein, N. D., Lyon, J. E., Sandman, P. M., & Cuite, C. L. (1998). Experimental evidence for stages of health behavior change: The Precaution Adoption Process Model applied to home radon testing. *Health Psychology, 17,* 445–453.

Wingood, G. M., & DiClemente, R. J. (2000). Applying a theoretical framework of gender and power to understand the exposures and risk factors for HIV among women. *Journal of Health Education and Behavior, 27,* 539–565.

Yin, R. K. (1989). *Case study methods: Design and methods* (2nd ed.). Thousand Oaks, CA: Sage.

Zaza, S. (Ed.). (2000). The guide to community preventive services. *American Journal of Preventive Medicine, 18* (Suppl. 1), 1–91.

Zaza, S., & Pickett, J. D. (2001). The guide to community preventive services: Update on development and dissemination activities. *Journal of Public Health Management Practice, 7,* 92–94.

Zucker, D., Hopkins, R. S., Sly, D. F., Urich, J., Kershaw, J. M., & Solari, S. (2000). Florida's "truth" campaign: A counter-marketing, anti-tobacco media campaign. *Journal of Public Health Management Practice, 6,* 1–6.

CHAPTER ELEVEN

CONSERVATION OF RESOURCES THEORY

Application to Public Health Promotion

Stevan E. Hobfoll
Jeremiah A. Schumm

In order to promote public health, communities and individuals must possess the resources necessary for engaging in healthy behavior. Conservation of Resources (COR) theory (Hobfoll, 1988, 1989, 1998a) offers a framework for implementing public health promotion strategies by focusing on the resources of individuals and communities. This theory provides a theoretical model for preventing resource loss, maintaining existing resources, and gaining resources necessary for engaging in healthy behaviors.

Origins of Conservation of Resources Theory

To introduce COR theory, we first describe the theoretical need within previously existing stress and coping paradigms that led to the development of COR theory. Second, we outline the theoretical types of coping resources and specific principles defined by COR theory.

Bringing the Environment into Focus

COR theory was developed in response to the need to incorporate more fully both the objective and perceived environment into the process of coping with stress. Homeostatic and transactional models of stress and coping (McGrath,

1970; Lazarus, 1966) define stress as the perception of imbalance between coping capacity and the environment. These theories emphasize that individuals' perceptions of imbalance are important.
Furthermore, these cognitively based models
suggest that individuals must perceive the
consequences of the imbalance as important,
asserting individual difference factors. By
emphasizing perceptions and values when
defining stress and coping capacity, secondary emphasis is placed on environmental contingencies.

COR theory was developed in response to
the need to incorporate more fully both
the objective and perceived environment
into the process of coping with stress.

In regard to developing public health promotion strategies, homeostatic and
transactional models of stress and coping present problems in their conceptualization of coping demand and coping capacity. In homeostatic and transactional
models, coping demand and capacity are not separately defined (Hobfoll, 1989).
Coping capacity is defined as that which offsets coping demand and demand as
that which challenges coping capacity (Lazarus & Folkman, 1984). Clearly, this
reasoning is circular and is solely a derivative of individual idiographic perception.
Because demand and capacity are not separately defined, they and the principles
relating to them are not amenable to empirical testing. Therefore, when left to individual appraisal, it is difficult to assert which resources target groups will require
and what common obstacles will impede their applying resources to goal-directed
efforts. In addition, anchor points for defining capacity and demand are objectively
nonexistent. Thus, it would be difficult for public health promotion efforts to define
and target coping resources necessary for improving public health. If we have to
wait for individuals to appraise what is stressful to them, it is difficult to develop
interventions that suit groups or communities, and we are forced to wait until after
stressful events occur in order to know where to assert our best efforts.

Along with the problems in defining demand and capacity, deemphasis of the
objective environment in transactional and homeostatic models might be particularly problematic for public health promotion. Focusing on perceptions without
closely considering the objective environment may lead to some demands remaining unnoticed since individuals may be successfully coping in the course of the
process. Individuals rich in resources may be unaware of stressful environmental
circumstances, and those lacking resources may feel overwhelmed in dealing with
the same situation. Because many threats to public health are a result of or are at
least strongly influenced by environmental sources, it would serve public health
promotion efforts to focus on objective environmental circumstances. Even when
perceptions are to be considered, it is group and broad-based social perceptions,
not individual differences, that must be considered foremost.

COR theory bridges the cognitive and environmental viewpoints. Unlike homeostatic and transactional models, COR emphasizes the environment in the coping process foremost and person-centered variables secondarily. Hobfoll (1988, 1989, 1998a) proposed that perceptions of most major stressful events of interest to public health promotion are universally held. For example, contraction of human immunodeficiency virus (HIV) and living through a natural disaster are events that are universally perceived as stressful. This is not to say that perceptions are unimportant in coping with such events. Perceptions can determine the strategies that one employs when attempting to offset the losses associated with these circumstances. However, COR theory argues that resources are the key components to determining individuals' appraisals of events as stressful, and resources define how individuals are able to cope with the situation.

COR emphasizes the environment in the coping process foremost and person-centered variables secondarily.

Description of Conservation of Resources Theory

COR theory proposes that individuals seek to create circumstances that will protect and promote the integrity of the individual, nested in the "tribe" (Hobfoll, 1998a). That is, the individual must always be viewed in social context and acts to protect and preserve the self and the attachments that establish self in social context relationship. The focus of this theory is on reactions toward the environmental events that affect resources. *Psychological distress* is thus defined as a reaction to the environment in which there is threat of net loss of resources, actual net loss of resources, or lack of resource gain following the investment of resources. Loss or threat of loss of resources is particularly stressful because individuals are faced with diminished coping capabilities in handling future challenges. Lack of resource gain following investment is stressful because individuals have failed to increase their coping capabilities following expenditure of resources. Because individuals have invested resources without an increase in return, this lack of gain, in essence, equates to resource loss. In each case, resources are the single unit necessary for understanding stress.

Resources are defined as objects, personal characteristics, conditions, or energies. Object resources are valued because of some aspect of their physical nature or because of their acquiring secondary status based on their rarity and expense. A small economy car has value because it provides transportation, whereas a BMW has increased value because it also indicates status. Conditions are resources that are valued and sought after; marriage and tenure are examples. Personal characteristics are resources in that they generally aid stress resistance. Personally held skills are a second type of personal resource, especially as these skills relate to acquiring or protecting valued resources. Mastery and optimism are personal resources that can affect resistance to stress. Energies are typically intrinsically valued in that they aid in the acquisition of other resources, such as time, money, and knowledge. In addition to resources being broadly defined, COR theory proposes that resources are interrelated, and changes in one or more types of resources can affect the availability of other resources. In summary, COR theory defines resources broadly and proposes that they are interrelated.

It has been argued that change in general is stressful. COR theory predicts that positive and negative changes in resources will have markedly differential effects. Evidence supports the theory supposition that when ferreting out positive and negative consequences of change, these consequences will have considerably different impacts (see Thoits, 1983, for a review). COR theory proposes that resource losses are psychologically stressful, whereas resource gains buffer against the effects of resource loss. Thus, loss and gain have discrepant outcomes for individuals.

In addition, COR theory proposes the following principles in relation to change in resources:

1. Resource loss is more powerful than resource gain.
2. Resources must be invested in order to gain resources or prevent their loss.

Furthermore, the theory proposes that those already lacking in resources will be more vulnerable to the experience of loss spirals, and those with ample resources will have more opportunity for resource gain. In other words, the theory suggests that initial loss leaves individuals, groups, and communities more vulnerable to the negative impact of ongoing resource challenges. Those endowed with greater resources will, of course, be more resilient, but ongoing resource loss will challenge even richly resource-endowed individuals or groups. Thus, loss spirals are a powerful force that is evident in individuals and communities already lacking resources.

COR theory proposes that those already lacking in resources will be more vulnerable to the experience of loss spirals, and those with ample resources will have more opportunity for resource gain.

COR theory provides not only a basis for approaching stress and coping at the individual level but also a framework for public health promotion. It also provides the agenda for conceptualizing the resources critical in promoting public health. In addition, public health promotion efforts that use COR theory can target loss spirals and prevent future loss in individuals and communities. Finally, the theory provides public health promotion with the framework to instill resources necessary to the individual and community for promoting public health.

Empirical Evidence for Conservation of Resources Theory

The studies that we examine cut across several domains and settings and provide broad evidence for the theory's principles. In addition, they offer empirical support for the theory in a variety of populations, thereby suggesting that the theory has been validated for application to assorted groups targeted by public health promotion. It is our contention that these studies have suggested not only that interventions based on COR theory are capable of reducing the negative psychological reactions but that resource-based interventions are a key intervention strategy.

Finally, we wish to reassert a point that is found between the lines rather than in them. That is, much health promotion work has focused on the mind and behavior, because the pathways and obstacles represented by people's availability of resources have often been taken by health psychologists and those in public health as a given. Poverty, low social status, racism, unavailability of health care, and other fundamental condition resources are often beyond the scope of many health promotion interventions. COR theory highlights that, minimally, these fundamental resources conditions should remain foremost on our minds, both because they are primary in the potential success of any program and because failing to refer to them opens the risk of blaming the victim. No health promotion program can sidestep the resource reservoir that is ultimately available to people and the pathways that are often denied those who lack resources or the status that allows them to use resources that they already possess.

> *No health promotion program can sidestep the resource reservoir that is ultimately available to people and the pathways that are often denied those who lack resources or the status that allows them to use resources that they already possess.*

Principle 1: Resource Loss Is More Powerful Than Resource Gain

COR theory proposes that resource loss is more salient than resource gain. Resource loss has been demonstrated to be a more powerful force than resource gain in a variety of cognitive, evolutionary, and psychosocial studies. Studies in the cognitive and evolutionary domain provide evidence for COR theory on a basic processing and evolutionary level. In turn, studies that focused on psychosocial outcomes provide evidence for the direct applicability of COR theory to outcomes of interest to public health.

In the cognitive processing domain, several studies have supported the primacy of resource loss. In Prospect Theory, Tversky and Kahneman (1974) noted the steeper gradient for loss when compared to gain. They also noted that an event involving loss engenders greater risk taking than a mathematical equivalent event involving gain. In this way, individuals seem predisposed toward deciding against initiating events that have the potential for loss as compared to the potential for gain. It is important to note that this cognitive bias is not represented in people's awareness; that is, they do not know that are making decisions based on the greater loss gradient.

In measuring brain activity, Cacioppo and colleagues (Cacioppo & Gardner, 1999; Ito, Larsen, Smith, & Cacioppo, 1998) provided evidence for a negativity bias when perceiving aversive, appealing, or neutral stimuli. These authors view positive and negative emotional systems as being separate neuroanatomical pathways and provide compelling evidence for greater processing energy elicited by negative stimuli. Their research suggests that negative or loss-related stimuli have a greater impact on processing efforts in the brain and supports the lopsided impact of loss primacy at the neuroanatomical level.

Additional evidence in cognitive psychology for the disproportional impact of resource loss can be found in recent work on immune neglect (Gilbert, Pinel, Wilson, Blumberg, & Wheatley, 1998). Learning theory would predict that people would become conditioned to the fact that negative life events are typically overcome. In other words, people should learn to perceive accurately the fact that adversity can be conquered and therefore cognitively weigh positive and negative events as generally equal. Contrary to this prediction, individuals continue to overestimate the duration and intensity of their affective reactions to aversive events. In other words, they ignore the robustness of their psychological immune system. This is significant for predicting people's actions because their behavior is largely derived from their predictions concerning the emotional consequences of the event. Research on immune neglect suggests that the primacy of loss is not overcome through conditioning to the subjective characteristics of the emotional reaction and overestimates of negative emotional consequences might lead to behaviors that would not otherwise be predicted by basic conditioning principles. What this suggests is that the impact of loss must be occurring on a biological level because it is resistant to environmentally based learning.

Although evolutionary explanations are generally unprovable, there is agreement among resource theorists that resource loss is primary because of its adaptive advantages for biological, attentional, psychological, and cultural systems

(Carver & Scheier, 1998). The deep-seated biological nature of psychological reactions in trauma events provides evidence for the evolutionary importance of losses as they relate to survival (van der Kolk, 1996a, 1996b). Specifically, traumatic events tend to imprint on the victim a memory for the event that alters the startle response to similar stimuli. In other words, whereas victims would normally exhibit an immediate, time-limited response that is accompanied by somatic and attentive arousal, this response is prolonged, is accompanied by the smells, sounds, and sights of the event, and is rekindled as if during the original event by associated stimuli. Such a trauma constellation has been argued to have a biological basis, since on a psychological level, this reaction would appear to be counterproductive to functioning. This imprinted hypervigilant reaction to trauma must serve the function of reminding the individual of the critical nature of the loss stimulus.

In addition to the cognitive-evolutionary evidence for the primacy of resource loss, evidence from psychosocial outcome literature also provides ample support for this principle. Studies have shown that resource loss in comparison to resource gain is a stronger predictor of negative psychological reactions such as anger, anxiety, and depression (Hobfoll & Lilly, 1993; Lane & Hobfoll, 1992; Wells, Hobfoll, & Lavin, 1997, 1999). For example, Lane and Hobfoll (1992) found in a longitudinal study of chronic obstructive-pulmonary disease patients that resource loss, but not resource gain, was predictive of outwardly expressed anger. Anger expression by these patients was concurrently related to anger expression of their significant others. Resource loss was found to be the major variable, compared to resource gain, in determining the anger of patients and subsequent anger of significant others. Thus, the amount of resources individuals acquire has less influence in preventing distress than the effect of resource erosion has on causing distress.

A particularly compelling series of studies by Holahan, Moos, Holahan, and Cronkite (1999, 2000) provided support for the powerful long-term impact of resource loss. In these studies, interpersonal and personality resource losses were directly predictive of depressive symptoms over the course of extended periods of years. This relationship existed after controlling for initial symptoms of depression, in the first case in a community sample and in the second instance in a clinically depressed sample. Critically, this study found that the impact of resource change entirely mediated the effect of life events on later depression. That is, only if resources were altered did life events influence changes in depression. This evidence again suggests the pervasive effect of loss on the psychological well-being of individuals. Taken together with other evidence for the primacy of resource loss in predicting distress, it would appear that public health promotion efforts should target loss to prevent immediate and long-term negative psychological reactions and the behavioral manifestations that accompany these reactions.

Loss Spirals

Loss spirals tend to occur among individuals already lacking adequate resources or when initial resource loss renders people's resource reserves inadequate to meet subsequent and ongoing demand. King, King, Foy, Keane, and Fairbank (1999) provided compelling evidence for the negative impact of long-term loss spirals. In this study, a large sample of Vietnam veterans provided information regarding prewar risk factors such as family instability, war-zone stressors such as perceived threat during combat, and postwar resiliency-recovery variables such as social support. Using structural equation modeling, King et al. (1999) developed a model for predicting symptoms of posttraumatic stress disorder (PTSD) that was consistent with the predictions made by COR theory (see Figure 11.1). The authors found that individuals experiencing prewar loss tended to lack the postwar resiliency-recovery variables to help offset the stressors experienced during combat. In other words, lifelong loss spirals in combination with war-zone stressors exacerbated symptoms of PTSD. Notably, the model was highly effective in predicting PTSD, accounting for the majority of the variance in PTSD symptoms.

In a second study, this one of middle-class pregnant women, Wells, Hobfoll, and Lavin (1999) found that women who had resource loss during later pregnancy were relatively unaffected by those events. In contrast, women who had resource loss both early and late in pregnancy were markedly negatively affected by the resource loss experiences. These findings indicate that these relatively well-

FIGURE 11.1. MODEL FOR PREDICTING POSTTRAUMATIC STRESS DISORDER.

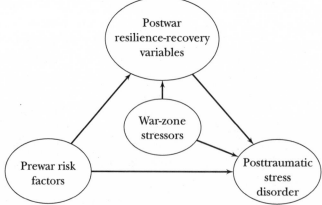

Source: Adapted from King et al. (1999).

resource-endowed women were resistant to resource loss if it was time limited. Their likely underlying resource pools were adequate to respond in their defense. However, as resource loss cycles continued, there was deterioration in their ability to defend themselves psychologically, and the negative sequelae in terms of increased anger and depressive mood were marked. This deterioration of defense has important public health implications because these same factors, increased anger and depressive mood, have been linked to infant health (Rini, Dunkel-Schetter, Wadhwa, & Sandman, 1999).

These studies suggest that public health promotion efforts would be most effective when applied early to those at risk for experiencing future loss. Children lacking the economic, familial, and psychological resources to buffer future trauma are already being set up for potential downward psychosocial spiral. Moreover, they suggest that even those possessing substantive resource reservoirs are vulnerable if loss cycles are ongoing. Interventions targeting one or more of these categorized risk factors have the potential for preventing the vicious snowballing loss cycle described in COR theory. For public health promotion efforts aimed at adult populations, an immediate focus in stopping resource loss would be extremely important in adults who have experienced a lifetime of resource loss. Specific strategies for prevention, especially as they relate to preventing and minimizing trauma reactions, will be discussed in greater detail later in this chapter. Comprehensive studies such as that of King et al. (1999) highlight the importance of interrupting or preventing loss spirals for interventions targeting psychological distress.

Principle 2: Resources Must Be Invested to Gain Resources or Prevent Their Loss

Resources do not simply fall from the sky. Yet most studies of resources as basic as self-efficacy and social support have uniformly ignored that circumstances had to occur that were facilitative of the growth and maintenance of these key resources. It follows from COR theory that individuals must invest in order to acquire the reservoirs needed for buffering future loss, or they must receive resource investment from outside sources, such as parents, loved ones, work, or a favorable social system. According to predictions made by COR theory, resource gains are important in the context of loss. However, the key to understanding the empirical prediction made by this principle is in the context of loss. Gain cycles are proposed to have an impact on stress-related responses principally in that such acquired resource reserves can serve to offset the losses.

A variety of personal resources have been shown to help offset the impact of resource loss. Self-efficacy is one such resource. Bandura (1997) defined self-efficacy as the view of self in the context of a specific challenge, such as the sense of mastering caretaking responsibilities with one's children. In prospective studies, self-efficacy has been found to be a personal resource that can help offset the losses associated with events ranging from minor hassles to major traumatic events (Bandura, 1997).

Another personal resource that has been shown to buffer resource loss is dispositional optimism. Scheier and Carver (1985, 1992; Carver & Scheier, 1998) have prospectively shown that surgery patients with higher dispositional optimism recover more quickly on both the physiological and the symptomatic levels. Thus, optimism might drive goal-oriented actions promoting health and have a more direct impact on people's well-being. Similar health-related outcomes have been found for self-esteem. People high in self-esteem are less likely to interpret difficulties as a function of their own inadequacies (Rosenberg, 1965). Women high in self-esteem, for example, have been found to be less negatively affected by complications of pregnancy (Hobfoll & Leiberman, 1987; Hobfoll, Nadler, & Leiberman, 1986). These studies suggest that public health promotion efforts would be wise to focus at the individual level on promoting gains in personal resources in order to provide a cushion for the powerful blow administered by resource loss.

Social resources have also been found to help buffer the effects of loss-related events. Social support has been an area of focus in this resource category. Social support is actually a complex construct that includes aspects such as the exchange of supportive interactions and the perception of the receipt of support (Sarason, Sarason, Shearin, & Pierce, 1986; Vaux, 1988). People higher in social support have been found to have better mental and physical health outcomes (Cohen & Wills, 1985; House, Landis, & Umberson, 1988; Vaux, 1988). Specifically related to physical health outcomes, recent experimental evidence convincingly shows that those with social support are less prone to infection (Cohen, Doyle, Skoner, Rabin, & Gwaltney, 1997). Thus, public health interventions should seek to increase not only the personal resources but also the social resources of the individual. Such efforts will become particularly important in the context of loss-related events such as physical illness or psychological trauma.

Although personal and social resources have been found to buffer loss, such resources have been found to have limited impact in the presence of major, ongoing loss cycles (Hobfoll & Lilly, 1993; Lane & Hobfoll, 1992). Although this notion was proposed in Principle 1 of COR theory, such reiteration serves to highlight the interaction in loss and gain cycles proposed by the theory. In addition to COR theory predictions that gain will not have opposite and equal impact, the prediction is made that impacts of gain are not independent of loss. Again, gain is important mainly in that it is directly related to the potential for offsetting loss.

Studies by Wells et al. (1997, 1999) provided empirical evidence for the importance of resource gain in the context of loss. Pregnant women were followed prospectively to examine the impact of potential loss and gain cycles in a population experiencing potentially stressful life change. Consistent with Principle 1 of COR theory, resource loss, but not resource gain, was found to be directly related to changes in anger and depressive mood. However, related to Principle 2 of COR theory, resource gain became very important in women experiencing a great deal of resource loss. Specifically, women who experienced substantive gains were significantly less affected by losses than were those who had experienced no resource gain. This study provided support for the prediction that resource gains are important in offsetting loss, but gains do not have appreciable direct impact as resource losses.

In another recent study by Billings, Folkman, Acree, and Moskowitz (2000), caretakers of people with acquired immunodeficiency syndrome (AIDS) who were experiencing severe resource loss cycles were found to be more psychologically resilient to the extent that they experienced resource gains with these same loved ones. One interpretation of this is that resource gains allowed resource replenishment at this critical period. A further interpretation harks back to early work of Frankl (1963), who noted that in the midst of tragedy, people seek to make positive meaning in order to sustain their plummeting psychological state. In making meaning, people attempt to create and focus on gains amid tragedy, and this may have a particularly sustaining effort. This would suggest that resource gain is both in itself recuperative and that individuals seek gains in order to sustain this recuperative impact.

Case Application of Conservation of Resources Theory as an Intervention

A case example will be used to provide a concrete model for applying COR theory to public health promotion. One area of public health in which little intervention research previously existed was HIV prevention with single inner-city women.

The studies presented in Table 1.11 focus on this area of prevention. They were generally well designed and followed prominent theoretical models, with the exception of two studies that were atheoretical. The approach to HIV prevention outlined in this chapter is similar to these studies in that a carefully planned methodological design was developed and theory was used in guiding the interventions. In addition, our case example has focused on many of the important outcomes as the studies presented in Table 11.1. However, we believe that our approach has provided several unique contributions in HIV prevention and health promotion. In particular, we propose that our case example demonstrates how public health promotion efforts can effectively target multiple resources. Specifically, the example demonstrates how to use the principles of COR theory in targeting multiple resources important to public health promotion. In addition, we propose that the use of objective measures of sex-related behavior change provides a potential advancement in designing and measuring the efficacy of sex-related public health promotion interventions.

We now present interventions reported in a series of publications by Hobfoll and colleagues in which COR theory is described as part of intervention strategies aimed at reducing HIV risk activity in this population (Britton et al., 1998; Hobfoll, 1998b; Hobfoll, Jackson, Lavin, Britton, & Shepherd, 1993, 1994a, 1994b; Hobfoll, Jackson, Lavin, & Schröder (submitted); Levine, Britton, James, Jackson, & Hobfoll, 1993; MacKenzie et al., 1999). We note at the outset that it is not our intent to show that our intervention was more effective than other excellent models in the literature. Rather, we hope to highlight how a resource approach informs intervention. Moreover, where our intervention is seen as similar to others that were derived from other theoretical perspectives, it may be argued that the resource perspective might be more fundamental to those perspectives than their authors have noted.

Specific Theoretical Assumptions of the Intervention

Several theoretical assumptions were used to guide the HIV prevention program.

1. *Change is resource driven, and resources are interrelated.* The HIV reduction intervention strategies that Hobfoll and colleagues used were based on several theoretical underpinnings. A general guiding assumption based on COR theory was that changes were resource driven (Hobfoll, 1998b). In order to produce changes in sexual behavior, it was assumed that individuals must be provided with the resources to produce those changes. In addition, personal, social, and socioeconomic resources were viewed as interconnected entities; that is, they tend to travel in caravans. This means that where one major resource is found, other key resources are likely to accompany it. Furthermore, these caravans tend to cross from the self to the social domains. Therefore, interventions were developed that would provide the women with the personal, social, and economic resources necessary to practice safer-sex behaviors.

Education about HIV and women's risk for contracting HIV was incorporated as an integral part of the interventions. It was assumed that if individuals

TABLE 11.1. HIV PREVENTION INTERVENTIONS
PUBLISHED BETWEEN 1996 AND 2000.

Authors	Theoretical Approach	Population	Outcomes of Focus
Carey et al. (2000)	Information-motivation-behavioral skills model	Mostly African American women from community-based organizations	Knowledge about HIV, motivation to reduce risky sexual behavior and risk-related behaviors
DiFranceisco et al. (1998)	Health belief model	Homosexual and bisexual males and severely mentally ill adults[a]	Completion of intervention[b]
Ickovics et al. (1998)	None	Women from community-based urban health clinics	Anxiety, depression, and sexual behavior
Pinkerton et al. (1998)	Theory of diffusion of innovations	Homosexual male bar patrons	Cost-effectiveness of intervention[b]
Guttmacher et al. (1997)	None	New York City and Chicago public school students	Sexual behavior and condom use
Klepp et al. (1997)	Social learning theory and theory of reasoned action	Tanzanian public primary school students	Sexual attitudes, beliefs, and behavior
Holtgrave & Kelly (1996)	Cognitive-behavioral model	Mostly African American women attending an urban primary health care clinic	Cost-effectiveness of intervention[b]
Kegeles, Hays, & Coates (1996)	Theory of diffusion of innovations	Homosexual male bar patrons and community members	Sexual behaviors
Fisher et al. (1996)	Information-motivation-behavioral skills model	Mostly Caucasian undergraduates	Knowledge about HIV, motivation to reduce risky sexual behavior and risk-related behaviors

Source: Based on a manual search of *Health Psychology* and *American Journal of Public Health.*

[a] Study based on two concurrent intervention programs.

[b] Results of intervention were reported in previous publications.

were not convinced of the need for change, they were likely to take cognitive shortcuts, such as minimizing their risk assessment (Hobfoll, 1998b). Efforts were made to relate the risk to a variety of outcomes for the women such as the consequences that HIV might have for their health and their children. The intervention focused on convincing women of the potential negative impact of HIV on a broad array of personal consequences.

If individuals did not have the resources necessary for change, they were also expected to engage in cognitive shortcuts (Hobfoll, 1998b). In other words, provision of education was viewed as necessary but not sufficient in changing women's decision making about their risk for contracting HIV. If women were provided with the information on their HIV risk but not the resources necessary to change this risk, it was expected that they would minimize their assessment of their perceived risk for contracting HIV. Therefore, provision of the personal, social, and economic resources for changing sexual behavior was necessary for the women to change their personal risk assessment.

2. *Empowerment increases the resources needed for change.* Similar to the approach used by Wingood and DiClemente (see Chapter Twelve, this volume), Hobfoll and colleagues viewed empowerment as a key to promoting safer-sex behaviors in inner-city pregnant women (Hobfoll, 1998b). The approach to empowerment they used was based on the Theory of Gender and Power (Connell, 1987) and defined empowerment as the interpersonal concept of relationships. In accordance with this theory, interventions emphasized ethnic and gender pride to increase women's sense of empowerment. It was assumed that such a strategy would increase the personal resources needed to instigate safer-sex behaviors such as the self-efficacy to negotiate with partners about using condoms. Thus, for example, increasing pride was assumed to be a facet of the intervention that would have an impact on the personal and social resources of women.

3. *Increasing sense of community and attachment helps change social norms.* For poorer inner-city women, raising the possibility of condom use with partners may raise the question of fidelity and endanger the women's romantic ties. In addition to being connected romantically to their partners, many of these women rely on their partners for economic support and a place to live. In order for women to implement condom use successfully, we encouraged them to engage support from both their partners and other women in the group. Interventions sought not only to raise women's sense of personal responsibility but also responsibility toward their partners, other women in the group, their parents, and their children (or future children). Women were encouraged to think about their health and well-being as part of their key social attachments. They were also provided skills for encouraging this perspective with their partners. In this way, a sense of community responsibility was used to change social norms about safer sex.

4. *Multiple sessions provide more opportunity for change.* A final theoretical assumption of Hobfoll and colleagues was that interventions should be spread over multiple sessions (Hobfoll, 1998b). Multiple sessions provided more opportunity for the women to increase their sense of community and empowerment. It was assumed that a single-session intervention would not allow the women to develop the social ties and pride necessary for producing adequate change in sexual practices. In addition, a multiple-session approach was assumed to provide more opportunity to increase the resources necessary for women to decide that safer-sex behaviors were necessary and achievable. In general, a multiple-session approach was assumed to be necessary for increasing the resources for change.

Of course, many interventions have used multiple sessions. The others, however, have tended to use multiple interventions to reach additional goals, with each session having a different objective. COR theory suggests that resource gain is slow and incremental. Hence, our intervention has tended to have fewer goals and to work on each resource gain more intensively. Indeed, if we could convince women to come for more sessions, we would still not increase our number of resource targets, but instead work on each in more depth.

Two Randomized Controlled Clinical Trials

Hobfoll and colleagues (1994a) applied COR theory in developing two generations of HIV prevention trials among inner-city women. To provide an example of how COR theory might guide the empirical progression of health promotion interventions, we describe each generation of these trials.

First-Generation Trial. Hobfoll and colleagues (1994a) conducted a randomized clinical trial of the first generation of their intervention. Participants in this first trial were single, pregnant inner-city women. The intervention was tailored toward affecting the specific resources necessary for these women to engage in safer sex.

The efficacy of the intervention was assessed through self-report and objective measures of behavior change. Participants completed a variety of self-report measures similar to those focused on in the HIV prevention efforts outlined in Table 11.1. In addition, the investigators provided participants with condom credit cards through which they could obtain free condoms and spermicide from several local pharmacies, and pharmacies provided reports on the number of condoms and spermicide tubes that participants obtained. Participants were randomly assigned to one of three groups: HIV prevention, health promotion, or no-intervention control. Intervention groups met for four sessions lasting one and a half to two hours each and included up to eight participants in addition to a female group leader. HIV prevention and health promotion interventions differed in that the prevention group focused on sexual behavior, and the health promotion group focused on more general health-related behaviors, such as turning down alcohol or not smoking. Consistent with theoretical assumptions, interventions were multi-session and provided the information and resources deemed necessary for change.

A variety of techniques were used to provide women with the social and personal resources necessary for initiating safer sex. Videotapes were created to support the curriculum and ensure the integrity of the intervention across group leaders and over time. They were used to demonstrate and facilitate discussion of assertiveness, negotiation, and planning. Videotapes included actors representative of the target population, which was thought to strengthen the effectiveness of the modeling techniques being demonstrated (Bandura, 1977). Consistent with the tenets of COR theory, videotapes were training based; that is, they encouraged participant skill practice rather than passive viewing and discussion. In addition, discussion and practice of the modeled behaviors were planned in order to contribute to the participants' sense of empowerment and community.

Related to the interactions based on modeled behavior, group discussion of previous sex-related mastery experiences was also viewed as essential to increasing the social and personal resources of women. These discussions helped group members develop a repertoire of strategies for engaging in safer sex or healthy behaviors and therefore broaden their personal resources. As with the videotape facet of the intervention, group discussions were thought to provide women with the resources necessary for enacting targeted behaviors, increase their sense of empowerment, and increase their sense of community.

Other facets of personal and social resources were also targeted through cognitive rehearsal and conditioning experiences. Participants cognitively rehearsed enacting target behaviors to help develop scripts for engaging in such behaviors in the future. Thus, cognitive rehearsal was another strategy used to increase women's personal resources necessary for engaging in safer sex. Interventions also incorporated aversive-conditioning (Wolpe, 1958) experiences paired with positive-conditioning experiences. For the aversive-conditioning experiences, participants were asked to imagine an unhealthy behavior (such as unprotected sex) and aversive outcome (for example, becoming infected with HIV). Aversive conditioning was followed by a positive-conditioning experience in which participants paired a healthy behavior with a healthy outcome. The goals of the conditioning experiences were to increase mastery and change the group norms for healthy and unhealthy behaviors. Thus, techniques were adopted from the cognitive and behavioral literature in order to target personal and social resources effectively.

A final component of the intervention was providing participants with condom credit cards, which allowed them to obtain free latex condoms and spermicide from several pharmacies near the clinic sites. Credit cards were valid from the time participants began the study until twelve months postintervention (yoked to time for the no-intervention control group). Provision of the means for engaging in protected sex was viewed as necessary for instigating safer-sex behavior change. Not only were participants provided with the personal and social resources necessary for changes in their sexual behavior, but the intervention also provided participants with the physical or economic resources necessary for instigating these changes.

Results provided strong support for the efficacy of the intervention. The HIV prevention group made greater overall gains within the outcome variables (HIV knowledge, safer-sex intentions and behaviors, discussion of HIV and HIV prevention with partners, and condom and spermicide use) than the health promotion or no-intervention control group, and these effects were maintained at the six-month follow-up. The results provided support for the effectiveness of this particular intervention in increasing self-reported sex behaviors that is commonly examined in HIV prevention studies.

The HIV-focused intervention was found to be especially effective for promoting changes in objective behavior: acquisition of condoms and spermicide. Women in the HIV intervention were found to be more likely to have used condom credit cards, obtained a greater number of condoms, and obtained a greater amount of spermicide. Similar effects were found for the health-focused group, although the effects were not as pervasive as with the HIV-focused group. The HIV intervention produced the strongest changes in objective measures of sex-related behavior.

Second-Generation Trial. In the second-generation randomized clinic trial, Hobfoll, Jackson, Lavin, and Schröder (December 2000) incorporated negotiation skills training more centrally into the interventions. Negotiation training was hypothesized to increase women's resources for engaging in safer sex by increasing women's abilities to engage their partners in safer sex. Interventions included nonpregnant and pregnant women, along with African American and European American women. Interventions also included facets tested in the previous generation of interventions (Hobfoll et al., 1994a), along with laboratory testing for sexually transmitted diseases (STDs). Thus, the second-generation trial sought to expand the applicability of the interventions and increase the resources of women, with major attention placed on the acquisition of negotiation skills.

Consistent with the first-generation trial, women in the HIV prevention group were found to exhibit pervasive changes in self-reported and objective sexual behavior. In addition, women in the HIV prevention and health promotion groups were found to improve in the efficacy of their negotiation skills. Such an effect was anticipated because both interventions targeted general negotiation skills. Finally, women in the HIV prevention group who had contracted an STD some-time earlier in their life showed reduction in incidence of laboratory-confirmed STDs, compared to women in the health promotion group, although no different from the no-intervention control. These results provided further objective evidence for the effectiveness of this public health promotion strategy. In summary, the second-generation trial provided support for the efficacy of increasing women's resources toward engaging in safer sexual behaviors.

Summary of Trials. The controlled clinical trials presented here highlight the importance of resource-driven change in public health promotion. Women were provided with the personal, social, and physical resources necessary for changing behavior. Interventions provided opportunities for increasing personal and social resources such as mastery, sense of community, and sense of empowerment. Furthermore, opportunities for obtaining the physical resources necessary for behavior change (condoms and spermicide in the study) were incorporated. In conclusion, a multifaceted intervention, guided by COR theory, was shown to be effective in targeting the multiple resources necessary for engaging in healthy behaviors.

What is also important to note is where we failed to produce change. In this regard, women often reported limitations to change that were due to resource constraints. Their lack of economic viability, associated with their poor education and poor availability of good work, often made them dependent on men whom the women themselves felt were undesirable or unsafe. On a more day-to-day basis, women would miss sessions due to day care limitations or last-minute changes in their employers' requirements for their work. Having few work-related benefits of insurance, guaranteed sick leave, or vacation time, they were often at the employers' whim. Furthermore, lack of transportation made attendance difficult for some women, especially in inclement weather. Major disruptions occurred when women lost their telephone or housing. As many as 40 percent of these women had no rights to their housing, but were living at another's behest, and often they lost their housing when interpersonal difficulties arose. Thus, at the same time as we attempt to alter women's resources, we must acknowledge greater social and economic factors that serve as obstacles to intervention.

Future Directions

A second promising direction for extending the application of COR theory is in the realm of traumatic stress.

Application to Traumatic Stress

Research has demonstrated the importance of resource loss in predicting psychological and physical health in victims of trauma. By evaluating efforts based on COR theory to date, we can also use this opportunity to explain how COR theory can be applied to community-level resources and move beyond the individual focus.

King et al. (1999) found strong support for COR theory in their study of PTSD in Vietnam veterans. Long-term losses over the course of the veterans' lifetimes were found to account for the large majority of variability in PTSD diagnoses. In a study of victims of Hurricane Andrew in 1992, Ironson and colleagues (1997) found resource loss to be the best of a wide array of cognitive and psychological predictors of PTSD and general psychological distress. Resource loss was also found to have biological correlates in hurricane victims. Specifically, resource loss predicted lowered natural killer cell cytotoxicity and increased white blood cell count, indicating an increase in immune system effort toward fighting infection. Predictions made by COR theory have implications not only in the prediction but also in the promotion of the psychological and physical health of trauma victims.

Research has also demonstrated that resource loss is the key variable in predicting ability to cope with natural disasters. Freedy and colleagues (Freedy, Saladin, Kilpatrick, Resnick, & Saunders, 1994; Freedy, Shaw, Jarrell, & Masters, 1992), in studying individuals in two types of natural disasters (hurricanes and earthquakes), found that resource loss was the most important variable in predicting motivation to cope with these natural disasters. This research suggests that public health promotion should focus, when possible, on minimizing or eliminating resource loss in order to increase individuals' motivation for coping and ability to cope with disasters.

The nature of losses during traumatic events makes the mobilization and provision of resources especially important (Kaniasty & Norris, 2001; Norris & Kaniasty, 1996). Traumatic stress involves rapid loss of highly valued resources (Hobfoll, 1991). Those with few existing resources prior to the trauma have greater difficulty in coping with the effects of the traumatic loss and are at greater risk for clinical trauma reactions such as PTSD or depression. In addition, the rapidity of losses during trauma, the unexpected nature of those losses, and the excessive demands of the traumatic event further burden those with few existing resources (Hobfoll, 1991). Therefore, the mobilization and provision of resources to offset the losses resulting from trauma is critical for intervention strategies.

The mobilization and provision of resources to offset the losses resulting from trauma is critical for intervention strategies.

Application to Trauma Interventions

At the community level, COR theory can capture and guide collective efforts for coping with large-scale traumatic events such as earthquakes or nuclear disasters. It is helpful to categorize community resources for the purpose of targeting multiple resources (Monnier & Hobfoll, 2000). Examples of personal characteristics of the community that might be targeted are community pride and cohesion (Monnier & Hobfoll, 2000). Increasing and mobilizing community pride and cohesion can help the community work together and increase collective coping efforts. Resources such as bridges, roads, and industries can be conceptualized as community object resources (Monnier & Hobfoll, 2000). The impact of object resources permeates the community's short-term and long-term coping ability. Along with community personal and object resources, communities' conditional resources such as availability of employment and emergency services might be important focuses of trauma intervention efforts. Finally, resources such as money, heating, and transportation and fuel costs are energy resources that community-level interventions can target. In all, COR theory provides interventionists with useful ways of organizing facets of the intervention into conceptual categories and helps interventionists arrange mobilization efforts directed at these conceptual categories.

In addition to conceptualizing which resource categories to target, interventionists should proceed through several steps when helping communities and individuals cope with trauma (Monnier & Hobfoll, 2000). First, the focus should be on estimating the extent of the loss. For community-level trauma, this step might center on measuring the loss of people and property. Second, the availability of resources for dealing with the loss should be assessed (Monnier & Hobfoll, 2000). Emergency services might be needed to limit immediate trauma-related loss, and mental health professionals might be mobilized to help individuals deal with the loss and limit clinical trauma reactions. Third, interventionists should consult with community leaders to become educated on the scope of the trauma and coping strategies that the community can use (Monnier & Hobfoll, 2000). Community leaders can help interventionists prioritize the most important community resources. Interventions can successfully be developed using COR theory to guide the categorization of resources and following descriptive steps in administering the intervention.

To help communities and individuals cope with trauma, prevention efforts need to involve initiating resource gain cycles prior to the traumatic event (Monnier & Hobfoll, 2000). For example, helping communities gain the emergency services needed to cope with disasters will provide them with immediate resources necessary for coping when disasters occur. Along with using the conceptual resource categories of COR theory for developing a strategy when trauma occurs, interventionists can use the conceptual categories in order to organize and target prevention efforts.

Theoretical Integration with Conservation of Resources Theory

Another promising direction is to investigate the efficacy of COR theory in combination with other theoretical approaches. COR theory provides a framework for ensuring the resources are in place for effectively integrating specific intervention approaches focused on specific interpersonal, cognitive, or behavioral strategies.

Integrating the Theory of Gender and Power with COR Theory. Hobfoll and colleagues have integrated the Theory of Gender and Power (Connell, 1987) along with the tenets of COR theory to develop an effective approach to help inner-city women increase safer-sex behaviors. The Theory of Gender and Power focuses on interpersonal resources, especially power within male-female relationships. Such an approach is especially important when considering the resource needs of historically disempowered groups such as minority inner-city women or women experiencing a lifetime of resource loss spirals.

Hobfoll et al. (2002) found that childhood resource loss in the form of abuse has long-term impact on women's risk for contracting STDs. This suggests that women experiencing the tragic interpersonal loss cycles associated with abuse might have lacked the opportunities to develop the interpersonal resources necessary for enacting safer sex. In this study, women with a history of childhood physical abuse also displayed higher levels of anger and depressive mood. This distress might have contributed to negative interactions between the women and their partners and further eroded the women's abilities to negotiate safer sex. In summary, childhood abuse appears to initiate loss cycles that counteract women's efforts to develop and use interpersonal resources and power within their romantic relationships that are necessary for engaging in safer sex.

Therefore, a promising area of future research is to help women who have experienced abuse gain the additional interpersonal resource strategies necessary for enacting safer-sex behaviors. Integrating the Theory of Gender and Power (Connell, 1987) into COR theory, future interventions should help women gain interpersonal power within the romantic relationship. Interventions should incorporate strategies such as increasing the women's assertiveness skills, along with increasing skills in negotiation and sense of mastery. This approach will provide women with a better stance within the relationship from which to negotiate safer sex effectively.

Integrating the IBM Model with COR Theory. Another model that can be combined with COR theory to formulate public health interventions is the Information-Motivation-Behavioral Skills (IBM) model (see Chapter Three, this volume). The IBM model can be used to conceptualize the important target variables necessary for change: possession of necessary information, motivation, and behavioral skills. COR theory can be used in conjunction with the IBM model to guide the provision of coping resources necessary for increasing the targets viewed to be necessary for behavior change.

For example, the IBM model predicts that in order for individuals to practice safer sex, they must possess the necessary information, motivation, and behavioral skills for engaging in safer-sex behavior. COR theory predicts that in order for individuals to become motivated to engage in safer sex, they must possess the necessary resources for such behavior. Public health promotion efforts using these combined strategies would focus on increasing the knowledge, motivation, and specific behavioral resources relevant to safer sex while eliminating loss or threat of loss to these resources. Interventionists using these two theoretical approaches will be provided with specific conceptual guidance regarding which constructs to target and how to provide the resources necessary for changing these target constructs.

Integrating Decision-Making Theories with COR Theory. Decision-making theories can also be used in conjunction with COR theory to guide specific techniques used for information and motivation delivery. For interventions using COR theory in conjunction with decision-making theories, COR theory can be used as the encompassing model for providing individuals with the resource necessary for change. The decision-making models can be used within the framework of COR theory to deliver the necessary personal and conditional resources for change (for example, making a decision to enact behavior change and maintaining the motivation for change).

Interventions combining Fischhoff's Behavior Decision Theory (1989) with COR theory can provide individuals with the guidance necessary for making logical decisions and the resources necessary for enacting those decisions. Behavior Decision Theory could be integrated into interventions to help individuals identify a list of options for changing their health, identify and weigh the consequences of those options, become informed on the probability of the consequences, and make a decision as to which option to pursue. COR theory can be used in conjunction to help individuals assess the resources necessary for changing their health and provide them the resources necessary for enacting logical options for changing health-related behavior.

In addition to incorporating Behavior Decision Theory with COR theory, public health promotion efforts might integrate the Elaboration Likelihood Model (see Chapter Four, this volume) with COR theory. This model provides predictions on how to frame information relevant to changing health-related behavior. Thus, the model can be used to guide efforts to encourage individuals to engage in healthy behaviors, while COR theory can be used to help provide individuals with the resources necessary for enacting and maintaining healthy behaviors.

A final example of a decision-making theory that can be combined with COR theory is the Precaution Adoption Process Model (PAPM) (see Chapter Two, this volume). The PAPM model provides descriptions of the stage processes through which individuals will progress when deciding to engage in health-related behaviors. According to the PAPM, interventions will be most effective when tailored to the current stage of the individual. Therefore, the PAPM can be used to provide and frame the appropriate information for helping individuals move toward making healthy choices. COR theory can be combined with the PAPM to provide people with the resources necessary for progressing through the decision-making stages and the resources necessary to act on health-conscious decisions. Resource realities must again always be considered because the motivation of individuals faced with difficult obstacles will decline. Therefore, paths of less resistance can be more effectively identified if people's resources and their resource needs in relation to their environment are acknowledged.

Resource realities must again always be considered because the motivation of individuals faced with difficult obstacles will decline. Therefore, paths of less resistance can be more effectively identified if people's resources and their resource needs fit.

In summary, decision-making approaches can provide interventionists with the specific techniques for encouraging individuals to engage in healthy decisions. COR theory can help interventionists provide individuals with the resources necessary for enacting and maintaining healthy decisions. A combination of decision-making theory with COR theory can also help interventionists develop the tools necessary for changing people's decisions, motivations, and resources for changing health-related behaviors.

Theoretical Overlap and Limitations of Conservation of Resources Theory

Although COR theory has many unique aspects and is increasingly well documented in the stress literature, it also has many properties that are overlapping with other theories and models. This in part stems from the fact that resource ideas have been pervasive since Rabkin and Streuning (1976) noted that stress itself accounted for relatively little variance in outcomes and that people's resources moderate the impact of stress. It is also the case that COR theory itself has been in the literature for nearly fifteen years and is quite well referenced as the leading pan-resource theory. As such, the implications of COR theory may have filtered down to many interventions that acknowledge the stressful nature of public health crises.

Finally, we would acknowledge the limitations of COR theory. The most germane one to this discussion is that this theory outlines a general process but does not specify which resources are most relevant in any given domain. For this, a study of that domain's ecology is critical (Kelly, 1966). In this regard, every health domain has a working ecology that defines how resources are naturally exchanged and interact prior to intervention. Furthermore, an understanding of such ecologies not only highlights what resources need to be altered to effect health changes but also what resources and ecological conditions are likely to be resistant to change or even implacable. COR theory emphasizes objective elements of the ecology and the resources available to individuals. Other theories and models are relevant for any intervention, as in our own efforts where we have incorporated cognitive-behavioral models and other theories in order to complement COR theory in practice. As is so often the case, marriage to any single model is typically too narrow for the real-world demands of health crises and responsive intervention efforts.

Conclusion

COR theory was developed as a response to the need to incorporate the environment as a more integral part of the stress and coping process. It emphasizes change in resources as the key to stress and suggests that resource losses are more powerful than resource gains. In addition, it states that resource gains serve to buffer against future loss. Predictions made by COR theory have been empirically supported in a variety of populations, and the theory has been shown to be an effective framework for HIV prevention. Application of the theory also appears promising in the area of developing interventions for coping with traumatic events. Another promising area of research appears to be in combining this theory with theories targeting specific variables important in public health promotion. COR theory sets out the conceptual framework for providing people with the necessary resources for coping with stress and engaging in and maintaining healthy behaviors.

References

Bandura, A. (1977). *Social learning theory.* Upper Saddle River, NJ: Prentice Hall.
Bandura, A. (1997). *Self efficacy: The exercise of control.* New York: Freeman.

Billings, D. W., Folkman, S., Acree, M., & Moskowitz, J. T. (2000). Coping and physical health during caregiving: The roles of positive and negative affect. *Journal of Personality and Social Psychology, 79,* 131–142.

Britton, P. J., Levine, O. H., Jackson, A. P., Hobfoll, S. E., Shepherd, J. B., & Lavin, J. P. (1998). Ambiguity of monogamy as a safer-sex goal among single, pregnant, inner-city women. *Journal of Health Psychology, 3,* 227–232.

Cacioppo, J. T., & Gardner, W. L. (1999). Emotion. *Annual Review of Psychology, 50,* 191–212.

Carey, M. P., Braaten, L. S., Maisto, S. A., Gleason, J. R., Forsyth, A. D., Durant, L. E., & Jaworski, B. C. (2000). Using information, motivational enhancement, and skills training to reduce the risk of HIV infection for low-income urban women: A second randomized clinical trial. *Health Psychology, 19,* 3–11.

Carver, C. S., & Scheier, M. F. (1998). *On the self-regulation of behavior.* Cambridge: Cambridge University Press.

Cohen, S., Doyle, W. J., Skoner, D. P., Rabin, B. S., & Gwaltney, J. M. (1997). Social ties and susceptibility to the common cold. *Journal of the American Medical Association, 277,* 1940–1944.

Cohen, S., & Wills, T. A. (1985). Stress, social support, and the buffering hypothesis. *Psychological Bulletin, 98,* 310–357.

Connell, R. W. (1987). *Gender and power.* Stanford, CA: Stanford University Press.

DiFranceisco, W., Kelly, J. A., Sikkema, K. J., Somlai, A. M., Murphy, D. A., & Stevenson, L. Y. (1998). Differences between completers and early dropouts from two HIV intervention trials: A health belief approach to understanding prevention program attrition. *American Journal of Public Health, 88,* 1068–1073.

Fischhoff, B. (1989). Making decisions about AIDS. In V. M. Mays, G. W. Albee, & S. F. Schneider (Eds.), *Primary prevention of AIDS* (pp. 168–201). Thousand Oaks, CA: Sage.

Fisher, J. D., Fisher, W. A., Misovich, S. J., Kimble, D. L., & Malloy, T. E. (1996). Changing AIDS risk behavior: Effects of an intervention emphasizing AIDS risk reduction information, motivation, and behavioral skills in a college student population. *Health Psychology, 15,* 114–123.

Frankl, V. E. (1963). *Man's search for meaning.* Boston: Beacon Press.

Freedy, J. R., Saladin, M. E., Kilpatrick, D. G., Resnick, H. S., & Saunders, B. E. (1994). Understanding acute psychological distress following natural disaster. *Journal of Traumatic Stress, 7,* 257–273.

Freedy, J., Shaw, D., Jarrell, M., & Masters, C. (1992). Toward an understanding of the psychological impact of natural disasters: An application of the Conservation of Resources stress model. *Journal of Traumatic Stress, 5,* 441–454.

Gilbert, D. T., Pinel, E. C., Wilson, T. D., Blumberg, S. J., & Wheatley, T. P. (1998). Immune neglect: A source of durability bias in affective forecasting. *Journal of Personality and Social Psychology, 75,* 617–638.

Guttmacher, S., Lieberman, L., Ward, D., Freudenberg, N., Rodosh, A., & Des Jarlais, D. (1997). Condom availability in New York City public high schools: Relationships to condom use and sexual behavior. *American Journal of Public Health, 87,* 1427–1433.

Hobfoll, S. E. (1988). *The ecology of stress.* New York: Hemisphere Publishing Corporation.

Hobfoll, S. E. (1989). Conservation of resources: A new attempt at conceptualizing stress. *American Psychologist, 44,* 513–524.

Hobfoll, S. E. (1991). Traumatic stress: A theory based on rapid loss of resources. *Anxiety Research, 4,* 187–197.

Hobfoll, S. E. (1998a). *Stress, culture, and community: The psychology and philosophy of stress.* New York: Plenum.

Hobfoll, S. E. (1998b). Ecology, community, and AIDS prevention. *American Journal of Community Psychology, 26,* 133–144.

Hobfoll, S. E., Bansal, A., Schurg, R., Young, S., Pierce, C. A., & Hobfoll, I. (2002). The impact of perceived physical and sexual abuse on Native American women's psychological well-being and AIDS risk. *Journal of Consulting and Clinical Psychology, 70,* 252–257.

Hobfoll, S. E., Jackson, A. P., Lavin, J., Britton, P. J., & Shepherd, J. B. (1993). Safer sex knowledge, behavior, and attitudes of inner-city women. *Health Psychology, 12,* 481–488.

Hobfoll, S. E., Jackson, A. E., Lavin, J., Britton, P. J., & Shepherd, J. B. (1994a). Reducing inner-city women's AIDS risk activities: A study of single, pregnant women. *Health Psychology, 13,* 397–403.

Hobfoll, S. E., Jackson, A. P., Lavin, J., Britton, P. J., & Shepherd, J. B. (1994b). Women's barriers to safer sex. *Psychology and Health, 9,* 233–252.

Hobfoll, S. E., Jackson, A. P., Lavin, J., & Schröder, K.E.E. *The effects and generalizability of communally-oriented HIV/AIDS prevention versus general health promotion groups for single, inner-city women in urban clinics.* Manuscript completed December 2000 and submitted for publication.

Hobfoll, S. E., & Leiberman, J. (1987). Personality and social resources in immediate and continued stress-resistance among women. *Journal of Personality and Social Psychology, 52,* 18–26.

Hobfoll, S. E., & Lilly, R. S. (1993). Resource conservation as a strategy for community psychology. *Journal of Community Psychology, 21,* 128–148.

Hobfoll, S. E., Nadler, A., & Leiberman, J. (1986). Satisfaction with social support during crisis: Intimacy and self esteem as critical determinants. *Journal of Personality and Social Psychology, 51,* 296–304.

Holahan, C. J., Moos, R. H., Holahan, C. K., & Cronkite, R. C. (1999). Resource loss, resource gain, and depressive symptoms: A ten-year model. *Journal of Personality and Social Psychology, 77,* 620–629.

Holahan, C. J., Moos, R. H., Holahan, C. K., & Cronkite, R. C. (2000). Long-term post-treatment functioning among patients with unipolar depression: An integrative model. *Journal of Consulting & Clinical Psychology, 68,* 226–232.

Holtgrave, D. R., & Kelly, J. A. (1996). Preventing HIV/AIDS among high-risk urban women: The cost-effectiveness of a behavioral group intervention. *American Journal of Public Health, 86,* 1442–1445.

House, J., Landis, K., & Umberson, D. (1988). Social relationships and health. *Science, 241,* 540–545.

Ickovics, J. R., Druley, J. A., Grigorenko, E. L., Morrill, A. C., Beren, S. E., & Rodin, J. (1998). Long-term effects of HIV counseling and testing for women: Behavioral and psychological consequences are limited to 18 months posttest. *Health Psychology, 17,* 395–402.

Ironson, G., Wynings, C., Schneiderman, N., Baum, A., Rodriguez, M., Greenwood, D., Benight, C., Antoni, M., LaPierre, P., Huang, H., Klimas, N., & Flether, M. A. (1997). Post-traumatic stress symptoms, intrusive thoughts, loss, and immune function after Hurricane Andrew. *Psychosomatic Medicine, 59,* 128–141.

Ito, T. A., Larsen, J. T., Smith, N. K., & Cacioppo, J. T. (1998). Negative information weighs more heavily on the brain: The negativity bias in evaluative categorizations. *Journal of Personality and Social Relationships, 75,* 887–900.

Kaniasty, K., & Norris, F. H. (2001). Social support dynamics in adjustment to disasters. In B. R. Sarason & S. Duck (Eds.), *Personal relationships: Implications for clinical and community psychology* (pp. 201–224). New York: Wiley.

Kegeles, S. M., Hays, R. B., & Coates, T. J. (1996). The Mpowerment project: A community-level HIV prevention intervention for young, gay men. *American Journal of Public Health, 86,* 1129–1136.

Kelly, J. G. (1966). Ecological constraints on mental health services. *American Psychologist, 21,* 535–539.

King, D. W., King, L. A., Foy, D. W., Keane, T. M., & Fairbank, J. A. (1999). Posttraumatic stress disorder in a national sample of female and male Vietnam veterans: Risk factors, war-zone stressors, and resilience-recovery variables. *Journal of Abnormal Psychology, 108,* 164–170.

Klepp, K. I., Ndeki, S. S., Leshabari, M. T., Hannan, P. J., & Lyimo, B. A. (1997). AIDS education in Tanzania: Promoting risk reduction among primary school children. *American Journal of Public Health, 87,* 1931–1936.

Lane, C., & Hobfoll, S. E. (1992). How loss affects anger and alienates potential supporters. *Journal of Consulting and Clinical Psychology, 60,* 935–942.

Lazarus, R. S. (1966). *Psychological stress and the coping process.* New York: Springer.

Lazarus, R. S., & Folkman, S. (1984). *Stress, appraisal, and coping.* New York: Springer, 1984.

Levine, O. H., Britton, P. J., James, T. C., Jackson, A. P., & Hobfoll, S. E. (1993). The empowerment of women: A key to HIV prevention. *Journal of Community Psychology, 21,* 320–334.

MacKenzie, J. E., Hobfoll, S. E., Ennis, N., Kay, J., Jackson, A., & Lavin, J. (1999). Reducing AIDS risk among inner-city women: A review of the collectivist empowerment AIDS prevention (CE-AP) program. *Journal of the European Academy of Dermatology and Venereology, 13,* 166–174.

McGrath, J. E. (1970). A conceptual formulation for research on stress. In J. E. McGrath (Ed.), *Social and psychological factors in stress* (pp. 10–21). New York: Holt, Rinehart, & Winston.

Monnier, J., & Hobfoll, S. E. (2000). Conservation of resources in individual and community reactions to traumatic stress. In S. Yehuda & K. McFarlane (Eds.), *International handbook of human response to trauma* (pp. 325–336). New York: Plenum.

Norris, F. H., & Kaniasty, K. (1996). Received and perceived social support in times of stress: A test of the social support deterioration deterrence model. *Journal of Personality and Social Psychology, 71,* 498–511.

Pinkerton, S. D., Holtgrave, D. R., DiFranceisco, W. J., Stevenson, L. Y., & Kelly, J. A. (1998). Cost-effectiveness of a community-level HIV risk reduction interventions. *American Journal of Public Health, 88,* 1239–1242.

Rabkin, J. G., & Streuning, E. L. (1976). Life events, stress and illness. *Science, 194,* 1013–1020.

Rini, C. K., Dunkel-Schetter, C., Wadhwa, P. D., & Sandman, C. A. (1999). Psychological adaptation and birth outcomes: The role of personal resources, stress, and sociocultural context in pregnancy. *Health Psychology, 18,* 333–345.

Rosenberg, M. (1965). *Society and adolescent self-image.* Princeton, NJ: Princeton University Press.

Sarason, I., Sarason, B., Shearin, E., & Pierce, G. (1986). A brief measure of social support: Practical and theoretical implications. *Journal of Social and Personal Relationships, 4,* 497–510.

Scheier, M. F., & Carver, C. S. (1985). Optimism, coping, and health: Assessment and implications of generalized outcome expectancies. *Health Psychology, 4,* 219–247.

Scheier, M. F., & Carver, C. S. (1992). Effects of optimism on psychology and physical well-being: Theoretical overview and empirical update. *Cognitive Therapy and Research, 16,* 201–228.

Thoits, P. A. (1983). Dimensions of life events that influence psychological distress: An evaluation and synthesis of the literature. In H. B. Kaplan (Ed.), *Psychosocial stress: Trends in theory and research* (pp. 33–103). Orlando, FL: Academic Press.

Tversky, A., & Kahneman, D. (1974). Judgement under uncertainty: Heuristics and biases. *Science, 185,* 1124–1131.

van der Kolk, B. A. (1996a). The body keeps the score: Approaches to the psychobiology of posttraumatic stress disorder. In B. A. van der Kolk, A. C. McFarlane, & L. Weisaeth (Eds.), *Traumatic stress: The effects of overwhelming experience on mind, body, and society* (pp. 214–241). New York: Guilford Press.

van der Kolk, B. A. (1996b). Trauma and memory. In B. A. van der Kolk, A. C. McFarlane, & L. Weisaeth (Eds.), *Traumatic stress: The effects of overwhelming experience on mind, body, and society* (pp. 279–302). New York: Guilford Press.

Vaux, A. (1988). *Social support: Theory, research and intervention.* New York: Praeger.

Wells, J., Hobfoll, S. E., & Lavin, J. (1997). Resource loss, resource gain, and communal coping during pregnancy among women with multiple roles. *Psychology of Women Quarterly, 21,* 645–662.

Wells, J., Hobfoll, S. E., & Lavin, J. (1999). When it rains, it pours: The greater impact of resource loss compared to gain on psychological distress. *Personality and Social Psychology Bulletin, 25,* 1172–1182.

Wolpe, J. (1958). *Psychotherapy by reciprocal inhibition.* Stanford, CA: Stanford University Press.

CHAPTER TWELVE

THE THEORY OF GENDER AND POWER

A Social Structural Theory for Guiding Public Health Interventions

Gina M. Wingood
Ralph J. DiClemente

Originally developed by Robert Connell, the Theory of Gender and Power is a social structural theory based on existing philosophical writings of sexual inequality, gender, and power imbalance (Connell, 1987). According to the theory, three major structures characterize the gendered relationships between men and women: (1) the sexual division of labor, which examines economic inequities favoring males; (2) the sexual division of power, which examines inequities and abuses of authority and control in relationships and institutions favoring males; and (3) cathexis, which examines social norms and affective attachments. The three structures are overlapping but distinct and serve to explain the gender roles that men and women assume (Connell, 1987).

In our adaptation of this theory, we postulate that the gender-based inequities and disparities in expectations that arise from each of the three structures (division of labor, division of power, and structure of cathexis) generate different exposures and risk factors that influence women's risk for disease. The exposures and risk factors inherent in each structure increase women's vulnerability for disease. Consequently, public health and social and behavioral science interventions targeting these exposures and risk factors can reduce women's risk of disease.

This chapter articulates an extended version of the Theory of Gender and Power, as we have developed it, to examine the exposures, the social and behavioral risk factors, and the biological properties that increase women's vulnerability for acquiring human immunodeficiency virus (HIV). Subsequently, it applies the theory to assist in the design of several interventions aimed at reducing women's HIV risk. Employing this theory marshals new kinds of data, asks new and broader questions regarding women and their risk of HIV, and, most important, creates new options for prevention.

Origin and Historical Roots of the Theory

The concept of power imbalances in the subordination of women was first articulated in the early twentieth century by Charlotte Perkins Gilman, who wrote in *The Man-Made World; or, Our Androcentric Culture* ([1911] 1971) that

> all our human scheme of things rests on the same tacit assumption; man being held the human type; woman a sort of accompaniment and subordinate assistant, merely essential to the making of people. She has held always the place of a preposition in relation to man. She has always been considered above him or below him, before him, behind him, beside him, *a wholly relative existence*—"*Sydney's sister*," "*Pembrokes's mother*"—*but, never by any chance Sydney or Pembroke herself* [p. 20].

Gilman emphasized that in our androcentric culture, man defines woman not in relation to herself but in relation to him. Simone de Beauvoir's groundbreaking book, *The Second Sex*, first published in 1949, also expounded on gender and power imbalances without using the term *androcentric* (de Beauvoir, 1974). Her book eloquently stated that in our culture, males are perceived as "real" and everything else, including women, is perceived as "other." One consequence of "otherizing" women is that they become defined in terms of their similarity and dissimilarity to men. Another consequence is that they become defined in terms of their functional significance to men rather than in terms of their own significance. De Beauvoir's appreciation for power and sexual inequality was at the very core of the feminist movement in the 1960s and 1970s (Chapman-Walsh, 1995). Throughout the 1980s, women tried to understand the interaction of ethnicity with gender and power as women of color organized around improving the health-related quality of life of African American and Latina women, particularly with regard to their sexual and reproductive health.

During the mid-1980s, R. W. Connell, an Australian sociologist, began examining the available theories on gender and power in search of an integrative theory that would reassemble the existing theories in this field (Connell, 1987). Several researchers have applied an elaboration of Connell's integrative Theory of Gender and Power to understand women's risk of developing lung cancer (Chapman-Walsh, 1995) and to determine the correlates of relationship abuse among African

American women (Raj, Silverman, Wingood, & DiClemente, 1999). During the 1990s, HIV prevention researchers noted that most of the theoretical models driving this field had an individualistic conceptualization and did not consider the broader context of women's lives.

By the turn of the century, researchers began applying our extended version of the Theory of Gender and Power to examine women's HIV-related risks and design more efficacious HIV prevention interventions (Wingood & DiClemente, 2000). We published a seminal article (2000) extending this social structural theory to examine women's risk for HIV. Using HIV as a case study, we (1) identify and operationalize gendered risk factors (individual level influences), (2) identify and operationalize exposures (influences external to a woman), (3) address important but understudied gender-specific biological processes, and (4) describe how interventions may be developed that target gendered risk factors and exposures that may affect women's risk for HIV.

Description of the Theory of Gender and Power

The Theory of Gender and Power is a social structural model that seeks to understand women's risk as a function of different structures. According to the theory, three major structures characterize the gendered relationships between men and women: the sexual division of labor, the sexual division of power, and the structure of cathexis (Connell, 1987; see Table 12.1). Both the sexual division of labor and the sexual division of power had been identified from previous research as two fundamental structures that partially explain gender relations. Connell devised the third structure, the structure of cathexis, to address the affective component of relationships. Wingood and DiClemente, in their extension of the theory, have renamed this structure *affective and social exposures,* to emphasize the important social factors that comprise this structure. These three overlapping but distinct structures serve to explain the gender roles that men and women assume. It is important to emphasize that none of the three structures is or can be independent of the others. Neither is there one structure from which the others are derived.

According to the Theory of Gender and Power, three major structures characterize the gendered relationships between men and women.

The three structures exist at two different levels: societal and institutional (Connell, 1987). The higher level in which the three social structures are embedded is the societal level. The three structures are rooted in society through numerous historical and sociopolitical forces that consistently segregate power and ascribe social norms on the basis of gender-determined roles. As society slowly

TABLE 12.1. PROPOSED MODEL CONCEPTUALIZING THE INFLUENCE OF THE THEORY OF GENDER AND POWER ON WOMEN'S HEALTH.

Societal Level	Institutional Level	The Social Mechanisms	Exposures	Risk Factors	Biological Factors	Disease
Sexual division of labor	Work site School Family	Manifested as unequal pay, which produces economic inequities for women	Economic exposures risk factors	Socio-economic		
Sexual division of power	Relationship Medical system Media	Manifested as imbalances in control, which produce inequities in power for women	Physical exposures	Behavioral risk factors		
					Douching Pregnancy Contraception	HIV
Structure of cathexis: Social norms and affective attachments	Relationships Family Church	Manifested as constraints in expectations, which produce disparities in norms for women	Social exposures	Personal risk factors		

evolves, these structures remain largely intact at the societal level over a long period of time.

The three social structures are also evident at a lower level, the institutional level (Connell, 1987). Social institutions include schools, work sites and industries, families, relationships, religious institutions, the medical system, and the media. The three structures are maintained within institutions through social mechanisms such as unequal pay for comparable work and discriminatory practices at school and work, in the imbalance of control within relationships and at work sites, and in the stereotypical or degrading images of women in the media. The presence of these and other social mechanisms constrains women's daily lifestyle practices by producing gender-based inequities in women's economic potential, women's control of resources, and gender-based expectations of women's role in society. Institutional changes occur more rapidly than societal changes, but changes at the institutional level are also gradual.

Structure Exposures and Risk Factors

In our adaptation of the Theory of Gender and Power, we postulate that the gender-based inequities and disparities in expectations that arise from each of the three structures generate different exposures and risk factors that influence women's risk for HIV. We define exposures as variables external to women that may influence their sexual risk behavior and, subsequently, their likelihood of being infected with HIV. Several HIV-related exposures are having limited family support, having an abusive male partner, and having less access to preventive health resources such as condoms and drug treatment (Wingood & DiClemente, 2000).

In the social and behavioral sciences, the term *risk factor* is traditionally used to denote any influence that increases the risk for HIV. In our adaptation of the Theory of Gender and Power, this term is reserved specifically to denote individual-level variables that emanate from within women and influence their risk for HIV. Examples are attitudes and beliefs nonsupportive of condom use, limited self-efficacy to use or negotiate condom use, and perceived normative beliefs that do not support maintaining HIV-preventive sexual practices.

Examining the Three Structures: Implications for Designing Interventions

To understand the Theory of Gender and Power, we cannot analyze one structure without also examining the other two because each structure constitutes different risk factors and exposures that increase women's vulnerability for adverse health outcomes. Thus, it is critical to assess the exposures and risk factors of all three structures as they interact to cause an adverse impact on women's health.

It is critical to assess the exposures and risk factors of all three structures as they interact to cause an adverse impact on women's health.

We discuss the three structures in depth and define potential exposures and risk factors generated by each structure (see Figure 12.1). Using HIV as a case study, we then examine for each structure many of the exposures and risk factors that increase women's HIV risk. For each structure, we review several public health HIV interventions aimed at reducing women's HIV risk. Subsequently, we discuss a new addition to the theory: the influence of biological risk factors on women's HIV risk.

The Sexual Division of Labor: Defining the Structure, Exposures, and Risk Factors. A fundamental structure in this theory is the sexual division of labor (Connell, 1987). At the societal level, this refers to the allocation of women and men to

FIGURE 12.1. THE THEORY OF GENDER AND POWER: EXPOSURES, RISK FACTORS, AND BIOLOGICAL PROPERTIES.

Sexual Division of Labor:

Economic Exposures—Women who:	Socioeconomic Risk Factors—Women who:
Live at the poverty level Have less than a high school education Have no employment or are underemployed Have a high demand–low control work environment Have limited or no health insurance Have no permanent home (are homeless)	Are ethnic minorities Are younger (less than eighteen years of age)

Sexual Division of Power:

Physical Exposures—Women who have:	Behavioral Risk Factors—Women who have:
A history of sexual or physical abuse A partner who disapproves of practicing safer sex A high-risk steady partner A greater exposure to sexually explicit media Limited access to HIV prevention (drug treatment, female-controlled methods, school-based HIV prevention education)	A history of alcohol and drug abuse Poor assertive communication skills Poor condom use skills Lower self-efficacy to avoid HIV Limited perceived control over condom use

Structure of Social Norms and Affective Attachments:

Social Exposures—Women who have:	Personal Risk Factors—Women who have:
A partner who is older A desire or whose partner desires to conceive Conservative cultural and gender norms A religious affiliation that forbids the use of contraception A strong mistrust of the medical system Family influences not supportive of HIV prevention	Limited knowledge of HIV prevention Negative beliefs not supportive of safer sex Perceived invulnerability to HIV/AIDS A history of depression or psychological distress

Biological Properties: Anatomical and biomedical properties

HIV is transmitted more efficiently from men to women than from women to men, as women are the receptive partner during sexual intercourse.

STDs, aside from HIV, are also transmitted more efficiently from men to women than from women to men; these STDs can increase women's vulnerability to HIV.

STDs are more asymptomatic in women; thus, women may be less likely to seek treatment for STDs and more likely to develop STD-related complications.

Biological characteristics such as having sex while menstruating, using oral contraceptives, history of cervical ectopy, and having an immature cervix may increase HIV risk among younger women).

certain occupations. Often women are assigned different and unequal positions relative to men. Women are often delegated the responsibility of "women's work," an assignment that constrains women because the nature and organization of this work limit their economic potential and confine their career paths.

At the institutional level, the sexual division of labor is maintained by social mechanisms such as the segregation of unpaid nurturing work for women, namely, child care, caring for the sick and elderly, and housework (Connell, 1987). Because this work is uncompensated, an economic imbalance occurs in which women often have to rely on men financially. Other social mechanisms occurring within the sexual division of labor are practices that favor male educational attainment and the segregation of income-generating work for men, allowing men control of the family income. Although women do participate in the paid labor force, their participation is often less than that of males and remains highly sex segregated. Furthermore, whereas "men's work" is often valued either directly through paid remuneration or indirectly through its high status, "women's work" often fails to be recognized as work and is viewed as lower status.

The inequities resulting from the sexual division of labor are manifested as economic exposures and socioeconomic risk factors. According to the sexual division of labor, as the economic inequity between men and women increases and favors men (making women more dependent on men), women will be at greater risk for HIV. After reviewing the literature examining factors associated with HIV risk and protective practices for women, we have categorized HIV-related economic exposures to include experiencing poverty, having limited or no health insurance, being homeless, and having a stressful work environment. Socioeconomic risk factors (factors emanating from within the individual) include being younger, being an ethnic minority, and having less than a high school education (Wingood & DiClemente, 2000).

The Sexual Division of Power: Defining the Structure, Exposures, and Risk Factors.

Another fundamental structure in this theory is the sexual division of power (Raj et al., 1999). At the societal level, inequalities in power between the sexes form the basis for the sexual division of power. Power has been conceptualized differently by several different disciplines (van Ryn & Heaney, 1997). The social-psychological literature defines it as having the capacity to influence the action of others, conceptualizing power in terms of power over others (Antonovsky, 1988). This ability resides primarily at the interpersonal level and occasionally at the institutional level. The empowerment literature defines power as having the ability to act or to change in a desired direction (Moser & Dracup, 1995). This ability can reside at the individual, interpersonal, institutional, and community level.

Thus, power can be defined as having the power to act or change or having power over others (Antonovsky, 1988; Moser & Dracup, 1995).

At the institutional level, the sexual division of power is maintained by social mechanisms such as the abuse of authority and control in relationships. Women in power-imbalanced relationships tend to depend on their male partner because men usually bring more financial assets (money and status) to the relationship. The sexual division of power is also maintained at the institutional level by social mechanisms such as the media, which disempower women through sexual degradation.

The inequities resulting from the sexual division of power are manifested as physical exposures and behavioral risk factors. As the power inequity between men and women increases and favors men, women's sexual choices and behavior may be constrained, thereby increasing their risk for HIV. After reviewing the literature examining factors associated with HIV risk and protective practices among women, we defined the HIV-related physical exposures as including interpersonal (partner-related) and institutional (media, medical system, work site) factors. Physical exposures include having a sexually abusive, physically abusive, drug-abusing, or high-risk (nonmonogamous) sexual partner; being exposed to sexually explicit media; lacking or having limited access to condoms or drug treatment; and having more occupational stressors. Behavioral risk factors include using alcohol or drugs, being less efficacious in negotiating and using condoms, and perceiving oneself as being powerlessness (Wingood & DiClemente, 2000).

The Structure of Cathexis: Defining the Structure, Exposures, and Risk Factors. The newest structure in this theory is the structure of cathexis (Connell, 1987). To emphasize the affective and normative components of this structure, we refer to this structure henceforth as the structure of affective attachments and social norms. At the societal level, this structure dictates appropriate sexual behavior for women and is characterized by the emotional and sexual attachments that women have with men. This structure constrains the expectations that society has about women with regard to their sexuality, and, as a consequence, it shapes women's perceptions of themselves and others and limits their experiences of reality. This structure also describes how women's sexuality is attached to other social concerns, such as those related to impurity and immorality.

At the institutional level, the structure of social norms and affective attachments is maintained by social mechanisms such as biases people have regarding how women and men should express their sexuality. These biases produce cultural norms, the enforcement of strict gender roles and stereotypical beliefs such as believing that women should have sex only for procreation, creating taboos regarding female sexuality (for example, being labeled as a bad girl for having premarital sex), restraining women's sexuality (being monogamous as opposed to having multiple partners, an accepted norm for men but not women; Fullilove, R. Fullilove, Bowser, Haynes, & Gross, 1990), and believing that women should refrain from touching their own body.

The inequities resulting from the social mechanisms occurring within the structure of social norms and affective attachments are manifested within the field of public health as social exposures and are manifested in the psychosocial domain as personal risk factors (see Figure 12.1). According to the structure of social norms and affective attachments, women who are more accepting of conventional social norms and beliefs will be more likely to experience adverse health outcomes. Therefore, we hypothesize that women who have more social exposures and more personal risk factors will be more burdened by the structure of social norms and affective attachments, compared to women not having these exposures and risk factors, and subsequently, they will experience poorer health outcomes. The social exposures and personal risk factors are conceptualized as variables and constructs, assessed by scales with demonstrated reliability, among diverse female populations.

Social exposures include women who have older partners, an interest or a partner's interest in conceiving children, family influences that are not supportive of HIV prevention, a mistrust of the medical system, conservative cultural and gender norms, and a religious affiliation that forbids the use of contraception. Personal risk factors include having limited knowledge of HIV prevention, negative attitudes and beliefs about condoms, and a history of depression or psychological distress (Wingood & DiClemente, 2000).

Empirical Evidence Supporting the Theory of Gender and Power

The utility of a theory for public health practice and research lies in its utility to explain behavior and guide the development of health-promoting behavior change interventions. Next we review some of the recent empirical findings that provide support for the theory and its constructs.

The Sexual Division of Labor: Exposures and Risk Factors That Influence Women's Risk of HIV

To illustrate how the sexual division of labor influences women's risk of HIV, we consider some of the relevant economic exposures and socioeconomic risk factors. These constructs are shown in Table 12.1.

Living in Poverty as an Economic Exposure. In the United States in the past decade, as poverty rates have increased, case rates of acquired immunodeficiency syndrome (AIDS) have also increased, (Swenson, 1992). The poverty rate is based on a set of income thresholds that vary by family size and composition (U.S. Department of Commerce, 1996). In 1995, the poverty rate among female heads of households in the United States was more than double the poverty rate among male heads of households—32.4 percent versus 14 percent, respectively (Orshansky, 1965). Several studies have demonstrated that having a lower income increases women's exposure to HIV. One notable study, conducted among a random probability sample of 580 women, found that relative to women having higher incomes, women having lower incomes were less likely to use condoms (Peterson et al., 1992). Women living in poverty may not be able to afford HIV prevention materials (condoms), thereby increasing their exposure to HIV.

Being Unemployed or Underemployed as Economic Exposure. The sexual division of labor illustrates how women's vulnerability to HIV should be considered within the context of occupational sex segregation, manifested as the assignment of more women than men to part-time and marginal jobs (Sorensen & Verbrugge, 1987). Women who are underemployed or unemployed may have to rely on their male partners economically. Some women who are economically dependent on their husbands or other male partners have few alternatives but to engage in HIV risk behaviors imposed by these partners. In a study conducted among African American women, compared to women who were employed, women who were receiving Aid to Families with Dependent Children were nearly three and a half times more likely never to use condoms (Wingood & DiClemente, 1998a). A closer examination of women's working environment can elucidate how women's occupations may increase their exposure to HIV.

Working in a High Demand–Low Control Environment as an Economic Exposure. The sexual division of labor is also manifested in women's participation in the paid labor force. The U.S. labor force is 45 percent female, yet it remains highly sex segregated. Women are 99 percent of secretaries but comprise only 19 percent of lawyers, 95 percent of nurses but only 20 percent of physicians, and 97 percent of child care workers (U.S. Department of Labor, 1994). According to Karasek and Theorell's job strain model (1990), jobs can be ranked by the demand or strain exerted on the worker, as well as the level of control that the worker has in the position. Several researchers believe that women's work is characterized by high demands and low control (Hall, 1991). Many studies demonstrate that workers in jobs characterized by high demands and low control report greater depression and anxiety (Karasek & Theorell, 1990; Baker, 1985). One occupation that exemplifies a high demand–low control position is prostitution. Some women, as a result of economic pressures, are forced into prostitution or occasional commercial sex work. Prostitution is not simply a rational choice by women to exchange sexual services for money. It may be better conceived of as an industry that exploits women sexually, forgoing safer-sex concerns for the gain of large financial returns that can be made by sex industry entrepreneurs (Adkins, 1995). Although prostitutes have historically been viewed as vectors of HIV, numerous studies have illustrated their vulnerability to the virus. Several researchers have shown that compared to professional prostitutes, novices are less likely to use condoms (Cohen, 1992). Prostitutes who are novices may be less likely to adopt HIV preventive practices because they may perceive these practices as threatening their opportunities to support themselves financially. Thus, women's work environment should be considered when understanding women's risk of HIV.

Having Limited or No Health Insurance as an Economic Exposure. For many women, health insurance either does not cover important preventive reproductive health services or STD-related services, or it requires copayments and deductibles for these services (Women's Research and Education Institute, 1994; Freeman et al., 1987). Women who are uninsured delay seeking care for health problems longer than women who have private insurance or Medicaid coverage (Schwartz, Colby, & Reisinger, 1991). In addition, although many women do have Medicaid, Medicaid often provides less effective coverage than private insurance since many physicians refuse to treat Medicaid beneficiaries, further restricting access to care. Because untreated STDs can facilitate the transmission of HIV (Wasserheit, 1992), women's limited health insurance or lack of insurance may decrease their access to STD services and potentially increase their exposure to HIV.

Being an Ethnic Minority Woman as a Socioeconomic Risk Factor. In the United States, a disproportionate number of ethnic minority women are living with HIV or AIDS. Among women with AIDS, 55 percent are African American and 21 percent are Hispanic (Centers for Disease Control and Prevention, 1997). One study observed that African American and Latina women were four and three and a half times less likely, respectively, to use condoms compared to white women (Catania et al., 1992). Ethnic minority women's lack of condom use may not simply be attributable to their ethnicity or race but probably is the result of their having to cope with more immediate survival needs, such as the provision of food and shelter for their children (Mays & Cochran, 1988). These needs may be more pronounced among ethnic minority women given that the poverty rates among African Americans and Hispanics are 33 percent and 29 percent, respectively, compared to 11 percent among whites (Williams & Collins, 1995). Thus, ethnic minority women may have fewer economic resources to assist in their HIV prevention efforts.

Being a Younger Woman as a Socioeconomic Risk Factor. Twenty-five percent of new HIV infections in the United States are estimated to occur among those aged thirteen to twenty (Office of National AIDS Policy, 1996). Two young people become infected with HIV every hour of every day; of these, more than one-third are female. In addition, adolescent females have higher STD rates than any other age or gender group (Cates, 1990). Several studies have identified a relationship between age and condom use, with younger woman reporting lower condom use (Upchurch et al., 1992; Fleisher, Senie, Minkoff, & Jaccard, 1994). One explanation may be that compared to older women, younger women often have less power to negotiate condom use and may have less control over the sexual relationship, further increasing their risk of HIV (EDK Associates, 1994).

Having Less Than a High School Education as a Risk Factor. Women's HIV risk behaviors should be considered in the context of educational attainment. In a national probability sample of women seventeen to forty-four years of age, having less than a high school education was associated with being less likely to use condoms (Anderson, Brackbill, & Mosher, 1996). Similar results were observed among women attending an STD clinic (Upchurch et al., 1992). Being less educated may limit women's comprehension of printed HIV prevention materials or restrict their access to HIV prevention programs, decreasing their ability to engage in safer-sex practices (de Bruyn, 1992). Closely related to women's educational level is their employment status.

HIV Interventions for Women Addressing the Sexual Division of Labor. A unique public health intervention that addresses the division of labor was designed to reduce the risk of HIV among women fishmongers by redefining their work environment (O'Reilly, 1993). Women fishmongers were being sexually exploited by male buyers because they had no other outlet to sell their fish and earn an income. To redress the economic pressures to engage in unwanted sex with male buyers, a women's cooperative was initiated that allowed women to bypass male buyers. Women's economic choices were no longer constrained because they were able to develop an alternative buying source.

Another innovative intervention targeting the structure of labor was conducted in rural Tanzania (Grosskurth et al., 1995). This intervention focused on (1) establishing an STD clinic, (2) training clinic staff in the diagnosis and treatment of STDs, (3) ensuring the continuous availability of medications to treat STDs, (4) conducting regularly scheduled visits to health facilities, and (5) providing health education about STD treatment. This study observed a 42 percent reduction in HIV incidence as a result of the intervention. One of the largest impacts was seen in women aged fifteen to twenty-four. The authors concluded that the availability of an aggressive STD screening and treatment intervention played an important part in reducing HIV transmission, particularly among women.

A third intervention that targets the structure of labor, known as the 100 percent condom program, has been pioneered in Phitsanuloke, Thailand (Hanenberg, Rojanapithaykorn, Kunasol, & Sokal, 1993). The key components of this program are the restructuring of women's work environment and improving women's access to STD screening and treatment. The components of this program include (1) requiring commercial sex workers to use condoms with all clients, thus reducing the potential coercion from their male sex partners to engage in high-risk sex; (2) forcing brothel owners to assist commercial sex workers with uncooperative clients, thus providing women with the resources to enforce safer sex laws; (3) monitoring condom use; (4) monitoring compliance with condoms through a regular review of women's gonorrhea rates; and (5) applying graduated sanctions for noncompliance, including closing brothel owners' establishments if repeated violations occur, thus increasing the owner's incentive for maintaining a safer sexual working environment. In the province in which this program was introduced, the STD incidence among sex workers decreased from 13 percent to 0.5 percent.

The structure of labor is not the only force influencing women's susceptibility to HIV. Women's vulnerability to HIV can also be viewed as a reflection of the distribution of physical, social, and economic power, that is, the sexual division of power.

The Sexual Division of Power: Exposures and Risk Factors That Influence Women's Risk of HIV

To illustrate how the sexual division of power influences women's risk of HIV, we consider some of the relevant physical exposures and behavioral risk factors. (These constructs are shown in Table 12.1.)

Having a History of Sexual and Physical Abuse as Physical Exposures. Women's lack of power in heterosexual relationships often translates into constraints on their sexual behavior (Wingood & DiClemente, 1995). The sexual division of power suggests that having a physically abusive partner increases a women's risk for HIV. A study conducted among African American women found that women with physically abusive partners were less likely to use condoms and more likely to experience

verbal abuse, emotional abuse, and threats of physical abuse when they discussed condoms with their male partners relative to women not in abusive relationships (Wingood & DiClemente, 1997). This investigation and a study conducted among Latina women reported that fear of the partner's anger in response to requests to use condoms was an important predictor of noncondom use (Marin, Tschann, Gomez, & Kegeles, 1993).

The act of being raped, as well as being a rape survivor, serves to increase women's vulnerability to HIV directly and indirectly. For many women, sex is often imposed, not voluntary. Although the risk of contracting HIV infection as a result of rape is unknown, cases of HIV infection resulting from rape have been reported (Claydon et al., 1991). In addition, women with a history of rape are less likely to use condoms, are less likely to negotiate condom use, and are more likely to engage in prostitution, increasing their risk for HIV (Wyatt, 1992; Wingood & DiClemente, 1998b). Rape survivors may be less likely to negotiate safer sex, fearing that such assertiveness may provoke a violent attack that threatens them with bodily harm and even threatens their survival.

Having a Steady High-Risk Sexual Partner as a Physical Exposure.
Women's sexual behaviors are highly dependent on the nature of their relationship with their male partner. For example, a number of studies have reported that compared to women who have casual and secondary partners, women who have a steady partner are nearly three to four times more likely never to use condoms, and when condoms are used, they are used less often (Wingood & DiClemente, 1988). Women with steady partners who fail to use condoms may increase their risk of HIV as sexual relationships outside the primary relationship are often not disclosed, particularly when these relationships are between two men. In one study, nearly two-thirds of men who had both male and female partners had not modified their sexual behaviors to protect their female partners from HIV (Weisman, Plichta, Nathanson, Einsminger, & Robinson, 1991). In addition, men who have multiple female sexual partners increase women's HIV risk because they have a greater probability of having sex with a partner who is STD positive and transmitting this infection to a steady female partner (Kalichman, Roffman, Picciano, & Bolan, 1997). Having a steady partner who injects drugs also increases women's HIV risk.

The majority of women who inject drugs have steady sexual partners who are also injecting drug users (Pivnick, Jacobson, Eric, Doll, & Drucker, 1994). A study conducted among women enrolled in methadone treatment reported that more than 50 percent of the women who lived with a steady sexual partner reported that their partner was using drugs. Men are often the initiators of women's drug use, play a role in the progression of their drug use, and are involved in women's drug-related crimes such as prostitution (Amaro, Zuckerman, & Cabral, 1989). Thus, being in a steady relationship with a high-risk sexual partner can increase women's HIV risk.

Viewing Sexually Oriented Media as a Physical Exposure. Women's sexuality can be manipulated through media exposures (D'Emilio & Freedman, 1988). Sexually oriented television shows, movies, music videos, and magazines often illustrate images of women as having to forfeit or at least limit their ability to determine the use of their body with little regard for safer-sex practices. Lowry and Shidler (1993) identified an average of ten references per hour to either an implied or direct sexual behavior on network prime-time television programs. There was only one reference to STD or pregnancy prevention for every twenty-five references to sexual behavior.

In addition to displaying women's lack of control over their sexuality, the media often depict women's value as inherently linked to their sexuality, as either sex objects or mothers, in a manner and to such a degree that men are not portrayed (D'Emilio & Freedman, 1988). These popular cultural prescriptions may subliminally cultivate a norm that women should fulfill the sexual obligations of men and disregard their concerns about safer sex. The media's portrayal of the actual and subliminal control of women's sexuality by men may increase women's vulnerability to HIV. Recently, a study conducted among African American female adolescents reported that nearly 30 percent of adolescents had recently viewed X-rated movies. Those adolescents who were exposed to X-rated movies were 1.4 times more likely to have negative attitudes toward using condoms, twice as likely to have multiple sex partners, 1.8 times more likely to have sex more frequently, more than twice as likely to have not used contraception in the past six months, and 2.3 times as likely to have a strong desire to conceive. Of most concern, exposure to X-rated movies was associated with being 1.7 times more likely to test positive for chlamydia (Wingood et al., 2001).

Having Limited Access to HIV Education, Drug Treatment, and Female Condoms as Physical Exposures. The sexual division of power is manifested by conservative policies that prohibit HIV prevention education and the distribution of condoms in schools. As of September 1995, twenty-two states and the District of Columbia had legal mandates that required schools to provide both sexuality and STD/HIV education, and fifteen states required schools to provide only STD/HIV education; thirteen states did not require schools to provide sexuality or HIV/STD education (National Abortion Rights Action League Foundation, 1995). Although many states require the provision of sexuality or HIV/STD education, this education is often restricted in its content and focuses primarily on abstinence promotion. The efficacy of abstinence-only programs has been questioned (DiClemente, 1998), particularly in the light of recent empirical findings (Jemmott, Jemmott, & Fong, 1998) demonstrating few differences in sexual activity among youth in an abstinence or an HIV prevention program. In the same study, however, youth in the HIV intervention were markedly more likely to use condoms at long-term follow-up. These data illustrate that a restrictive focus on abstinence as opposed to HIV prevention may increase female adolescents' risk of HIV. Unfortunately, recent federal funding supports programs that focus on promoting sexual abstinence (Eng & Butler, 1997).

Conservative drug treatment policies also increase women's HIV risk. Unfortunately, women have had less access to drug treatment programs than their male counterparts (Heimer, Kaplan, O'Keefe, Khoshnood, & Altice, 1994). Drug treatment programs are particularly limited for women who have children and women who may be pregnant (Heimer et al., 1994). Moreover, compared to men, women have less access to needle exchange programs. Given the efficacy of needle exchange programs in preventing HIV (Normand, Vlahov, & Moses, 1995), women's limited access to these programs may further increase their HIV risk.

The limited access that women have to female-controlled barrier methods, such as the female condom, also increases their HIV risk. For many women, the female condom is inaccessible because the cost is prohibitive (Shervington, 1993). Moreover, many women object to using it due to aesthetics, insertion difficulties, reduced sensation, partner objections, and other concerns regarding its acceptability (Shervington, 1993). Women's limited access to HIV education, drug treatment, needle exchange programs, and female-controlled STD/HIV preventive methods, such as the female condom, further increases their vulnerability to HIV.

Having a History of Alcohol and Drug Abuse as Behavioral Risk Factors. In the United States, 45 percent of women acquire HIV from injecting drugs (Centers for Disease Control, 1997). Other drugs can also increase women's risk of HIV. Several studies have reported an association of crack use with an increase in partner exchange, prostitution, poorer condom use, and STDs (R. Fullilove, Fullilove, Bowser, & Gross, 1990). Use of alcohol has also been associated with HIV risk taking and STDs. One study reported that compared to women who were not problem drinkers, women who were problem drinkers were four and a half times more likely to have had an STD (Ericksen & Trocki, 1992).

Several theories attempt to explain the relationship of alcohol and drug use to risky sex. One interpretation is that alcohol and drugs are sexual disinhibitors that may place individuals at risk of becoming infected with HIV through unsafe sex. Another interpretation is that alcohol and drug use may serve as a marker for individuals who practice a constellation of high-risk behaviors. Both explanations stress the effects of alcohol and drug use as influencing high-risk sexual behaviors (Leigh & Stall, 1993).

Limited Self-Efficacy in Negotiating and Using Condoms as Behavioral Risk Factors. Self-efficacy is the confidence one has in the ability to effect change in a specific practice (Bandura, 1994). Having the self-efficacy to communicate and negotiate condom use means having the confidence to bargain for safer sex in the light of the social cost of such negotiations. Women's inability to negotiate condom use is one of the strongest correlates of poor condom use (Wingood & Di-Clemente, 1988; R. Fullilove et al., 1990; Peterson et al., 1992; Catania et al., 1992). Their ability to negotiate safer sex may be particularly difficult when the partner is older (Miller, Clark, & Moore, 1997) or abusive (Wingood & Di-Clemente, 1997), and when women are in committed relationships (Wingood & DiClemente, 1988; R. Fullilove et al., 1990; Peterson et al., 1992). Having low self-efficacy adversely affects a number of HIV prevention strategies. Several studies have reported that women who have low self-efficacy for using condoms, women who were less efficacious about their ability to avoid HIV (Peterson et al., 1992; R. Fullilove et al., 1990), and women who perceived themselves as having less confidence in controlling condom use (Wingood & DiClemente, 1988) are more likely to engage in HIV-related sexual risk taking. Increasing women's self-efficacy in using and negotiating condom use can be an effective HIV prevention approach for women (Exner, Seal, & Ehrhardt, 1997; Wingood & DiClemente, 1996).

HIV Interventions for Women Addressing the Structure of Power. HIV prevention programs addressing the structure of power may include enforcement of legal statutes prosecuting perpetrators of violence against women, banning pornography, and developing HIV prevention social marketing programs. In Zaire, a television miniseries employed soap opera stars as role models to enhance the status of women and promote safer sex (Ferreros, Mivumbi, Kakera, & Price, 1990). The miniseries was seen by two-thirds of the young couples targeted and included a dramatic bedroom scene in which the partners negotiated condom use. This condom marketing and mass media campaign increased the number of condoms sold by 443 percent from 1988 to 1989. In a study of fifteen hundred people in a region of Zaire, the proportion of respondents who said they practiced mutual fidelity increased from 28.9 percent to 45.7 percent following introduction of the program.

Another intervention that targets the structure of power focuses on strengthening women's control over their sexuality by increasing the acceptability and accessibility of the female condom. To date, there have been no studies on the efficacy of the female condom in reducing HIV infection among women. However, an efficacy study has been conducted among women diagnosed with another STD, vaginal trichomoniasis (Soper et al., 1993). In this study, rates of reinfection of vaginal trichomoniasis were 15 percent, 14 percent, and 0 percent, respectively, among women who never, inconsistently, and consistently (during every intercourse occasion) used the female condom. This study illustrates that making the female condom acceptable and accessible and using the female condom consistently can have a protective effect against the recurrence of a highly prevalent STD, vaginal trichomoniasis. Given that untreated STDs can facilitate the transmission of HIV (Terrell & Terrell, 1995), this study has potentially important implications for the prevention of HIV.

A third intervention that targets the structure of power is an HIV prevention program conducted among incarcerated women. This study compared interventions driven by two different theories: Social Cognitive Theory and the Theory of Gender and Power (St. Lawrence et al., 1997). The Gender and Power intervention focused on fostered discussion of HIV prevention for women but did not provide modeling or practice, while the Social Cognitive Theory intervention provided modeling of condom use and negotiation skills. At six-months follow-up, both interventions produced increased self-efficacy and self-esteem, fostered attitudes supportive of condom use, and increased AIDS knowledge, communication, and condom application skills. Participants in the intervention based on Social Cognitive Theory showed greater improvement in condom application skills, and women in the program based on the Theory of Gender and Power evidenced greater commitment to change. It is of considerable interest that the intervention based on the Theory of Gender and Power was equally effective in changing behavior compared to the skills-based intervention, although presumably by different mechanisms (fostering self-empowerment). Although these programs are effective in enhancing women' practice of safer sex, for women to have true equality in protecting themselves from unsafe sex, societal norms and practices structured to preserve male power and regulate female sexuality will have to change. Closely bound up with the division of power is the structure of affective attachments and social norms.

For women to have true equality in protecting themselves from unsafe sex, societal norms and practices structured to preserve male power and regulate female sexuality will have to change.

The Structure of Affective Attachments and Social Norms: Exposures and Risk Factors That Influence Women's Risk of HIV

To illustrate how affective attachments and social norms influence women's risk of HIV, we consider some of the relevant social and affective exposures and personal risk factors. (These constructs are shown in Table 12.1.)

Having a Relationship with an Older Male Partner as a Social Exposure. The structure of social norms and affective attachments manifests itself in the sexual and emotional connections that we feel toward other people, including those involved with sexual desire, sexual attraction, and sexual arousal. This structure is manifest in stereotypes—for example, men are more sexually attracted to younger women and younger women are more attracted to older men (Rienzo, 1985). Congruent with this belief is the finding from one study reporting that adolescent females were less likely to use condoms with older heterosexual male partners than with same-age male partners (Miller et al., 1997). Furthermore, female adolescents are less likely to use condoms if they are more attracted to their partner (Sheer & Cline, 1994). These studies illustrate how safer-sex practices may be influenced by the sexual attraction that partners have for one another, as well as the imbalances of power in relationships.

Family Influences as Social Exposures. Family values, whether they emphasize a more individualistic approach, as is prevalent among European Americans, or cooperation and interdependence, as is prevalent among ethnic minority families, are often viewed as protective factors in health (Chapman-Walsh, 1995). Two studies conducted by our research team address some of these familial influences on adolescent females' sexual health. In the first study, we examined associations between parent-adolescent communication about sex-related topics and African American adolescent females' sex-related communication and practices with partners, as well as their perceived ability to negotiate safer sex.

A theory-guided survey and structured interview were administered to 522 sexually active African American females (fourteen to eighteen years old) recruited from neighborhoods with high rates of unemployment, substance abuse, violence and STDs. Analyses, which controlled for observed covariates, identified less frequent parent-adolescent communication as being associated with nonuse of contraceptives in the past six months and nonuse of contraceptives during the past five sexual episodes (DiClemente et al., 2001c). Less frequent parent-adolescent communication also increased the odds of never using condoms in the past month, during the past five sexual episodes, and at last intercourse. Less frequent parent-adolescent communication was also associated with less communication between adolescents and their male sex partners and lower self-efficacy to negotiate safer sex.

In another report, we examined the influence of less perceived parental monitoring on a spectrum of adolescent health-compromising behaviors and outcomes (DiClemente, Wingood, Crosby, Sionean, Cobb, Harrington, et al. 2001b). In logistic regression analyses, controlling for observed covariates, adolescents perceiving less parental monitoring were 1.7 times more likely to test positive for an

STD, 1.7 times more likely to report not using a condom at last sexual intercourse, twice as likely to have multiple sexual partners, 1.5 times as likely to have risky (nonmonogamous) sex partners, 3 times as likely to have a new sex partner in the past thirty days, and almost twice as likely not to use any contraception during the last sexual intercourse episodes. Furthermore, adolescents perceiving less parental monitoring were more likely to have a history of marijuana use and use marijuana more often in the past thirty days, a history of alcohol use and greater alcohol consumption in the past thirty days, and a history of arrest. There was also a trend toward having engaged in fights in the past six months.

Overall, the findings from these two studies demonstrate a consistent pattern of health risk behaviors and adverse biological outcomes associated with less perceived parental monitoring and less parent-adolescent communication about sex. The findings demonstrate the importance of involving parents in HIV/STD and pregnancy prevention efforts directed at female adolescents. Further research needs to focus on developing theoretical models that help explain the influence of familial environment on adolescent health and developing and evaluating interventions to promote the health of adolescents.

Conversely, family influences may also increase women's sexual risk. Early initiation of sexual intercourse among adolescents is associated with having a single-parent family (Newcomer & Udry, 1987), having parents with lower educational attainment (Udry & Billy, 1987), and having parents who were either too strict or too permissive (Miller, McCoy, Olson, & Wallace, 1986). HIV-related risk taking is also associated with familial relationships (Amaro et al., 1989). In a study of women enrolled in methadone treatment, drug use and HIV permeated household relationships. Nearly one-third of the study participants' siblings were drug users, and 70 percent of women stated that at least one of their siblings also used drugs. Women who have family networks in which HIV risk taking occurs may be more vulnerable to HIV.

Mistrust of the Medical System as a Social Exposure. Fueled by the legacy of the Tuskegee syphilis study, the African American community has had a long history of distrusting the public health system (Thomas & Quinn, 1991). In addition, many women of color have apprehensions about the public health system, since the medical establishment has had a history of sterilizing African American, Native American, and Hispanic women without their knowledge or consent (Davis, 1981). Thus, women of color may be less inclined to seek traditional health care and may prefer more culturally sanctioned approaches.

This mistrust of the medical system may motivate women to rely on alternative practices that may in fact increase their exposure to HIV. Douching, a traditional practice used to cleanse the vagina, is prevalent among African American women, particularly those living in the South (Snow, 1983; Aral, Mosher, & Cates, 1992). Many African American women believe that douching is an effective contraceptive practice. Unfortunately, douching may be associated with increased risk of STDs (Wølner-Hanssen et al., 1990).

Conservative Gender and Cultural Norms and Traditional Beliefs as Social Exposures.

Several studies have shown that women who adhere to traditional norms are more likely to engage in behaviors that increase their risk of HIV. One study reported that adolescent females who believed that there is a double standard between how young men and women should act were less likely to practice safer sex (Moore & Rosenthal, 1992). In another study, women who believed that asking a sex partner to use condoms implied that he was unfaithful were four times more likely never to use condoms compared to women who did not believe that asking a sex partner to use condoms implied infidelity (Centers for Disease Control, 1997). These gender norms interact with cultural norms to increase ethnic minority women's HIV risk.

It has been suggested that African American women may be less likely to negotiate safer sex given the African American community's sex ratio imbalance, defined as the existence of fewer economically self-sufficient and available men compared to women (Guttentag & Secord, 1993). The sex ratio for the American population as a whole is 0.95, indicating a slight excess of women. In contrast, the sex ratio of men to women among African American, white, and Latina women living below the poverty level is 0.69, 0.73, and 0.84, respectively (U.S. Department of Commerce, 1996). Such gender imbalances afford men greater opportunity to have multiple female partners. As such, the sex ratio imbalance is associated with high STD rates (Aral & Wasserheit, 1995) and may be associated with increased risk of HIV among women.

Adherence to conservative religious values among ethnic minority women also serves to increase their HIV risk. Religious institutions serve as a foundation for community values and norms, which are often culturally determined and socially sanctioned. For example, among Latin Americans, Catholicism is the predominant religion, and Catholics forbid the use of birth control (Marin, 1989). The social identity and acceptability of Latina women is often culturally determined by their fertility, and this may account for the poorer contraceptive use among Latina women compared with white women (Marin et al., 1993). Furthermore, among Latina women, having unprotected anal sex may be considered an effective contraceptive strategy and a viable way to preserve their virginity. Regrettably, this practice increases the risk of HIV. Another study was conducted among three hundred Muslim women living in Kuwait. Muslims also forbid the use of contraception. In this study, only 1 percent of women reported that they were currently using condoms (Al-Gallaf, Al-Wazzan, Al-Namash, Shah, & Bahbehani, 1995). Gender-based rules, cultural norms, and religious institutions may instill expectations in ethnic minority women that constrain their options, thereby increasing ethnic minority women's vulnerability to HIV.

Limited HIV Knowledge, Negative Beliefs About Condom Use, and Lower Perceived Risks for HIV as Personal Risk Factors. The structure of affective attachments and social norms is further manifested in the limited knowledge that women have regarding the protective effect that condoms have on sex, which may increase their risk for HIV. A number of investigations have shown that women who are less knowledgeable about HIV prevention are also less likely to engage in HIV prevention activities (Nyamathi, Bennett, Leake, Lewis, & Flaskerud, 1993). In addition, women harbor many beliefs associated with not using condoms—for example, believing that condoms have a negative impact on sexual enjoyment (Peterson et al., 1992; Catania et al., 1992), feeling that using condoms during sex is embarrassing (Peterson et al., 1992), and having limited beliefs in the efficacy of condoms (Helweg-Larson & Collins, 1994). In one study, Latina women who did not use condoms did not perceive themselves as being at risk of HIV/STDs (Ramirez-Valles, Zimmerman, & Newcomb, 1998). Increasing women's knowledge about HIV, reducing their negative beliefs about condoms, and decreasing their perceived invulnerability toward HIV are effective HIV prevention efforts for women (Wingood & DiClemente, 1996).

Having a Desire to Conceive as a Personal Risk Factor. The structure of social norms and affective attachments is clearly related to the desire to conceive. To date, there is no method for women to protect themselves from HIV if they desire to bear a child. Although it is important to stress using condoms for both pregnancy and HIV prevention, the desire to become pregnant will, of necessity, undermine conscientious use of condoms. Moreover, in African American and Latin cultures, the status of motherhood is highly valued, and the procreational value of sex is synonymous with motherhood (Marin, 1989). One study conducted among African American women has shown that compared to women who did not desire children, women who wished to conceive were nearly 8.5 times less likely to use condoms (Wingood & DiClemente, 1988). Research is needed to develop a technology that will allow women to bear children without the threat of HIV.

Depression as a Personal Risk Factor. Women are at high risk of depression during the same years when they are at high risk of acquiring HIV. Prior research has shown that among women, the highest risk of depression occurs from twenty-five to forty-five years of age (Weissman, 1987). One study reported that women between the ages of twenty-five and forty-five who reported a high number of depressive symptoms, as measured by the Center for Epidemiology Depression (CES-D) scale, were more likely to engage in HIV risk taking (Orr, Celentano, Santelli, & Burwell, 1994). Another study reported that women experiencing significant psychological distress were also less likely to use condoms (Kennedy et al., 1993). One study by our team directly addressed this issue.

We prospectively examined the association between adolescents' psychological distress and their STD/HIV-associated sexual behaviors and attitudes using an abbreviated version of the CES-D (alpha = .84). (DiClemente, Wingood, et al., 2001c). In multivariate analyses and controlling for observed covariates, adolescents with significant distress at baseline were, at six-month follow-up, 2.1 times more likely to be pregnant, 1.9 times more likely to have had unprotected vaginal sex, 1.7 times more likely to have nonmonogamous male sex partners, and 1.5 times more likely not to use any form of contraception. In addition, they were 2.2 times more likely to perceive more barriers to condom use and twice as likely to be fearful of the adverse consequences of negotiating condom use, twice as likely to perceive less control in their relationship, 2.4 times as likely to have experienced dating violence, and twice as likely to have norms nonsupportive of a healthy sexual relationship. These findings suggest that mental health factors can influence women's HIV risk behaviors.

HIV Interventions for Women Addressing the Structure of Social Norms and Affective Attachments. The structure of social norms and affective attachments informs us that women might be better served by a closer examination of the role that male partners can play in influencing women's risk of HIV infection. One strategy that recognizes males' power moves beyond gender-segregated prevention efforts and focuses on couples. Although little research has been conducted on the effectiveness of HIV primary prevention programs for heterosexual couples, substantial risk reduction has been achieved in counseling and testing programs involving serodiscordant couples, that is, couples in which one partner is HIV infected and the other is HIV negative. Following couple and group counseling with serodiscordant couples residing in Kigali, Rwanda, condom use increased from 3 percent at baseline to 57 percent at one-year follow-up (Kamenga et al., 1991).

In addition to couples interventions, several scientists funded by the National Institutes of Health are now testing the efficacy of family-based HIV interventions. One such study is intervening with both the mother and daughter (DiIorio et al., 2000), and another is intervening with both the mother and son (Jemmott et al., 2000). These interventions are designed to reduce the families' HIV risk practices.

Biological Factors Increasing Women's Susceptibility to Sexually Transmitted HIV. A theoretically innovative contribution to the Theory of Gender and Power is the specification of gender-specific biological processes or anatomical differences that may influence women's risk for HIV. Although the theory comprises structures and their respective exposures and risk factors, the biological processes represent a separate domain of influence, beyond the structures (see Table 12.1).

Compared to men, women are biologically more likely to become infected if they are exposed to a sexually transmitted pathogen. Biologically, women are at greater risk for HIV because they are the receptive sexual partner in heterosexual intercourse. The risk of acquiring HIV from a single act of intercourse is at least eight times higher from men to women than from women to men (Padian et al., 1987; De Vincenzi, 1994). Also, several female-specific biologic characteristics may increase the efficiency of heterosexual HIV transmission. Although limited research has been conducted in these areas, gender-specific biologic characteristics that may increase women's HIV risk include having sex during menstruation, using oral contraceptives, and cervical ectopy (Clemetson et al., 1993). Moreover, as discussed earlier, douching, a hygienic practice that many African American women use, alters the biological ecology of a woman's vagina by reducing the bacteria that protect against genital pathogens, which may increase women's susceptibility to STDs, including HIV (Snow, 1983; Aral et al., 1992). Further research is needed to examine gender-specific factors that may increase women's HIV risk and how these factors may interact with risk factors and exposures that also serve to increase women's vulnerability to HIV.

Case Application of the Theory of Gender and Power: HIV Infection Among Women

Using the case of HIV prevention for women to examine the application of the Theory of Gender and Power is appealing for several reasons. First, AIDS is the fourth leading cause of death among women and men between the ages of twenty-five and forty-four (Centers for Disease Control, 1993). Second, in the United States between 1991 and 1995, the number of women between ages eighteen and forty-four with AIDS increased by 63 percent, more than any other group, making women the fastest-growing sector of people with AIDS (Wortley & Fleming, 1997). Globally, women account for 40 percent of the estimated 30.6 million adults infected with HIV. Third, HIV and AIDS affect not just younger women; 14 percent of women with AIDS in the United States are over 45.3 years old (Centers for Disease Control, 1997). Fourth, because women infected with HIV are the primary source of infection for infants, preventing the spread of HIV infection in women will reduce vertical transmission (Ehrhardt, 1992). Fifth, at the National Institutes of Health Consensus Development Conference on Interventions to Prevent HIV Risk Behaviors, the panel reported that it is essential to continue developing multilevel interventions to reduce HIV among women (National Institutes of Health, 1997).

Two published reports have reviewed HIV sexual risk-reduction interventions for at-risk women from the beginning of the AIDS epidemic. One study, published in 1997 by Exner et al., reviewed all interventions that were conducted in the United States, Canada, and Puerto Rico. The other study, published in 1996 by Wingood and DiClemente (1996), focused on randomized controlled HIV prevention interventions that were conducted in the United States. Both reviews suggest that the most efficacious HIV prevention programs for women (1) are guided by social psychological theories; (2) include only women; (3) emphasize gender-related influences, such as gender-based power imbalances and sexual assertiveness; (4) are peer led; and (5) require multiple sessions. Both reviews suggest that future research needs to address the environmental conditions impeding women's ability to protect themselves against HIV. Thus, theories such as the Theory of Gender and Power are quite applicable because they can address these environmental constraints that are so prevalent and prominent in the lives of women.

This case study shows how we designed an HIV prevention program for African American women using the Theory of Gender and Power (DiClemente & Wingood, 1995). Because this intervention was designed for African American women, the topic of HIV prevention was contextualized within a framework that addressed African American cultural pride, gender awareness, and values prioritized by African American women. Women in the HIV intervention received five two-hour weekly group sessions implemented by two African American women peer health educators. The five-session HIV sexual risk-reduction program is known as SISTA (Sisters Informing Sisters About Topics on AIDS). The acronym SISTA was chosen because it represents the sisterhood that African American women share with one another.

The project motto—"SISTA love is strong. SISTA love is safe. SISTA love is surviving."—was also designed to be culturally appropriate for young African American women. "SISTA love is strong" is reflective of the strong pride and dignity that African American women possess. "SISTA love is safe" refers to the desire to create a norm of safer sex and the establishment of safer relationships. "SISTA love is surviving" refers to the legacy of African American women surviving through hardship. Woven throughout the entire intervention are issues that personally address African American young women when attempting to protect themselves from HIV infection. The intervention addresses barriers that African American women face when practicing or attempting to practice safer sex.

Furthermore, the intervention discussed those aspects of the African American culture that act as facilitators and may make practicing safer sex more of a norm for this population. HIV prevention activities and structural factors were incorporated into the intervention to enhance its appropriateness for young African American women. Financial constraints are prevalent with this population; thus, bus tokens were provided to all participants, and child care was available on-site for all women needing this service. Before each session, participants read and discussed a poem by an African American female artist that related to the theme of that particular session. And each session was tailored to be culturally relevant for young African American women.

The first session emphasized gender and ethnic pride. Prior to imparting risk-reduction knowledge, skills, and norms onto women, we listened to the women talk about their lives, their goals, and their dreams and had them assert their self-worth. We felt that it was essential for the participants to build their self-esteem and personal self-confidence before discussing issues related to sexuality and HIV. This process allowed us to embed the values of young African American women within the HIV prevention messages and vignettes. During this session, the women discussed the positive attributes of being an African American woman, identified personal African American women role models, and engaged in values clarification exercises. At the end of this session, the participants framed postcards designed by African American female artists, and the peer and health educators discussed how these artists served as positive role models for African American women.

The second session emphasized HIV risk-reduction information by increasing participants' knowledge about HIV-associated risk behaviors and preventive strategies. To increase their perceived risk of HIV, the session also discussed how the HIV epidemic disproportionately affects African American women compared with white women. Participants viewed and discussed an HIV educational video, *AIDS: Me and My Baby,* that encouraged women to take responsibility for sexual decision making. This session also emphasized staying safe not only for oneself but also for one's children and family, because unity and family values are highly prioritized by many African Americans. This session discussed the social relations that place African American women at greater risk for acquiring HIV. During this activity, the women discussed the consequences of having a sexual partner who injected drugs or had been in jail and may have had sex with other men.

The third session emphasized sexual assertiveness and communication training. Participants were first taught the difference between and the consequences of being assertive, passive, and aggressive in a relationship. The women were taught to distinguish between these communication styles in nonsexual vignettes using scenarios common to African American women. For example, one nonsexual scenario modeled how a young African American women assertively communicated to her beautician the need to restyle her hair braids prior to leaving the salon such that they appeared more attractive. Women were then taught an assertiveness model to assist them in managing risky sexual situations. The assertiveness model known as the SISTAS Assertiveness Model had six steps: including, thinking of one's *self* first, using the *information* they gained to practice safer sex, assessing the *situation*, stating the *trouble* to their partner, informing the partner of their concern in an *assertive* manner, and *suggesting* alternatives that both partners can be comfortable with if safer sex is not an option. Subsequent to learning the SISTAS Assertiveness Model, the women applied the model to assist them in negotiating the safer-sex vignettes. All exercises modeled by the peer health educators were role-played by participants in several practice situations, with the peer health educators providing corrective feedback.

The fourth session emphasized enhancing proper condom use skills and fostering positive norms toward consistent condom use. The health educator first sought to dispel many of the myths and misconceptions that many African American women have regarding condoms and their use. Then the peer educators conducted condom use demonstrations with African American phallic replicas. The condom application skills were subsequently role-played by participants. Norm-setting exercises focused on establishing the perception of consistent condom use as becoming more normative with young adult African American males and females.

The fifth session emphasized coping skills. During this session, the health educator defined coping and discussed adaptive and maladaptive coping styles. The vignettes focused on refining women's assertiveness skills to avoid sex when under the influence of alcohol, if a condom was not accessible, or if one's sexual partner was abusive. At the end of this session, the participants read a poem or story that illustrated how they had grown as African American women from the SISTA project. At the end of the fifth session, women received a certificate of empowerment, signed by the project director congratulating the women on their achievement.

Evaluation of the SISTA intervention revealed that participants in the social skills intervention, compared to the control condition, were twice as likely to practice consistent condom use, nearly twice as likely to have greater sexual self-control, four times as likely to engage in sexual communication, nearly twice as likely to be sexually assertive, and twice as likely to have a sex partner whose norms were supportive of consistent condom use (DiClemente & Wingood, 1995).

Since 1999, the Centers for Disease Control and Prevention has included the SISTA Program in its *Compendium of HIV Prevention Interventions with Evidence of*

Effectiveness (Centers for Disease Control and Prevention, 1999). Nationally, community-based organizations interested in implementing HIV prevention programs for African American women have adopted the SISTA program.

Strengths, Limitations, and Future Directions

Applying the Theory of Gender and Power to understand the influences that affect women's health can be challenging. Social structures are often abstract and difficult to operationalize, and they do not take into account variations across different cultures. Moreover, when applying the Theory of Gender and Power, it can be difficult to isolate and quantify the influence of a particular social structure on women's health. Furthermore, the social structures are so deeply rooted in our culture and so routinely taken for granted that they often go unnoticed. In some ways, these situations make it difficult to test the model empirically. This is the primary reason that it is difficult to construct a cogent empirical case that patriarchy is damaging to women's health.

Notwithstanding these caveats, using the Theory of Gender and Power to understand women's health specifies a range of gender-based exposures and risk factors for examining women's risk of disease. Employing the Theory of Gender and Power marshals new kinds of data, asks new and broader questions regarding women's health, and creates new options for prevention. Focusing on the social construction of health encourages designing, implementing, and evaluating larger social interventions. Women's social risk for disease can be addressed through a variety of public health strategies, from education to policy. Interventions for women are destined to be less than optimally effective if they ignore the social environment. Similarly, strategies that lack practical programs for social change seem equally shortsighted and, in the long run, futile. Social structural theories such as Theory of Gender and Power can help to chart a course between the two extremes (Chapman-Walsh, 1995).

References

Adkins, L. (1995). *Gendered work*. Bristol, PA: Open University Press.

Al-Gallaf, K., Al-Wazzan, H., Al-Namash, H., Shah, N. M., & Bahbehani, J. (1995). Ethnic differences in contraceptive use in Kuwait: A clinic-based study. *Social Science and Medicine, 41*, 1023–1031.

Amaro, H., Zuckerman, B., & Cabral, H. (1989). Drug use among adolescent mothers: Profile of risk. *Pediatrics, 84,* 144–151.

Anderson, J. E., Brackbill, R., & Mosher, W. D. (1996). Condom use for disease prevention among unmarried U.S. women. *Family Planning Perspectives, 28,* 25–28.

Antonovsky, A. (1988). *Unravelling the mystery of health.* San Francisco: Jossey-Bass.

Aral, S. O., Mosher, W. D., & Cates, W. (1992). Vaginal douching among women of reproductive age in the United States: 1988. *American Journal of Public Health, 82,* 210–214.

Aral, S. O., & Wasserheit, J. N. (1995). Interactions among HIV, other sexually transmitted diseases, socioeconomic status, and poverty in women. In A. O'Leary & L. S. Jemmott (Eds.), *Women at risk* (pp. 13–41). New York: Plenum.

Baker, D. (1985). The study of stress at work. Annual Review of Public Health, 6, 367–381.

Bandura, A. (1994). Social Cognitive Theory and exercise of control over HIV Infection. In R. J. DiClemente & J. Peterson (Eds.), *Preventing AIDS: Theories and methods of behavioral interventions* (pp. 25–59). New York: Plenum.

Catania, J. A., Coates, T. J., Kegeles, S., Fullilove, M. T., Peterson, J., Marin, B., Siegel, D., & Hulley S. (1992, February). Condom use in multi-ethnic neighborhoods of San Francisco: The population-based AMEN (AIDS in Multi-Ethnic Neighborhoods) study. *American Journal of Public Health, 82*(2), 284–287.

Cates, W. (1990). Epidemiology and control of sexually transmitted diseases in adolescents. In M. Schydlower & M. A. Shafer (Eds.), *AIDS and other sexually transmitted diseases* (pp. 409–427). Philadelphia: Hanly & Belfus.

Centers for Disease Control and Prevention. (1993). *Facts about women and HIV/AIDS, October, 1993.* Atlanta, GA: Author.

Centers for Disease Control and Prevention. (1997). *HIV/AIDS surveillance report: Year-end edition, 1997.* Atlanta, GA: Author.

Chapman-Walsh, D. (1995). Gender, health and cigarette smoking. In B. C. Amick, S. Levine, A. R. Tarlov, & D. Chapman-Walsh (Eds.), *Society and health* (pp. 131–171). New York: Oxford University Press.

Claydon, E., Murphy, S., Osborne, E. M., Kitchen, V., Smith, J. R., & Harris, J. R. (1991). Rape and HIV. *International Journal of STD and AIDS, 2,* 200–201.

Clemetson, D. B., Moss, G. B., Willerford, D. M., Hensel, M., Emonyi, W., Holmes, K. D., Plummer, F., Ndinya-Achola, J., Roberts, P. L., & Hillier, S. (1993). Detection of HIV DNA in cervical and vaginal secretions: Prevalence and correlates among women in Nairobi, Kenya. *JAMA, 269,* 2860–2864.

Cohen, J. (1992, July). Different types of prostitution show wide variation in HIV and other sexually-transmitted disease risk. Paper presented at the Eighth International Conference on AIDS, Amsterdam.

Connell, R. W. (1987). *Gender and power.* Stanford, CA: Stanford University Press.

Davis, A. Y. (1981). Women, race and class. New York: Random House.

de Beauvoir, S. (1974). *The second sex.* New York: Vintage Books.

de Bruyn, M. (1992). Women and AIDS in developing countries. *Social Science and Medicine, 34,* 249–262.

De Vincenzi, I. (1994). A longitudinal study of human immunodeficiency virus transmission by heterosexual partners. European Study Group on Heterosexual Transmission of HIV. *New England Journal of Medicine, 331,* 341–346.

D'Emilio, J., & Freedman, E. B. (1988). *Intimate matters: A history of sexuality in America.* New York: HarperCollins.

DiClemente, R. J. (1998). Preventing sexually transmitted infections among adolescents: A clash of ideology and science. *JAMA, 279,* 1574–1575.

DiClemente, R. J., & Wingood, G. M. (1995) A randomized controlled trial of an HIV sexual risk-reduction intervention for young adult African American women. *JAMA, 274,* 1271–1276.

DiClemente, R. J., Wingood, G. M., Crosby, R., Sionean, C., Brown, L., Rothbaum, B., Zimand, E., Cobb, B. K., Harrington, K., & Davies, S. (2001a). A prospective study of psychological distress and sexual risk behavior among African American adolescent females. *Pediatrics, 108*(5), 1–6.

DiClemente, R. J., Wingood, G. M., Crosby, R., Sionean, C., Cobb, B. K., Harrington, K., Davies, S., Hook, E. W., III, & Oh, M. K. (2001b). Parental monitoring: Association with adolescents' risk behaviors. *Pediatrics, 107*(6), 1363–1368.

DiClemente, R. J., Wingood, G. M., Crosby, R., Sionean, C., Cobb, B. K., Harrington, K., Davies, S., Oh, M. K., & Hook, E. W., III (2001c). Parent-adolescent communication and sexual risk behaviors among African American adolescent females. *Journal of Pediatrics, 139*(3), 407–412

DiIorio, C., Resnicow, K., Denzmore, P., Rogers-Tilman, G., Wang, D. T., Dudley, W. N., Lipana, J., & Fisher Van Marter, D. (2000). Keepin' It R.E.A.L.! A mother-adolescent HIV prevention program. In W. Pequegnat & J. Szapocznik (Eds.), *Working with families in the era of HIV/AIDS* (pp. 113–132). Thousand Oaks, CA: Sage.

EDK Associates. (1994). *Women and sexually transmitted diseases: The dangers of denial.* New York: EDK Associates.

Ehrhardt, A. A. (1992). Trends in sexual behavior and the HIV pandemic. *American Journal of Public Health, 82,* 1459–1461.

Eng, T. R., & Butler, W. T. (Eds.). (1997). *The hidden epidemic: Confronting sexually transmitted diseases.* Washington, DC: National Academy Press.

Ericksen, K. P., & Trocki, K. F. (1992). Behavioral risk factors for sexually transmitted diseases in American households. *Social Science and Medicine, 34,* 843–853.

Exner, T. M., Seal, D. W., & Ehrhardt, A. A. (1997). A review of HIV interventions for at-risk women. *AIDS and Behavior, 1,* 93–124.

Ferreros, C., Mivumbi, N., Kakera, K., & Price J. (1990, June). Social marketing of condoms for AIDS prevention in developing countries: The Zaire experience. Paper presented at the Sixth International Conference on AIDS, San Francisco.

Fleisher, J. M., Senie, R., Minkoff, H., & Jaccard, J. (1994). Condom use relative to knowledge of sexually transmitted disease prevention, method of birth control, and past or present infection. *Journal of Community Health, 19,* 395–407.

Freeman, H. E., Blendon, R. J., Aiken, L. H., Sudman, S., Mullinix, C. F., & Corey, C. R. (1987). Americans report on their access to health care. *Health Affairs Millwood, 6,* 6–18.

Fullilove, M. T., Fullilove, R., Bowser, B. P., Haynes, K., & Gross, S. A. (1990). Black women and AIDS: Gender rules. *Journal of Sex Research, 27,* 47–64.

Fullilove, R. E., Fullilove, M. T., Bowser, B. P., & Gross, S. A. (1990). Risk of sexually transmitted disease among black adolescent crack users in Oakland and San Francisco, California. *JAMA, 263,* 851–855.

Gilman, C. P. (1971). *The man-made world; or, our androcentric culture* (pp. 20–22). New York: Johnson Reprint. (Original work published 1911)

Grosskurth, H., Mosha, F., Todd, J., Mwijaubi, E., Klokke, A., Senkoro, K., Mayaud, P., Changalucha, J., Nicoll, A., ka-Gina, G., Newell, J., Mugeye, K., Mabey, D., & Hayes, R.

(1995). Impact of improved treatment of sexually transmitted disease on HIV infection in rural Tanzania: Randomized controlled trial. *Lancet, 346*(8974), 530–536.

Guttentag, M., & Secord, P. F. (1993). *Too many women?* Thousand Oaks, CA: Sage.

Hall, E. (1991). Gender, work control and stress. A theoretical discussion and an empirical test. In J. V. Johnson & G. Johansson (Eds.), *The psychosocial work environment: Work organization, democratization and health* (pp. 89–108). Amityville, NY: Baywood.

Hanenberg, R., Rojanapithaykorn, W., Kunasol, P., & Sokal, D. (1993). Impact of Thailand's HIV-control programme as indicated by the decline of sexually transmitted diseases. *Lancet, 344,* 243–245.

Heimer, R., Kaplan, E. H., O'Keefe, E., Khoshnood, K., & Altice, F. (1994). Three years of needle exchange in New Haven: What have we learned? *AIDS and Public Policy Journal, 9,* 59–74.

Helweg-Larson, M., & Collins, B. E. (1994). The UCLA multidimensional condom attitudes scale: Documenting the complex determinants of condom use in college students. *Health Psychology, 13,* 224–237.

Jemmott, J. B., Jemmott, L. S., & Fong, G. T. (1998). Abstinence and safer sex HIV risk-reduction interventions for African American adolescents: A randomized controlled trial. *JAMA, 279,* 1529–1536.

Jemmott, L. S., Outlaw, F. H., Jemmott, J. B., Brown, E. J., Howard, M., & Hopkins, B. (2000). Strengthening the bond: The Mother-Son Health Promotion Project. In W. Pequegnat & J. Szapocznik (Eds.), *Working with families in the era of HIV/AIDS* (pp. 133–154). Thousand Oaks, CA: Sage.

Kalichman, S. C., Roffman, R. A., Picciano, J. F., & Bolan, M. (1997). Continued high-risk sex among HIV-seropositive gay and bisexual men seeking HIV prevention services. *Health Psychology, 16,* 369–373.

Kamenga, M., Ryder, R. W., Jingu, M., Mbuyi, N., Mbu, L., Behets, F., Brown, C., & Heyward, W. L. (1991). Evidence of marked sexual behavior change associated with low HIV-1 seroconversion in 149 married couples with discordant HIV-1 serostatus: Experience at an HIV counseling center in Zaire. *AIDS, 5*(1), 61–67.

Karasek, R., & Theorell, T. (1990). *Healthy work: Stress, productivity, and the reconstruction of working life.* New York: Basic Books.

Kennedy, C. A., Skurnick, J., Wan, J. Y., Quattrone, G., Sheffet, A., Quinones, M., Wang, W., & Louria, D. B. (1993). Psychological distress, drug and alcohol use as correlates of condom use in HIV-serodiscordant heterosexual couples. *AIDS, 7,* 1493–1499.

Leigh, B. C., & Stall, R. (1993). Substance use and risky sexual behavior for exposure to HIV: Issues in methodology, interpretation, and prevention. *American Psychologist, 48,* 1035–1045.

Lowry, D. T., & Shidler, J. A. (1993). Prime time TV portrayals of sex, "safe sex" and AIDS: A longitudinal analysis. *Journalism Quarterly, 70,* 628–637.

Marin, B. V., Gomez, C. A., & Tschann, J. M. (1993). Condom use among Hispanic men with secondary female sexual partners. *Public Health Reports, 108,* 742–750.

Marin, B. V., Tschann, J. M., Gomez, C. A., & Kegeles, S. M. (1993). Acculturation and gender differences in sexual attitudes and behaviors: Hispanic vs. non-Hispanic white unmarried adults. *American Journal of Public Health, 83,* 1759–1761.

Marin, G. (1989). AIDS prevention among Hispanics: Needs, risk behaviors and cultural values. *Public Health Reports, 104,* 411–415.

Mays, V. M., & Cochran, S. D. (1988). Issues in the perception of AIDS risk and risk reduction activities by black and Hispanic/Latina women. *American Psychologist, 43,* 949–957.

Miller, B. C., McCoy, J. K., Olson, T. D., & Wallace, C. M. (1986). Parental discipline and control attempts in relation to adolescent sexual attitudes and behavior. *Journal of Marriage and the Family, 48,* 503–512.

Miller, K., Clark, L., & Moore, J. S. (1997). Heterosexual risk for HIV among female adolescents: Sexual initiation with older male partners. *Family Planning Perspectives, 29,* 212–214.

Moore, S. M., & Rosenthal, D. A. (1992). The social context of adolescent sexuality: Safe sex implications. *Journal of Adolescence, 15,* 415–435.

Moser, D. K., & Dracup, K. D. (1995). Psychosocial recovery from a cardiac event: The influence of perceived control. *Heart and Lung, 24,* 273–280.

National Abortion Rights Action League Foundation. (1995, September). *Sexuality education in America: A state-by-state review* (Rev ed.). Washington, DC: Author

National Institutes of Health. (1997). *NIH consensus development conference on interventions to prevent HIV risk behaviors.* Washington, DC: U.S. Government Printing Office.

Newcomer, S., & Udry, J. R. (1987). Parental marital status effects on adolescent sexual behavior. *Journal of Marriage and Family, 49,* 235–240.

Normand, J., Vlahov, D., & Moses, L. E. (Eds.). (1995). *Preventing HIV transmission: The role of sterile needles and bleach.* Washington, DC: National Academy Press.

Nyamathi, A., Bennett, C., Leake, B., Lewis, C., & Flaskerud, J. (1993). AIDS-Related knowledge, perceptions, and behaviors among impoverished minority women. *American Journal of Public Health, 83,* 65–71.

Office of National AIDS Policy. (1996). *Youth and HIV/AIDS: An American agenda: A report to the president.* Washington, DC: White House.

O'Reilly, K. R. (1993, August). An international view of intervention approaches to prevent HIV. Paper presented to the Third Science Symposium on HIV Prevention Research: Current Status and Future Directions, Northern Arizona University, Flagstaff.

Orr, S. T., Celentano, D. D., Santelli, J., & Burwell, L. (1994). Depressive symptoms and risk factors for HIV acquisition among black women attending urban health centers in Baltimore. *AIDS Education and Prevention, 6,* 230–236.

Orshansky, M. (1965, January). Counting the poor: Another look at the poverty profile. *Social Security Bulletin, 28,* 3–29.

Padian, N., Marquis, L., Francis, D. P., Anderson, R. E., Rutherford, G. W., O'Malley, P. M., & Winkelstein, W. (1987). Male-to-female transmission of human immunodeficiency virus. *JAMA, 258*(6), 788–790.

Peterson, J. L., Grinstead, O. A., Golden, E., Catania, J. A., Kegeles, S., & Coates, T. J. (1992). Correlates of HIV risk behaviors in black and white San Francisco heterosexuals: The population-based AIDS in Multiethnic Neighborhoods (AMEN) study. *Ethnicity and Disease, 2*(4), 361–370.

Pivnick, A., Jacobson, A., Eric, K., Doll, L., & Drucker, E. (1994). AIDS, HIV infection and illicit drug use within inner-city families and social networks. *American Journal of Public Health, 84,* 271–273.

Raj, A., Silverman, J., Wingood, G. M., & DiClemente, R. J. (1999). Prevalence and correlates of relationship abuse among a community-based sample of low income African American women. *Violence Against Women, 5,* 272–291.

Ramirez-Valles, J., Zimmerman, M. A., & Newcomb, M. D. (1998). Sexual risk behavior among youth: Modeling the influence of prosocial activities and socioeconomic factors. *Journal of Health and Social Behavior, 39,* 237–253.

Rienzo, B. A. (1985). The impact of aging on human sexuality. *Journal of School Health, 55,* 66–68.

Schwartz, A., Colby, D. C., & Reisinger, A. L. (1991). Variation in Medicaid physician fees. *Health Affairs Millwood, 10,* 131–139.

Sheer, V. C., & Cline, R. J. (1994). The development and validation of a model explaining sexual behavior among college students: Implications for AIDS communication campaigns. *Human Communication Research, 21,* 280–304.

Shervington, D. O. (1993). The acceptability of the female condom among low-income African American women. *JAMA, 85,* 341–347.

Snow, L. F. (1983). Traditional health beliefs and practices among lower class black Americans. *Western Journal of Medicine, 139,* 820–828.

Soper, D. E., Shoupe, D., Shangold, G. A., Shangold, M. M., Gutmann, J., & Mercer, L. (1993). Prevention of vaginal trichomoniasis by compliant use of the female condom. *Sexually Transmitted Diseases, 20,* 137–139.

Sorensen, G., & Verbrugge, L. M. (1987). Women, work and health. *Annual Review of Public Health, 8,* 235–251.

St. Lawrence, J. S., Eldridge, G. D., Shelby, M. C., Little, C. E., Brasfield, T. L., & O'Bannon (1997). RE: HIV risk reduction for incarcerated women: A comparison of brief interventions based on two theoretical models. *Journal of Consulting and Clinical Psychology, 65,* 504–509.

Swenson, R. M. (1992). The lessons of Belle Glade. *Annals of Internal Medicine, 116,* 343–346.

Terrell, F., & Terrell, S. L. (1995). The Cultural Mistrust Inventory: Development, findings and implications. In R. L. Jones (Ed.), *Handbook of tests and measurements for black populations* (Vol. 2, pp. 321–331). Hampton, VA: Cobb & Henry Publishers.

Thomas, S. B., & Quinn, S. C. (1991). The Tuskegee syphilis study, 1932 to 1972: Implications for HIV education and AIDS risk education programs in the black community. *American Journal of Public Health, 81,* 1498–1504.

Udry, J. R., & Billy, J. (1987). Initiation of coitus in early adolescence. *American Sociological Review, 52,* 841–855.

Upchurch, D. M., Ray, P., Reichart, C., Celantani, D. D., Quinn, T., & Hook, E. W. (1992). Prevalence and patterns of condom use among patients attending a sexually transmitted disease clinic. *Sexually Transmitted Diseases, 19,* 175–180.

U.S. Department of Commerce. (1996, September). Poverty in the United States: 1995. In *Current population reports of consumer income* (pp. 60–194). Washington, DC: Economics and Statistics Administration, Bureau of the Census, U.S. Department of Commerce.

U.S. Department of Labor. (1994). *Employment and earnings.* Washington, DC: U.S. Government Printing Office.

van Ryn, M., & Heaney, C. A. (1997). Developing effective helping relationships in health education practice. *Health Education and Behavior, 24,* 683–702.

Wasserheit, J. (1992). Epidemiological synergy: Interrelationships between human immunodeficiency virus infection and other sexually transmitted diseases. *Sexually Transmitted Diseases, 9,* 61–77.

Weisman, C. S., Plichta, S., Nathanson, C. A., Einsminger, M., & Robinson, J. C. (1991). Consistency of condom use for disease prevention among adolescent users of oral contraceptives. *Family Planning Perspectives, 23,* 71–74.

Weissman, M. (1987). Advances in psychiatric epidemiology: Rates and risks for major depression. *American Journal of Public Health, 77,* 445–451.

Williams, D. R., & Collins, C. (1995). U.S. socioeconomic and racial differences in health: Patterns and explanations. *Annual Review of Sociology, 21,* 349–386.

Wingood, G. M., & DiClemente, R. J. (1988). Partner influences and gender-related factors associated with noncondom use among young adult African American women. *American Journal of Community Psychology, 26,* 29–53.

Wingood, G. M., & DiClemente, R. J. (1995). Understanding the role of gender relations in HIV prevention research. *American Journal of Public Health, 85,* 592.

Wingood, G. M., & DiClemente, R. J. (1996). HIV sexual risk reduction interventions for women: A review. *American Journal of Preventive Medicine, 12,* 209–217.

Wingood, G. M., & DiClemente R. J. (1997). Consequences of having a physically abusive partner on the condom use and sexual negotiation practices of young adult African American women. *American Journal of Public Health, 87,* 1016–1018.

Wingood, G. M., & DiClemente, R. J. (1998a). Relationship characteristics associated with noncondom use among young adult African American women. *American Journal of Community Psychology, 26,* 29–53.

Wingood, G. M., & DiClemente, R. J. (1998b). Rape among African American women: Sexual, psychological and social correlates predisposing survivors to HIV infection. *Journal of Women's Health, 7,* 1–8.90.

Wingood, G. M., & DiClemente, R. J. (2000). Application of the theory of gender and power to examine HIV-related exposures, risk factors, and effective interventions for women. *Health Education and Behavior, 27,* 539–565.

Wingood, G. M., DiClemente, R. J., Harrington, K., Davies, S., Hook, E. W., III, & Oh, M. K. (2001). Exposure to X-rated movies and adolescents' sexual and contraceptive-related attitudes and behaviors. *Pediatrics, 107,* 1116–1119.

Wølner-Hanssen, P., Eschenbach, D. A., Paavonen, J., Stevens, C. E., Kiviat, N. B., Critchlow, C., DeRouen, T., Koutsky, L., & Holmes, K. K. (1990). Association between vaginal douching and acute pelvic inflammatory disease. *JAMA, 263,* 1936–41.

Women's Research and Education Institute. (1994). *Women's Health Care Costs and Experiences.* Washington, DC: Author.

Wortley, P. M., & Fleming, P. L. (1997). AIDS in women in the United States: Recent trends. *JAMA, 11,* 911–916.

Wyatt, G. E. (1992). The sociocultural context of African American and white American women's rape. *Journal of Social Issues, 48,* 77–91.

CHAPTER THIRTEEN

THE BEHAVIORAL ECOLOGICAL MODEL

Integrating Public Health and Behavioral Science

Melbourne F. Hovell
Dennis R. Wahlgren
Christine A. Gehrman

Prevention of morbidity and mortality in populations is a public health goal that can be achieved by behavior change. Behavior change is dependent on valid theory. We believe the Behavioral Ecological Model (BEM) is consistent with natural sciences in its reliance on environmental and selectionist explanations of behavior and that it is more likely to result in changes and maintenance of a population's health-related behavior than cognitive models of behavior and in this sense is face valid.

Philosophy of Science

A century ago, the primary cause of death was infectious disease, such as tuberculosis (Elder, Geller, Hovell & Mayer, 1994). Life expectancy increased with water treatment, waste disposal, increased income, education, and development of antibiotics and immunization. The primary cause of death in developed nations is now chronic disease (Murphy, 2000). Although disease etiology is multifactorial, chronic diseases are due largely to lifestyle. For example, increasing access to

This research was supported by grants funded by the University-wide AIDS Research Program, University of California, number IS99-SDSUF-206; Maternal Child Health Bureau, number R4O MC 00185; and National Institutes of Health, number 1 R01 HD37749.

tobacco and access to the diet and labor-saving technology of developed nations predicts increases in morbidity and mortality in these nations (Elder, 2001).

Infectious disease, attributed to a virus, bacteria, or a parasite, can also be attributed to behavior. We transmit colds when we cough, transmit hepatitis and enteric infections when we fail to wash our hands, spread sexually transmitted diseases (STDs) by engaging in unprotected sexual intercourse, and increase malaria-carrying mosquitoes and hantavirus-carrying mice in populated areas with deforestation practices and rural development. Thus, all diseases are caused in part by individual or community practices—and they are thus preventable by changes in those same practices. As Kaplan (1990, 1994) asserted, behavior is the central outcome of concern for health care. Change in lifestyle could save thousands of lives per year.

Objectivity and Manipulable Variables

Following models provided by physics and natural sciences, it is important to apply objective science to understanding behavior. We must assume a priori that behavior is orderly and determined. People are part of nature, and so our behavior is as lawful as the universe around us. To assume otherwise limits objective science and our ability to understand or influence behavior, including health-related behavior. To "control" behavior, we must focus on manipulable influences of behavior. Manipulable influences are found only in an individual's environment. These mandates for objectivity and examination of manipulable parts of the environment may be self-evident for all science. However, not all models of behavior reflect these mandates.

To "control" behavior, we must focus on manipulable influences of behavior. Manipulable influences are found only in an individual's environment.

Because all people are also observers of their own and others' behavior, individual and cultural explanations of behavior arise. Some of these are illogical. Our approach is designed to avoid the most common logical errors made in accounting for behavior:

• *Reification.* Concepts are reified when they are treated as equivalent to objective events. Reference to "minds" represents ontological errors that are reified in our language and culture. Thus, some investigators observe behavior from which inferences about a person's mind are made. This is "mentalism," that is, treating a hypothetical entity as an objective physical event.

• *Circular logic.* Psychologists and laypeople have a tradition of using descriptions as explanations for behavior. A child who fights with his sibling is labeled "aggressive," and the explanation often given for fighting is that he or she is "aggressive." The circularity is obvious. Often this is combined with a reification error: "He fights because he has an aggressive personality." The transformation of verbs into nouns extends this error. "Remembering" (which is behavior) may become "memory" (a hypothetical structure). "Learning" (change in behavior) becomes "information" stored somewhere in the hypothetical "memory." These errors do a disservice to science by halting investigation or causing endless creation of ever more elaborate models of how these hypothetical mental structures interrelate.

• *Errors of association.* Psychology (and our general culture) has a longstanding tradition of committing errors of association. The most common is the attribution of cause to subjective feelings that occur close in time to behavior of interest. Reaction to a snarling dog may include feelings of terror, fight or flight syndrome, and running. Often the explanation for running is feeling fear. We could equally conclude that the dog causes both the fear and running. Yet all too often psychology attributes behavior to private feelings. This invents a higher-order variable as the theoretically causal agent for behavior. Association error and the inability to manipulate feelings directly make these explanations far from satisfactory. We must ask how to elicit fear to cause running; the answer to this always returns us to the environment. Many "cognitive" processes presumed to mediate behavior share this liability. At best, their usefulness is limited to predictions, as environmental determinants that can be manipulated in order to change behavior remain to be identified. While physiological mediators must be involved in causal explanations of behavior, the assignment of subjective emotions as mediating variables, which are not directly manipulable, may delay identification of environmental explanations of behavior.

• *Teleological error.* The last common error often made in explaining behavior is teleological explanation, that is, putting the effect before the cause. Teleological errors are usually found with terminology such as "in order to," "trying to," "wanting to," and "so she can." The young man approaches a young lady because he wants to meet her. The child climbs the counter to get a cookie. However, the meeting and the cookie are future events; they have not yet happened and cannot function as a cause. Modern evolutionary models no longer talk about giraffes "wanting to or trying to" grow long necks "in order to" reach leaves (Guerin, 1994). The cause of long necks was the past selective environment that enabled only giraffes with long necks to survive. The cause must be an antecedent.

A Selectionist Model

The behavioral sciences that avoid these errors are called "behavior analysis," the "experimental analysis of behavior" (basic science), or "applied behavior analysis" (applied science). The philosophy of science underlying these specialties is referred to as functional contextualism (Biglan & Hayes, 1996) or radical behaviorism (Skinner, 1953). In these fields, behavior is the outcome, and the presumed explanation is found in the environment. The study of environment-behavior interactions parallels ecology and rests on a hierarchical selectionist model. Variation and selection are the mechanism for change. At the first level, natural selection (that is, evolution) accounts for biological structure and physiology and, to some extent, behavior. However, this level prepares a species only for an environment that resembles the past selecting environment. Environments change within an individual's lifetime. Fortunately, one trait that was selected for in most species was the ability of behavior to be shaped by its current environment (that is, learning). Some variants of behavior tend to produce effective consequences, and these consequences select for, or make more likely, those variants in behavior. The third and final level of variation and selection is proposed to lie at the cultural level, in which practices engaged in by groups of people may be selected by the consequences produced and thereby alter (or sustain) the whole group's behavior—that is, culture.

Basic Principles as a Foundation of the Behavioral Ecological Model

The foundation of the BEM consists of the basic principles of respondent and operant conditioning.

Respondent Conditioning

Pavlov, a Russian physiologist, showed that certain types of physiological behavior could be learned. Most people can recite his studies of dogs conditioned to salivate in response to a bell (Pavlov, 1927). His work demonstrated that a neutral stimulus (a conditional stimulus) paired with a stimulus that naturally elicits a response (an unconditional stimulus) will acquire the eliciting properties, yielding a new response (a conditioned response). The key relation is the contextual antecedent pairings with food powder.

Following Pavlov's classic research paradigm, more recent investigators have shown that the immune system of mice can be taught to respond to neutral stimuli, thereby making it possible for trained mice with autoimmune disease to live about 50 percent longer when treated with a lower dosage of medication than untrained mice (Ader, Felten, & Cohen, 1991). Siegel (1975) demonstrated that drug tolerance is learned in the same manner: drug-opposing effects are elicited by environmental cues reliably paired with drug administration and may account for dependence. When Siegel (1982) showed that heroin-tolerant rats were more likely to die of overdose when the narcotic was given in a novel environment, he showed that an unknown but reliable physiological protective process kept addicted rats alive when injected in familiar environments. This type of conditioning may explain overdose among drug addicts.

These studies suggest that physiological responses can respond differentially to specific external environments. The findings provide manipulable environmental variables and basic principles that may serve as the foundation for designing effective interventions (Poulos, Hinson, & Siegel, 1981). Also, the respondent learning that accounted for changes in physiology and subsequent survival of rats and people was identified without reference to inferred mentalistic functions.

Operant Conditioning

Skinner is credited with cogent descriptions of operant conditioning as a model of gross motor and social behavior (Skinner, 1953). He defined an operant as behavior that operates on the environment, or produces consequences. The controlling relation was in the postcedent contingent consequence that a response produces. However, the response is not caused by its consequence, as this would be teleological. Rather, the class of similar future responses is "caused" by the contingent reinforcement of past responses. Thus, the causal agent remains prior to the behavior caused.

Avoiding a stubbed toe reinforces lifting one's foot to avoid a curb when walking. Similarly, physiological and social reinforcers from a partner may reliably reinforce sexual behavior. Thus, physical and social contingencies are responsible for operant behavior.

Discriminative Stimuli

Aspects of the context for behavior may be reliably correlated with contingent reinforcement, and responses previously reinforced are likely to increase in their presence. These stimuli occasion (or "cue") responses previously learned. Noticing that it is time for lunch can cue "going to lunch." The time serves as a discriminative stimulus for going to lunch, based on past reinforcement for going to lunch at the same time. Furthermore, a discriminative stimulus can serve as a reinforcer for other behavior. This happens in chained behavior in which the consequence for one behavior (for example, walking to another room—behavior—and seeing an interesting magazine there—reinforcing consequence) occasions another behavior (sitting and flipping through the magazine). Thus, in the operant model, antecedent stimuli have evoking effects on the timing or topography of a behavior but are dependent on the response-consequence contingency. Respondent behavior, by contrast, is elicited as a function of previous pairings of antecedent events. However, strongly established discriminative stimuli can evoke operants so reliably as to appear reflexive in nature. They also can cause operant behavior to appear falsely as if it were independent of consequence contingencies.

Operant-Respondent Interactions

Pairing a stimulus with an operant reinforcer can bring the stimulus to function as conditioned reinforcer. Pavlov's bell eventually elicited salivation; used as a consequence, it might have been a reinforcer to teach dogs to sit. Use of a conditioned stimulus as an antecedent can elicit a physiological response, such as salivation; the same stimulus applied as a contingent consequence can increase the rate of operant behavior. The timing and contingent history define the function or effect of the environment on behavior. Thus, both cues and conditioned eliciting stimuli can function as reinforcers when provided contingent on a response. The same stimulus can have multiple effects on different responses in sequence.

Pavlov and Skinner codified principles of two distinctly different kinds of behavior: respondent and operant. However, it is most important to note that these classes of behavior, although often topographically similar, are functionally defined. An eye-blink can be elicited by dust—that is, respondent behavior. However, rewarding a child for blinking when asked may increase blinking-operant behavior. Thus, the class of behavior can be determined only by its functional relationship to contingent antecedent and consequent events, not by its topography.

The Selectionist Model

The operant model draws on biology, especially evolution (Darwin, 1936). In both the evolutionary and the operant model, variability and extinction are key concepts. The evolution of complex species is a shaping process by which the environment selects out ever more subtle or refined physical variants for which their unique character provides survival advantages. Similarly, complex forms of behavior can be shaped.

Operant conditioning relies on concepts of shaping in order to select differentially ever more refined or complex behavior. An infant's babbling produces mother's attention, feeding, and other desired behavior. With repeated babbling, mother's attention wanes, until the infant, perhaps at random, emits a sound similar to a word in the community's language. This might simply be "mah." To this response, the mother may shout with joy, reinforcing "mah." The process of withholding reinforcing consequences (that is, extinguishing the earlier and more rudimentary form of behavior) and then providing them only as the behavior changes in subtle but important ways can shape "mah" to mother and ultimately complex language (Skinner, 1957). However, shaping requires considerable time. Learning complex skills can be speeded by learning imitative skills.

More Complex Principles

To understand some of the more interesting aspects of our behavior requires that we move beyond the basic principles we have already introduced. Generalized response classes, such as imitation, rule-governed behavior, and schedules of intermittent reinforcement add to the basic foundations of the BEM.

Generalized Response Classes

Response classes are defined by common contingencies of reinforcement. "Door opening" as a class may include twisting and pulling a knob, depressing thumb-lever and pushing, and knocking and waiting, all of which can lead to opening doors. Thus, these behaviors are topographically different but functionally similar, if not equivalent.

Parents shape imitation as a generalized response class (Baer, Peterson, & Sherman, 1967; Gewirtz & Stingle, 1968). When imitation occurs, it is likely to be reinforced. When a baby imitates, parents and others react, reinforcing the imitative response. Imitation also can yield natural reinforcers. Imitating a sibling who asks for candy is likely to result in obtaining candy as well as attention. These processes establish a generalized imitative response class.

Once an imitative response class is established, some types of behavior never before reinforced may be imitated. Thus, a child might hear a parent curse and imitate the behavior. These generalizations may be sustained without explicit reinforcement, possibly in the context of criticism. Ongoing reinforcement of some types of imitation may sustain the imitation of other members (cursing) of the same behavior class. Thus, reinforcers for some imitative responses can sustain never-reinforced imitations.

The value of a generalized imitative repertoire is that many behaviors are likely to be imitated, and many of these will subsequently come under the influence of other contingencies of reinforcement. If a child imitates a teacher's simple addition, it speeds the development of computation skills that will lead to other practical outcomes (that is, "natural reinforcers"). Thus, imitation may be an especially efficient means of learning complex behavior.

Imitation and Mentalistic Explanations

Social Learning Theory was closely related to operant conditioning (Bandura, 1965; Bandura & Walters, 1963). The early research was strong science, with direct observations of children and systematic manipulations of models and reinforcing contingencies. These experiments showed that children were more likely to be aggressive after seeing a peer's aggression. Bandura attributed the effects of modeling to cognitive or "vicarious" reinforcement. His view is that children (and adults) imagine similar consequences for their own future behavior. This was to explain why children who had seen models were more likely to imitate them, hours later and in the absence of apparent reinforcement. However, the verifiable explanation resides in a generalized imitation response class and ongoing reinforcement for some members of the class. The former presumes unverifiable events; the latter has been verified empirically.

Bandura's Social Cognitive Theory (1986) and his recent Moral Disengagement Model (Bandura, Barbaranelli, Caprara, & Pastorelli, 1996) presume that the individual "selectively (cognitively) disengage(s) from detrimental conduct by converting harmful acts to moral ones . . . obscuring personal causal agency by diffusion and displacement of responsibility . . . and vilifying the recipients of maltreatment" (Bandura et al., 1996, p. 364). This view emphasizes cognitions and inner self-controllers as causal agents. It begs the question of what determines the actions of the inner controllers. Although this model has been supported by correlational evidence (Orpinas, Parcel, McAlister, & Frankowski, 1995), the one controlled trial of violence prevention based on it resulted in null outcomes (Orpinas et al., 2000). This might be because the intervention did not change students' social contingencies.

Reinforcement Schedules

Reinforcement contingencies need not be continuous to sustain behavior (Ferster & Skinner, 1957). Behavior that has been reinforced episodically but contingently will continue for extended periods of time in the absence of reinforcement and will be more resistant to extinction (that is, non-reinforcement) than when continuously reinforced. Gamblers may persist for hours and after cumulative financial loss before another small win may take place, sustaining the gambling behavior and guaranteeing financial loss in the long run. An observer unaware of the intermittent schedule would see consistent gambling seemingly independent of reinforcement. Gamblers may insist that they can stop when they want to, implying internal control. However, high rates of gambling behavior may be best explained empirically by intermittent reinforcement.

Rule-Governed Behavior

The development of language leads to rule-governed behavior. Individuals come under the influence of rules—instructions, advice, commands, and so forth. With experience, individuals acquire a generalized rule-governed response class. This means that we respond to verbal instructions given by a wide variety of people, instructions that often stipulate (or imply) specific contingencies (see Hayes, 1989, for details of three distinct types of rule following). Usually, these take the form of, "If you do X, consequence Y will follow." If you follow the instructions and put the nut on the correct bolt, the training wheels will support the child's bicycle. Thus, rule-governed behavior provides a chain of cues that, when responded to correctly, often will be followed by reinforcing consequences. Health education and counseling can also be viewed as attempting to modify patients' rule-governed behavior.

Rules and Competitive Contingencies

The problem that arises with rule-governed behavior is that promised reinforcers are often not true, are delayed, or are unreliable (that is, not contingent). Telling youth that sex will cause pregnancy loses credibility when few get pregnant. Advising youth to use seat belts to avoid injury results in no apparent change in injury experience for the majority of youth. The injury protection consequences are both delayed and too infrequent to be reinforcing for most youth. Rules also suffer from competition with more immediate reinforcement. The immediate relief from taking another puff sustains smoking, even if the smoker has been warned of cancer. Most smokers will not quit as a function of information about delayed health effects. However, instructions may provide another class of more immediate social reinforcement for health-protective practices.

Clinicians as Sources of Social Reinforcement

Following instructions may result in praise or other reinforcers from the clinician. Patients who return to the physician and are praised for having taken medication as prescribed may be reinforced by the contingent attention. However, it is quite likely that the rule-following behavior (for example, taking medication as prescribed) will falter as soon as treatment is completed and the reinforcers from the physician are discontinued. Maintenance requires at least intermittent and ongoing contingent reinforcement. This principle contrasts with cultural views of behavior as under the control of the patient and leads to repeated study of short-term education or counseling and little study of systems of sustaining reinforcing contingencies. For certain health problems, such as diabetes, it has been accepted that patients must have ongoing support. Clinicians provide attention for adherence, and this might be sufficient to help most diabetic patients adhere to their insulin regimen.

However, similar support for adhering to their diet, even if they can regulate their insulin as instructed, may not be effective. To alter their diet involves greater compromise in reinforcing consequences, and adherence to diet advice results in delayed improvements in health at best. Thus, rule-governed behavior or following instructions works just well enough to sustain the entire culture in the practice of providing advice and instructions. This works often enough to be highly reinforcing to the person giving advice. However, it does not work well for changing many health-related behaviors. Although it can sustain behavior, there are few health care delivery systems available to provide ongoing social reinforcement.

Overgeneralizations

The logical errors inherent in cognitive models of behavior are culturally based. Most societies use a language and logic system that implicitly, if not explicitly, places the explanation of behavior within the behaving person. The community reinforces explanations of why one is studying math when the student indicates that he or she "wants" to become a scientist. The community, however, rarely asks what causes one to want to become a scientist. Both types of behavior may be better explained by community contingencies of reinforcement than by the internal explanations. However, verbal explanations are consistent with cultural standards for cognitive models and are socially reinforced. This pattern tends to delay empirical investigations.

Extension of the Operant Model to Culture and Populations

Public health differs from clinical medicine in a variety of ways, the most obvious of which is the focus of the former on groups of people, or populations, as opposed to the clinical model of treating individuals. Therefore, to study behavior as it applies in public health requires that the operant model be extended to large groups.

Public Health and Clinical Models

The purpose of the public health profession is to improve the population's health. This contrasts with the clinical model, which focuses on improving the health of individuals. Behaviorally, it is easy to see how clinical services evolved. Individuals who are in pain or cannot function seek assistance. This can result in consolation and possibly relief or restoration of function. However, clinical services to individuals do not normally provide attention to the prevention of the problem, let alone prevention for whole communities. With few exceptions, people rarely seek out preventive services.

The advent of clinical services is an important development within a larger societal response to the control of morbidity and mortality. With effective medical care, key individuals in the society can be assisted in recovering from otherwise permanently disabling disease or injury, and their death may be postponed. Restoring the function of leaders, hunters, and others in a primitive society may contribute to the society's survival. Since delivery of medical services is expensive, services have always been rationed. Most societies limit services to the privileged among the small portion (5 to 10 percent) of the population who may be ill or injured at any one time. For instance, fewer than 5 percent of the U.S. population as a whole is infected with tuberculosis and fewer still have active disease. Yet medical care for tuberculosis is well established and routinely directed to the acutely ill. Alternatively, relatively few resources have been directed to prevention of tuberculosis, guaranteeing the recurrence of epidemics that demand expensive medical care. In fact, the U.S. investment in tuberculosis control has usually increased in times of epidemic and then dropped after relative control has been achieved. This cycle of funding is a function of contingencies derived first from the rates of disease and then from the competing demands for resources in the society—culturally based contingencies that emphasize short-term over long-term costs.

Medical and other clinical services require highly sophisticated training of specialists and technicians who can deliver intensive treatments. For many ills, it is impossible to train sufficient numbers of clinicians to repair the flood of the ill and injured. This is true for classic diseases such as tuberculosis and newer epidemics, such as acquired immunodeficiency syndrome (AIDS) (Rugg, Hovell, & Franzini, 1989) and type II diabetes in Western societies. The recognition that clinical services must be rationed and the recognition that increasing the size of the clinical fields is both expensive and cannot ultimately return all ill and injured to reasonable function leads to a search for prevention. This has led to the public health model, which focuses on the attention of population-wide effects and inherently emphasizes preventive interventions relatively more than does a clinical approach. The public health model directs attention to precursors of illness and injury. Public health professionals are concerned with providing screening of high-risk subpopulations in order to identify those infected with tuberculosis but not yet ill and then provide them with medications that prevent subsequent active disease. This relies on medical services to effect prevention and in the process prevents infection in the many individuals who would come in contact with a person with active tuberculosis. Screenings and prevention interventions move society resources from other uses, such as acute care, to treating well individuals who are at risk of becoming ill or injured.

When the public health model is extended to completely nonclinical interventions, it usually affects larger groups of people for less cost per person than clinical services. This is seen in chlorination of water systems, water fluoridation, sewage treatment systems, and air quality control. Even the provision of public education, making it possible for most people to obtain employment from which all other resources are derived, including medical care, will improve the population's health. Thus, public health interventions tend to be structural, such as investing in sewage systems, or in large-scale systems of social change, such as public education. These systems of communitywide intervention require change in culture based on recognition of short- and long-term risks and means of protecting the population from risks. Public health interventions also require establishing unique cultural contingencies designed to change these structural or social systems to protect whole populations. Because all forms of morbidity and premature mortality involve behavioral risk factors, the public health model necessarily requires intervention to change whole populations' behavior (Hovell, Elder, Blanchard, & Sallis, 1986).

Glenn and others (Skinner, 1953, 1987; Malagodi, 1986; Glenn, 1988, 1991; Malagodi & Jackson, 1989; Glenn & Malagodi, 1991; Lamal, 1991, 1997; Guerin, 1994; Biglan, 1995) proposed cultural contingencies of reinforcement as critical for understanding behavior. This advance in the operant model approximates ecological models of behavior that stem from biology. In both, the causal factors responsible for behavior are found in the environment.

Cultural Practices

A cultural practice is defined as a repetition of operant behavior across individuals, within and across generations (Glenn, 1988; Malagodi & Jackson, 1989). The practice involves two or more people whose interactions produce consequences for each and whose joint behavior produces an outcome that is reinforcing (Glenn, 1991). Glenn draws on anthropological concepts of the idioclone (a "scene," or interaction, between people at one place and time), the nomoclone (the event repeated over time with the same people), and the permaclone (the event repeated over time with some of the participants replaced with new people). She illustrates this with a birthday party that repeats year after year but with different participants. In addition, the participants attend other people's birthday parties at other times.

The key feature of the permaclone is the "interlocking reinforcement contingencies" for the behavior of the participants. The behavior of each participant in a permaclone is "maintained by contingencies provided by the behavior of others and the products of that behavior" (Glenn & Malagodi, 1991, p. 8). Thus, the cultural practice includes the social processes that maintain the practice. For example, attendees at a birthday party may bring gifts for the person whose birthday is being celebrated, thus reinforcing "throwing a birthday party for oneself." The guest of honor provides fun activities that reinforce attendance by guests. The guest of honor may be more likely to have another party the following year and invite more or different guests; the guests may be more likely to attend other people's birthday parties, expanding the permaclone.

Glenn suggests a hierarchy of contingencies of reinforcement, where an individual's behavior is under the influence of many proximal to distal contingencies simultaneously. Glenn's theoretical model suggests that cultural contingencies include such things as likely reinforcement from members of a culture, without collusion. Bowing instead of shaking hands in Japanese culture is acquired almost immediately by immigrants. Yet no one insists that newcomers bow. Rather, the density of models and subtle reinforcement provided in social settings quickly shape bowing when greeting another individual.

One of the many features of cultural contingencies is that they are widespread throughout a culture, and therefore the administration of models, instructions, and social consequences is not dependent on collusion, planning, or a professional service provider. These contingencies are not limited to short periods of time, but tend to be ongoing over long periods and over wide geographical areas. Thus, whether one visited northern or southern Japan, ten years ago or now, the promotion of bowing as a means of greeting would be about the same. In their consistency over time and wide geographical distribution, cultural contingencies may also approximate physical contingencies, such as moving from sunlight to shade to avoid heat.

Metacontingent Functional Relations

Glenn (1988) defined *metacontingency* as a contingent relation between a cultural practice and its aggregate outcomes to the group. Just as operant contingencies select adaptive responses within an individual, metacontingencies and their aggregate outcomes select for adaptive interlocking contingencies in groups of people: "Cultural outcomes . . . do not select the behavior of individuals; they select the interlocking contingencies comprising the cultural practice. Likewise, the behavior of any specific individual has little effect on cultural outcomes" (Glenn, 1988, p. 169). This defines a separate level of analysis, as distinct from that of the behavior of the individual (shaped by selection by reinforcement) and behavior and structure of the species (natural selection). Behavioral phenomena are built on physiological phenomena but cannot be explained well by physiological princi-ples. In the same way, cultural phenomena are built on behavioral phenomena but cannot be explained well by reduction to individuals' contingencies (Glenn & Malagodi, 1991).

The focus on the group as the unit of analysis follows research in applied behavior analysis that focuses on group contingencies of reinforcement. If the majority of the group performs in concert with the contingency, the reinforcer will be obtained for the whole group. This requires only that a proportion of the group be responsive to the contingency, while others may fail or thwart the group's practices.

Metacontingencies beget social reinforcement contingencies. Legislative rules and laws work this way. When legislators taxed cigarette sales in California, tobacco control efforts supported by taxes resulted in antitobacco education, restrictions on smoking in public, restrictions on points of sale to minors, and restrictions for advertising. These contingencies changed social reactions to smok-ing. It is common now for a smoker to be asked by a complete stranger not to smoke or not smoke around others. Thus, a law or regulation will yield a cascade of other contingencies and represents a metacontingency. Again, these tend to be cultural contingencies insofar as they are widely distributed throughout the com-munity and operate over long periods of time.

Group and Cooperative Contingencies

As a more discrete example of interlocking social contingencies, studies have shown that teacher-initiated group contingencies of reinforcement can be used effectively to reduce disruptive behavior and promote study and attending prac-tices (Wilson & Williams, 1973). These studies illustrate a simple form of meta-contingencies in the class population. Figure 13.1 shows a simplified or limited metacontingency model.

In this model, students in a classroom are told that they will get an extra ten minutes of recess if the class remains quiet and attentive to the assignment. This promised reinforcer is contingent on the whole group's behavior of remaining quiet and looking attentive, which is likely to generate social reinforcement con-tingencies among many of the students. If one child speaks to another, the re-maining students—possibly including the one spoken to—will frown, look away, hold their finger over their lips, and hush the speaker. These consequences sup-press talking. These practices take place without the class's discussing the means by which they will influence one another to be quiet. This is a simple model where a positive reinforcing group contingency may establish negatively reinforcing social contingencies by the class members.

FIGURE 13.1. CLASSROOM METACONTINGENCY EXAMPLE.

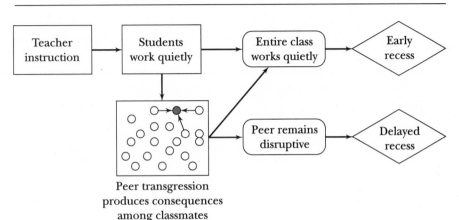

Peer transgression
produces consequences
among classmates

When the same students move to a different class, where the teacher has no group contingency, their behavior may be different. Over time, one teacher may have a quiet and attentive class, and the other may have a disruptive class, even though both classes consist of the same students. It would be possible to describe these differences as different cultures, generated by the interaction of normal youth socializing in the context of different metacontingencies.

Group contingencies have also proved valuable for promoting cooperative learning among youth. Reinforcement made contingent on average group performance (typically, academic performance) sustains supportive helping and within-group teaching and positively reinforces interactions among individuals in the group (Lloyd, Eberhardt, & Drake, 1996; Slavin, 1987). Natural group contingencies work the same way. When an individual is unable to move his or her vehicle to the side of the road, cooperation among multiple individuals working as a team will successfully move the vehicle. Cooperation among individuals, who jointly obtain reinforcing consequences as a result of cooperation, describes a simple metacontingency.

Population Change, Density of Encounters with Contingencies, and Inescapable Contact

The degree to which one or a set of interlocking contingencies is established throughout a given population will determine the probability of all members of the population coming in direct contact with the contingencies. It also will determine the probability of most individuals coming into contact with the contingencies repeatedly. In principle, for metacontingencies to be effective for changing or sustaining behavior in the majority of the population, the interlocking reinforcement contingencies between individuals must be densely distributed throughout the population. If almost everyone you meet bows, the likelihood of your bowing is almost 100 percent. Conversely, the degree to which the density of the contingency is limited in time, space, and across members of the society, the more attenuated its likely effects population wide.

In principle, for metacontingencies to be effective for changing or sustaining behavior in the majority of the population, the interlocking reinforcement contingencies between individuals must be densely distributed throughout the population.

Intermittent penalties for speeding set up a gambling schedule. It is virtually certain that most drivers will exceed the posted speed frequently, especially when late, when police are absent, when others are observed successfully speeding (thus modeling the behavior), and when traffic and other conditions permit. If speed were automatically recorded and relayed to the police, fines could be guaranteed for each instance of speeding. Timed traffic lights that turn green just before a driver approaches only when he or she has been traveling the correct speed will reinforce driving the correct speed. This type of contingency is easily engineered and can yield very reliable speeds for the majority of drivers. Yet most communities do not install timed street signals; most collect fines from traffic citations and pay the costs of trauma that might have been prevented from more precise behavioral engineering. These examples fit the definition of metacontingencies because they involve physical interlocking contingencies that produce group behavior that yields aggregate outcomes, such as decreased morbidity.

Redistributing the contingencies such that the density of reinforcement is high for driving slowly would guarantee lower speeds. In turn, this would increase the density of models driving within the speed limit. Indeed, once the density of models is sufficient, most drivers would adopt similar speeds, even if electronic sensing devices were not operating at the time. The theoretical extension of operant conditioning to populations and concepts of hierarchical contingencies has led to the Behavioral Ecological Model of health behavior.

The Behavioral Ecological Model

The BEM assumes an interaction among both physical and social contingencies to explain and ultimately control behavior (see Figure 13.2). Sallis and coworkers (Sallis & Owen, 1996, 1999; Sallis, Bauman, & Pratt, 1998) have described these interactions for physical activity. In one study, we showed that persons who lived

FIGURE 13.2. RANGE OF REINFORCEMENT CONTINGENCIES AFFECTING AN INDIVIDUAL'S BEHAVIOR AT ANY GIVEN TIME.

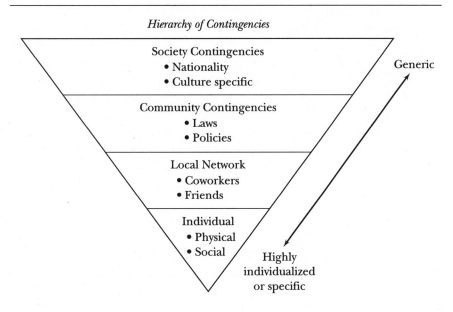

Hierarchy of Contingencies

Society Contingencies
- Nationality
- Culture specific

Community Contingencies
- Laws
- Policies

Local Network
- Coworkers
- Friends

Individual
- Physical
- Social

Generic

Highly individualized or specific

near fee-for-service exercise facilities, such as fitness centers, were more likely to engage in physical activity (Sallis et al., 1990). We hypothesized that these facilities served as cues—that people entering, leaving, and exercising in and around fitness centers serve as models for exercising and that the incidental interaction with individuals who exercise in the fitness center or nearby might provide social reinforcement for physical activity. Thus, the density of models and social contingencies may account for the relationship between activity and exercise centers.

These types of associations raise questions about the chicken or the egg. It is difficult to know whether fitness centers cause people to be more active or whether already active people are more likely to live where fitness centers are located. Both are likely. Experiments can disentangle these relationships by introducing sedentary individuals to a neighborhood with fitness centers, or vice versa. The BEM calls for these types of interventions.

Cohen and colleagues used this ecological approach to health promotion, based partially on the operant model (Cohen, Scribner, & Farley, 2000). They have shown that change in the physical environment can be associated with change in health risks, presumably mediated by changes in the interlocking social contingencies promoted by physical environments. As with the BEM, she notes this approach does not rely on cognitive processes but emphasizes physical, social, policy, and legal contingencies applicable to whole populations. Cohen's work is consistent with metacontingencies and supports the BEM (Cohen et al., 2000).

This environmental perspective was demonstrated in distribution of condoms and decrease in sexually transmitted diseases (STDs) and human immunodeficiency virus (HIV) risks (Hanenberg, Ronanapithayakorn, Kunasol, & Sokal, 1994; Cohen et al., 1999). The distribution of condoms was interpreted as reducing barriers, such as price and convenience, as well as altering the social acceptability (that is, praise or criticism) of carrying condoms, and it may have increased social support for condom use. The wide distribution of condoms may have rearranged the hierarchical series of contingencies (that is, metacontingencies) operating cumulatively to effect change in condom use for important subgroups of the larger community. It is important to note that change in the environment—in the example, condom distribution—resulted in change in risk behavior and disease outcomes (Cohen et al. 1999). This has not been true for many clinical or educational models of condom use. These demonstrations are far from proof of a theory, but they support the BEM. We believe it provides sufficient support to warrant formal experimental analyses across different cultures and health behaviors and for manipulation of more varied and powerful contingencies.

Social Institutions

The community can be divided into many units, such as church, business, government, clinical service providers, and educational institutions. These institutions represent unique metacontingencies or separate cultures. In these various institutions, the same person behaves differently under significantly different contingencies, and often very different groups of people are involved. The pattern of behavior is a function of experience unique to the individual, as well as a function of the various cultural units to which the individual belongs. Since individuals move from one institution to another, their behavior changes as a function of immersion in new cultural contingencies (subgroups or institutions within a given society).

Three institutions are aimed at systematically changing people's behavior. These are schools, media, and clinical services, and they provide unique contingencies that define the behavior of groups of teachers, principals, students, advertisers, actors, audiences, physicians, nurses, and patients. These institutions can be examined for how they can increase health-related behavior.

Engineering Limited Metacontingencies in Schools and Families

The daily or weekly report card system is an example of a behavioral intervention that involves the establishment of interlocking contingencies among parents, their children, and their children's teachers. For predelinquent youth, the use of a report-card-based contingency system has been shown to increase academic performance and reduce disruptive and delinquent behavior (Schumaker, Hovell, & Sherman, 1977). The system works by enabling teachers to assess a student's academic and disruptive practices. The teacher ranks the frequency of disruption and appropriate study behavior or the degree to which performance meets standards, such as passing an exam. This report is then relayed to the parents. Parents must be trained to provide positive feedback for improvement in performance based on the report card. They also must provide or restrict their child's access to privileges, such as watching television or visiting friends. This system ties the monitoring and praise contingencies from the teacher to the more powerful privilege contingencies managed by the parents in order to promote higher rates of homework completion, attendance, and attentiveness in school and to decrease disruptive behavior. Parents are also tied to the incidental notes from teachers about homework and how to assist the child in completing academic exercises. This interlocking process reinforces teacher participation when it decreases disruption in class. It also enables the teacher to contribute to the student's learning. It is reinforcing to parents for many of the same reasons, and it enables parents to provide positive reinforcers as the behavior improves instead of delivering threats or punitive consequences.

Although most adolescents are not initially happy with having to earn privileges that normally were not contingent on academic performance, they too like the report card system once they obtain privileges and begin achieving academic success. As math, reading, and other academic skills increase, the student can obtain other social reinforcers. Use of a report card contingency system with its use of external reinforcement may be able to improve a student's performance to the point that natural contingencies of reinforcement may sustain academic performance without the use of special privileges. Thus, the daily report card system represents a metacontingency insofar as it generates a cascade of interlocking contingencies for parents, teachers, and students.

This system requires cultural acceptance of the use of contingent reinforcement to shape academic practices and professional counselors who can organize and train parents, teachers, and students to employ the system. Many school professionals reject the use of external rewards, assuming that the motivation for academic achievement should come from within the child. Despite philosophy to the contrary, evidence supports the efficacy of reinforcement contingencies without compromise to intrinsic motivation (Eisenberger & Cameron, 1996; Cameron, Banko, & Pierce, 2001). Most schools, however, do not provide the funds needed to establish such a system, relying on suspensions and expulsion as a means of controlling delinquent youth. Thus, a valid, engineered metacontingency remains underused, primarily due to a larger set of cultural contingencies. Attention to the larger metacontingencies is required to effect change in educational systems, even when a valid technology is available for adoption.

Media

Media, ranging from interpersonal communication to mass media, are among the most important institutions that set and reflect cultural norms. They provide models, prompts, and instructions and rules, and sometimes reinforcing consequences that change behavior.

Unidirectional Media. Entertainment programs, advertisements, and most public relations campaigns are designed to evoke behavior, elicit emotions, and ultimately to pay for the entertainment or product sold. These efforts present vignettes that convey entertaining stories that can function as complex models and instructions to promote imitation and other action. Philip Morris, the top U.S. tobacco manufacturer, has created several television ads describing its charitable and humanitarian acts, clearly with the goal of reducing public criticism for causing so much death and disease through its tobacco products.

Media influence the initial and repeat purchase of products by promising reinforcers for purchase. They can promote repeat purchase by targeting an audience predisposed to buy and use the product, in effect tapping a unique subset of the community for whom reinforcing contingencies for using the product or service are already in place. For instance, selling ice cream is more likely to be successful in a warm and humid climate than in a cold climate. Thus, media are not solely responsible for selling ice cream. The most important variable is the ongoing reinforcement contingency: the context (heat) establishes cold foods as effective reinforcers. Media can promote specific brands and products, but it is the reinforcement contingency that sustains the behavior.

The most powerful media are likely to be the entertainment industry and feature-length television and movies and certain magazines with recurring stories. These provide models of seemingly real life with attractive characters that engage in behavior and experience consequences for their acted behavior. When violence, cigarette smoking, alcohol use, and other health-risk practices are illustrated in such media, some observers will imitate it. Inherent reinforcement may be forthcoming immediately, as in drinking a beer on a warm day or from social reactions from peer audiences. The television and other media can assist industries in the promotion of repeat purchases. However, sustained changes in lifestyle practices are much more likely for actions that are inherently reinforcing. When studies have examined movies and television, they often find that cigarettes, alcohol, and violence are displayed far more often than is true in real life. They also are displayed as resulting in reinforcing consequences and rarely with any evidence of illness or other untoward consequences. Thus, these models promote inaccurate estimates of the population's true practices and imply social reactions that support risk behavior. This constitutes an inaccurate depiction of metacontingencies (for example, a higher density of models engaging in the behavior and receiving reinforcement for doing so) and may function similarly to having actually been exposed to such a high density of contingencies in person.

Social Marketing. Social marketing includes media directed to changing behavior in socially important directions (Maiback & Parrot, 1995), for example, to promote lifestyles that protect health or the environment. Although the use of media affects health-related behavior every day, it is not a guaranteed means of changing or maintaining behavior.

Media can be employed to instruct communities to change, such as current efforts aimed at reducing power consumption in California. It can do this by announcing the problem, asking all consumers to conserve, and explaining how to conserve. Media also can increase their power to change practices by alerting the audience to probable reinforcing consequences. This may be to alert the public to rolling blackouts that will disrupt the community. They also can add references to fines. Media can promise rewards for those who conserve. These contingencies were operating in the northern California drought in 1976–1978 (Agras, Jacob, & Lebedeck, 1980).

Media may include reinforcing features directly. For example, when the newspaper prints an article showing that the funds raised for a local charity have reached the target, that feedback may be reinforcing. If the names and pictures of men who frequent sex workers are published, avoiding publicity may reinforce avoiding sex workers. If a picture is included in an article about how a businessperson has contributed civic services to the community, the attention may reinforce charitable services for all who seek to obtain such recognition.

These uses of media are most powerful when directed to behavior already reinforced in population subgroups. We conducted a demonstration experiment to show the possible effects of tailored print media on businesses' social and political action directed toward ensuring clean ocean waters off the California coast. Businesses that made money by selling services or products to tourists and others who used the beaches were recruited. Half the businesses were provided with a weekly newsletter that contained articles about ocean ecology and its likely impact on business income. It also included suggestions about how to contact friends, civic leaders, and elected officials to promote cleaner water and thereby protect their businesses. Businesses that received this newsletter significantly increased their political action directed to cleaning the California coast, as compared to controls that did not receive the newsletter (Schroeder, 1999). This study is important because it targeted social activism or practices that might influence policies and laws about ecology. Thus, this was designed as a simple experimental test of how to promote metacontingencies. To do so, we relied on market segmentation, selecting businesses likely to be reinforced by protecting water quality.

It is easy to imagine the use of media in a more interactive fashion. With more individualized information available for members of the community, it will be possible to tailor messages to individuals, and it will be possible to tailor the selection of subsets of the population, perhaps down to single individuals, in order to present messages that capitalize on or set new contingencies of reinforcement. For instance, grocery stores now promote purchases by club cards. This provides them with identifying information and purchasing history of the buyer. Personalized coupons, based on this history, are printed and included with the purchase receipt. With ongoing purchases from the same store or chain, it should be possible to track performance and institute contingencies and shaping procedures for sustained or increased buying practices. Thus, technology and media may be combined, following principles of behavior to establish interlocking contingencies for all individuals in a population simultaneously.

If mass media are employed and sustained alongside individualized media programs and if these begin to effect change in a critical proportion of the population, the density of the population who change become another important source of change for the rest of the population. Thus, if grocery stores promoted the sustained purchase of fruits and vegetables and a sufficient number of people began doing so, their interactions with other shoppers, family members, friends, and casual acquaintances would be a source of additional possible influence for more of the population to adhere to what may be a growing norm for the culture. This defines a hierarchical set of interlocking contingencies aimed at the same behavioral practices. However, can economic contingencies direct store managers to engineer change that promotes health?

Risks and Economic Contingencies. Unfortunately, the use of media to set norms and establish social contingencies that promote healthy behavior competes with reinforcing contingencies for risk practices. Consumption of alcohol, cigarettes, sweets, and high-fat foods involves inherent reinforcement. For addictive cigarette use, media may be directed to promoting initial use in order to establish the addiction or to promote brand loyalty. Countermedia are not likely to be as successful without investing in more powerful media programs that include competing reinforcing consequences. Similarly, for media to promote lifestyles such as physical activity, the reinforcing context in the community must be considered. The use of media to promote physical activity, a behavior that can be aversive to those who are ill, injured, or unfit, may lead some to try physical activity, only to experience aversive consequences. It can be socially aversive if physical activity results in perspiration under conditions that are not acceptable to others, such as at work. This suggests that context, such as access to showers at work, must be considered in addition to messages promoting activity. Understanding the interlocking metacontingencies is required to engineer efficacious media and other interventions that promote healthy lifestyles.

Reinforcing Contingencies for Medical Services

Hovell and coauthors have examined the probable metacontingencies influencing clinical medical care and delivery of preventive medicine services (Hovell, Kaplan, & Hovell, 1991; Hovell, Wahlgren, & Russos, 1997). The evidence reviewed suggests that physicians provide clinical services when compensated and not primarily due to their beliefs about helping people. When managed care insurance systems changed the capitation model for compensation, reducing the amount paid for knee surgery, most surgeons scheduled more operations to sustain their income despite increasing risks to patients. Russos et al. (1997, 1999) also showed that patient feedback to clinicians influenced the clinicians' smoking prevention counseling. Thus, the contingencies instituted by formal payment processes as well as the social contingencies define the type and quality of care delivered.

Instituting Metacontingencies for Injury Prevention

We had an opportunity to increase the use of child safety seats in Colorado (Lavelle, Hovell, West, & Wahlgren, 1992). Police were reluctant to ticket young mothers for failing to transport their child in a safety seat. We established a free training and loaner program that taught mothers how to use a seat and provided a free seat if needed. Attendance to training by ticketed mothers was reinforced by avoiding financial penalties and by obtaining a loaner seat. We explained to the police that they were making it possible for mothers to be educated and to obtain a car seat by issuing tickets. This enabled the police to provide a helping service instead of punishing mothers who failed to use a car seat and made the provision of tickets a less aversive, if not reinforcing, event for police officers. The established interlocking metacontingencies significantly increased the rate of ticketing.

These examples are limited in scope to fit the practical constraints of experimental tests. However, the BEM suggests that interlocking contingencies from the greatest number of institutions in society and from the greatest number of individuals within each institution (that is, high-density contingencies) would provide the strongest means of ensuring performance from almost all members of a population. If tax accountants, stockbrokers, bankers, pharmaceutical businesses, waste disposal businesses, and all other institutions in the community directed attention to the promotion of car safety seats, academic achievement of adolescents, delivery of preventive medicine services, and so forth, far more powerful effects should be achieved. This has been approximated in the California Tobacco Control Program.

Case Applications of the Behavioral Ecological Model

The California Tobacco Control Program provides a natural experiment that can be interpreted within the framework of the BEM and for which the BEM provides direction for further refinements. The BEM also provides a relatively novel and informative approach to increasing rates of physical activity and decreasing rates of behavior that places individuals at risk of sexually transmitted diseases.

California Tobacco Control Program

Tobacco smoking and environmental tobacco smoke (ETS) exposure are the first and third most preventable causes of premature death in the United States (U.S. Department of Health and Human Services [USDHHS], 1989; Glantz & Parmley, 1991). Several U.S. surgeon general reports and interventions, including health warnings on cigarette packs, have been ineffective against the momentum gained by over five hundred years of tobacco use in the New World (Breed, 2001) and a multibillion-dollar industry. As a consequence, smoking rates have declined only slowly. Given tobacco's impact on health and the inadequate reduction in tobacco use to about 25 percent prevalence, states have started aggressive approaches to increase smoking cessation, prevent new smokers, and prevent passive smoking.

Perhaps the best example of real-life metacontingencies for health behavior is the California Tobacco Control Program, based on the Standards for Comprehensive Smoking Prevention and Control of the National Cancer Institute (NCI) through "policy, media, and program interventions using community coalitions . . . to push tobacco use out of the charmed circle of normal, desirable practice to being an abnormal practice; in short, to de-normalize smoking" (Tobacco Control Section, 1998, p. 3). This objective emphasized changing the public's reactions from support to criticism for tobacco use, consistent with metacontingencies.

The California program includes media campaigns, laws restricting advertising by the industry, laws restricting sales to minors, and laws restricting ETS exposure in public buildings, and promotion of clinical services for smoking cessation. The program advocates policy and legislative restrictions. California led the way in 1988 with a voter initiative (Proposition 99) that added a pack tax of twenty-five cents, of which five cents was allocated to antitobacco education activities. This created the largest antitobacco program ever (Fichtenberg & Glantz, 2000). Of the $90 million spent annually for antitobacco activities, one-third was allocated for school programs and two-thirds to statewide media, local programs, and evaluations. Multiple initiatives now tax cigarettes. The funds generated by these have been directed to tobacco control efforts, restrictions of sales to minors, restrictions on advertising, and other social services. The most recent initiative, Proposition 10, added a pack tax of fifty cents, which will generate about $700 million per year in the first few years, with the funds to enhance child development and promote smoking cessation in pregnant mothers (Children and Families First, 2001). Thus, multiple interlocking contingencies have been initiated.

The tobacco control program is hierarchical and consistent with metacontingencies. Taxes increased the price of cigarettes, and for every 10 percent increase in price, consumption decreases by about 4 to 8 percent, while state revenues increase from both the tax revenue and decreased costs to Medicaid and other health entitlement programs (National Cancer Policy Board, 2000).

California's media campaign was designed to attack the tobacco industry as cold, manipulative, and deceptive and eschewed the reliance on health-risk scare tactics that were less effective among youth (Goldman & Glantz, 1998; USDHHS, 2000). The media campaign focused on denormalizing tobacco use by emphasizing consequences such as bad breath, yellow teeth, and bad-smelling clothes. These consequences are more powerful than health risks because they are immediate and because adults and youth have experienced them. They have exposed industry manipulation by explaining clearly the intent of the industry's public relations media, such as television ads that show charitable acts by the Phillip Morris companies. If autonomy and rebellion are important reinforcers for youth, these illustrations may decrease tobacco use because they indicate that youth are being manipulated and can "rebel" by choosing not to smoke.

The program contributed to the Synar amendment that prohibited sale of tobacco to minors and set the stage for the program to add to the media campaign support for enforcement of this amendment. Operation Storefront collected data on industry marketing to youth and point-of-sale tactics and exposed these through the media (Tobacco Control Section, 1998). This presumably reduced public and political support for the industry, increasing the public's voting support for additional taxes and other restrictions on the industry. Reduced public support probably changed social encounters between smokers and nonsmokers, including youth.

The program also includes infrastructure components to facilitate and encourage tobacco control activities at the local level, such as establishing tobacco control programs in local health departments, providing grants for local programs, establishing a clearinghouse for educational materials, and instituting a smoking cessation help line that links smokers to clinical services.

The program includes ongoing surveillance and science. Surveillance has been extended to tracking the tobacco industry's promotion of tobacco sales and its attempt to reverse tobacco control laws. These data will be used to counter these efforts. Counter-efforts will be based on the latest public health policies and science. The Tobacco Related Disease Research Program (TRDRP) is part of California's tobacco control program, funded by 5 percent of the twenty-five-cent tax. It funds basic and applied science that informs tobacco control efforts, including policies. The addition of surveillance and formal research efforts provides an ongoing feedback system that enables the statewide program to adjust to changes in the society and in industry promotional efforts. This represents a reciprocal, and self-correcting, metacontingency system.

The program is designed to change the culture of California with respect to tobacco use, ETS exposure, and sentiments toward the industry. The goal is to change not only the behavior of smokers and would-be (or susceptible) smokers, but to change the behavior of the nonsmoking community with respect to smokers and the industry. This goes beyond increasing the rates at which medical and public health professionals advise the public not to smoke. The California program is innovative by explicitly targeting the whole population in the attempt to create a social climate in which social reinforcers are shifted away from smoking and toward nonsmoking and away from the industry completely.

The ETS issue has been particularly effective; it clearly countered the industry assertion that smoking is a choice. The program has increased interlocking social contingencies such as asking smokers to refrain from smoking indoors where it is prohibited, such as bars, asking bar and restaurant staff to enforce indoor smoking regulations, and asking others to refrain from smoking around children. In some instances, this avoided a penalty (for example, being asked to leave a public establishment). In others, compliance on the part of the smoker caused the asking party to express gratitude. Similar negative and positive reinforcers may be produced among onlookers in such scenes too; disapproving frowns on the part of others nearby may become brief nods of acknowledgment or even "thank yous." This begins the culture change.

The sentiments against the industry and against tobacco use in California are remarkable and increasing nationwide. Several other states, including Massachusetts, Arizona, Oregon, and Florida, have followed California's model. This represents the development of a national metacontingency and the potential for establishing an efficacious antitobacco culture throughout the country. Moreover, there is evidence that the California program is working. The California program reduced smoking rates three times faster than the national average, reducing per capita consumption, and recently demonstrated greater reductions in tobacco-related disease than in other states (Traynor & Glantz, 1996; Tobacco Control Section, 2000; Fichtenberg & Glantz, 2000). These are particularly impressive results given that the program was outspent by the industry by tenfold (Tobacco Control Section, 2000) and in the light of political maneuvers that crippled the program during the Pete Wilson administration (Balbach, Traynor, & Glantz, 2000). However, the story is not yet complete.

The program is theoretically strong; however, complete eradication of tobacco may be dependent on change in critical contingencies supporting the foundation of the program. The first problem is that the program is operating with less financial support than the industry (Tobacco Control Section, 2000). Since the industry is promoting an addicting product, it has to get a small proportion of the youth and young adults to try it in order to establish new smokers and in order for these smokers to become agents for promoting acceptance of tobacco use. These countercontingencies are supported by media and by legislative efforts, as certainly as has been the case for the California Tobacco Control Program. If the industry directs more resources to this end, they may overwhelm the California program.

The second and more serious problem is the program's dependence on tobacco sales, which inherently weakens the program. As it is successful in reducing sales in California, the resources diminish, and interventions must be curtailed. Because controlling an ongoing business requires ongoing vigilance, the loss of financial support just as the program begins to produce beneficial effects is likely to severely undercut its ability to eliminate tobacco use in California. This is especially likely as the industry enjoys resources from sales in other states and countries. Future legislation may need to establish tax support that is not contingent on tobacco sales.

Because reductions in smoking can increase savings due to lower disease rates, perhaps general tax revenue should be employed to support the program based on estimated savings as the smoking rates drop. This would enable the program to be financed well past the last smoker's cessation and enable a system by which to prevent tobacco use indefinitely.

To make matters more worrisome, the financial contingencies supporting the California Tobacco Control Program might cause the program to support the industry inadvertently. Because the program's survival and effectiveness are dependent on income and the income is dependent on tobacco sales, the effort to control sales might be diverted (by emphasizing basic science instead of prevention and cessation policies) to activities that are not likely to eliminate tobacco use in the state. Use of funds to support basic science aimed at finding cures for lung cancer or medical care for low-income families, for instance, would obtain the support of the California Medical Association and most of the public. Thus, metacontingencies are available to support the divergence of the program to a system that might sustain smoking and disease, tobacco sales, and tax revenue. This risk is due to misunderstanding the correct use of contingencies.

The California Tobacco Control Program, similar tax-based programs in other states, and the recent Master Settlement Agreement (MSA) between forty-six states and the tobacco industry provide millions of dollars per year for tobacco control and related medical and other clinical services. With over $1 billion in new funds to California from the MSA award, in addition to tax revenues already available, the resources to establish effective countercontingencies to those promoting smoking would seem to be available. However, less than 4 percent of these funds have been directed to tobacco control. As Givel, Dearlove, and Glantz (2001) have asserted, it appears that the efforts to control tobacco use and the industry in California have stalled. Even the relatively protected research program in California, TRDRP, suffered the transfer of millions of dollars of potential antitobacco research funds from the research account to the general fund and the state health department. This severely limited the number of studies that met standards for support from obtaining awards. This type of damage to the tobacco control effort prevents the discovery of practical and effective means of changing tobacco use or countering industry promotional tactics. The diversion of funding from tobacco control to other public services costs the state thousands of lives each year to tobacco-related disease.

The majority of funds from tobacco taxes or settlement funds have been directed to services other than tobacco control in California and all other states, which magnifies the risk of inadvertently supporting the industry. This type of financial contingency, codified by legislation and court order, runs the risk of having to sustain tobacco sales in order to sustain support for education, medical care, city infrastructure and roadway maintenance, and other services. Cumulative state and national programs that generate revenue from tobacco sales for the purpose of supporting antitobacco programs and those that also fund other critical community services represent complex financial contingencies that effect change in legislators' and voters' behavior. These might reduce tobacco sales and use in the short term but not eliminate them. These types of contingencies may preclude the elimination of tobacco-related disease. Understanding metacontingencies might contribute to refinements in these systems. If the existing financial system can change a sufficient proportion of the public sentiments against tobacco and the industry, it might be possible to obtain public support for financing the war on tobacco from sources independent of tobacco sales. It might also be possible to obtain public support for avoiding the use of tobacco taxes to fund any critical social or health services. In a social evolutionary sense, the existing system may be a precursor to a more refined version that can stop tobacco use and the industry supporting it.

Physicians Changed Teams

As early as the 1930s, science indicated that smoking was harmful to health, and by the 1960s, ever-increasing disease and death became unavoidably attributed to smoking (Borio, 2001). The surgeon general's reports (USDHHS, 2001) summarized the best evidence, which has been accumulating exponentially since 1964 (USDHHS, 1964). Incidental observations among the public that friends and family who smoke are dying of tobacco-related disease and that smoking is highly addictive have slowly changed the public's behavior with respect to smoking. Early in the process, not surprisingly, physicians, who saw the morbidity and mortality most clearly, were among the first organized group to quit smoking. Ironically, this was after serving for years as spokespersons for the tobacco industry (National Cancer Institute, 1994). Most recently, medical associations have denounced all association of members with the tobacco industry (Martin, 2001). Medical surveillance of lung disease and related tobacco research probably set in motion contingencies that led to the development of the California Tobacco Control Program.

Cognitive Versus Ecological Models

Lawsuits asserted that the tobacco industry was responsible for disease and death of smokers. The industry argued successfully that smokers knew the risk, chose to smoke, and decided to continue smoking. This placed the responsibility on the individual and implied that the individual decided (that is, used a cognitive process) to smoke. This logic freed the industry from moral and fiscal responsibility in another example of the cognitive model of human behavior serving to divert attention from ecological models.

The California Tobacco Control Program established an alternate conceptual model that we believe is consistent with the BEM and is implicitly an ecological model. This represents a huge shift in the theoretical underpinnings for human behavior, in this case for tobacco use, and sets in motion an alternative conceptual model to that of individual responsibility and cognitive processes. Although it is not yet clear whether California and other states will be successful, they have contributed to the change in culture with respect to theoretical models of health behavior. It remains to be seen whether the public and government institutions can engineer strong enough metacontingencies to counter the competitive engineering from the industry.

The tobacco industry has not been curtailed in its ability to make profits. The industry enjoyed one of its most profitable years in 2000–2001, even as it recovered from the largest litigation charges in history. Clearly, the industry has not been stopped; it continues to market tobacco nationally and even more so internationally and continues to lobby for policy changes and reversal of existing laws. For example, the recently passed Proposition 10 in California was fought with Proposition 28, which called for the abolition of Proposition 10. The California voters passed Proposition 10 and defeated Proposition 28, but this may not be so likely as increasing public resources are directed to outlets other than tobacco control. This process shows that the industry remains active in setting contingencies that support tobacco sales and weaken community control efforts. With increasing profits, the industry's ability to wage a counterattack on the public is almost limitless.

Directions for Refining the Antitobacco Program

To counter this, state and federal governments as well as nongovernment organizations may need to invest nearly the same amount in antitobacco efforts as the industry does. These efforts also need to be supported by funds derived by taxes independent of the sale of tobacco in order to ensure sufficient support to prevent all tobacco use. We believe attention to metacontingencies and the BEM, as a guide to these refinements in the war against tobacco, will increase efficacy. The jury remains out.

Applications to Other Health-Risk and Health-Promoting Behavior

The BEM is the same for all behavior. However, the application will be unique to the circumstances that apply for each type of behavior. For instance, physical activity is performed in direct proportion to the development of labor-saving technology and sedentary recreational technology. It is easy to see the history of people from hunter-gatherers to modern societies, where physical activity is no longer required to obtain food, shelter, or protection from predators. To this shift in contingencies can be added the development of television, movies, videotapes, and Internet content that requires sedentary behavior, such as sitting and watching. These shifts in contingencies have played a role in the epidemic of sedentary behavior and the corollary increase in calories consumed relative to calories spent. Sedentary lifestyles are responsible for over 300,000 premature deaths per year (McGinnis & Foege, 1993) and account for one-third of deaths due to coronary heart disease, colon cancer, and diabetes (Powell & Blair, 1994).

These contingencies are not likely to be reversed, and calls for more education for promotion of exercise and for promotion of healthy diets are not likely to be sufficient to offset the march of technology. However, it might be possible for the metacontingencies illustrated in the California Tobacco Control Program to serve as models for the development of metacontingencies that reestablish physical activity among whole populations. This will require structural changes in the way we engineer physical and social environments.

Environmental Contingencies for Physical Activity

A few examples illustrate environmental influence on physical activity. Three observational studies found significant correlations (r = .74) between being outdoors or in play spaces and activity level (Sallis et al., 1993; Klesges, Eck, Hanson, Haddock, & Klesges, 1990). For example, Blamey, Mutrie, and Aitchison (1995) and Brownell, Stunkard, and Albaum (1980) showed that low-cost signs in public places increased stair use instead of escalators. Characteristics of community environments were significantly related to walking (Replogle, 1995). Walking has been shown to be higher for both work and nonwork trips in neighborhoods that included mass transit versus those that were designed more for automobile use (Cervero & Gorham, 1995). Traditional neighborhoods in the San Francisco area were associated with 2.7 to 5.5 times as many walking trips to a store compared to auto-oriented neighborhoods (Handy, 1995).

Vuori, Oja, and Paronen (1994) added showers and changing rooms, disseminated information, included lotteries for physical activity, and lobbied the city government to improve safety and increased the rate of walking and bicycling to work. Consequently, rearranging the natural reinforcers, including the avoidance of aversive consequences, increased physical activity. This is a promising direction for future research concerning the promotion of physical activity and departs importantly from the more traditional education interventions. With the advancement of ecological studies, it should be possible to engineer metacontingencies that tie together multiple systems of reinforcement for supporting physical activity in whole populations. Affirmative investment in engineering solutions to reverse the current epidemic of sedentary behavior will be critical to reverse the consequential chronic disease burden now present and largely due to advancing technology that makes physical activity unnecessary and sometimes impossible.

Prevention of Sexually Transmitted Disease

Relative to physical activity, control of certain lifestyle risks may be especially difficult to alter. Among these, sexual practices figure prominently. The prevention of AIDS, other STDs, and unplanned pregnancies requires modification of sexual behavior. For many reasons, it is fortunate that sexual behavior is highly reinforcing; the survival of the species depends on it. However, the fact that it is inherently reinforcing also complicates the community's ability to alter sexual practices. To complicate matters more, the social contingencies on sexual practices make the behavior exceptionally private, even covert. Even talking about sex is socially discouraged in most communities. Thus, communities' ability to assess the frequency and types of sexual practices actually performed by individuals or selected groups are fraught with problems of reporting error. Cultural contingencies are complex and often contradictory. Most communities do not approve of sexual practices in public, with the very young, and with same-sex partners. These social restrictions might result as much in false reporting and covert practices as they do in suppression of the behavior. Thus, public health efforts to alter these risk practices are compromised by inaccurate and incomplete estimates of risk practices and peoples' willingness to participate in safer-sex programs.

Most AIDS prevention interventions have been educational or counseling services provided to small groups or individuals, supplemented by limited media programs. Unfortunately, the evidence of efficacy for these approaches is equivocal. Some have reported decreases in risk behavior or sexually transmitted infections (Ickovics, Morrill, Beren, Walsh, & Rodin, 1994; Perry et al., 1994). Others have found no effects or increased disease rates (Wenger, Greenberg, & Hillborne, 1992; Otten, Zaidi, Wroten, Witte, & Peterman, 1993). The discrepancies among these studies may be due to our relative inability to measure the behavior and thereby provide precise contingencies. It also may be due to the many competing contingencies for practicing the risk behavior versus use of condoms or avoiding certain types of behavior (such as anal intercourse) or types of partners.

Ecological approaches to AIDS prevention may offer more, or at least make an important addition, to individual counseling or small-group education (Hovell et al., 1994). Distribution of condoms throughout a community might contribute to change in condom use and the social contingencies that could support such use. Changes in physical environments might include decreasing privacy in public settings where casual sex is possible, such as adding lighting in public parks. The means by which such a covert practice can be modified by use of meta-contingencies will require creativity. Public health professionals might have to emphasize group contingencies to alter the behavior, including reporting behavior, of confidants who are observers of the private practices. This might be possible by placing group contingencies on sexually transmitted infection rates, including HIV. For defined communities, such as localized neighborhoods where a high proportion of males who have sex with males reside, it might be possible to offer communitywide economic incentives for decreased infection rates. This could be in the form of tax relief, lottery or other payments, or free media exposure for local businesses, for example. These types of group incentives might generate communitywide change in interpersonal risk practices and social contingencies for decreasing risk and increasing protective behavior, such as condom use. Infection rates are potentially measurable and therefore could serve as a marker for risk practices and for putting outcome contingencies in place. However, this will be workable only with changes in policies to enable routine monitoring of sexually transmitted infections. To employ such procedures will require considerable engineering to ensure protection from undue aversive control and appropriate levels of confidentiality. Given evidence that cohorts of young men repeatedly engage in sexual risk practices, as seen in San Francisco, something more than individual counseling or media instructions is needed to control the AIDS epidemic in the United States. Applying the BEM to this problem appears justified by the evidence in other applications and by the relatively limited effects of prevention efforts to date.

Conclusion

We have outlined the learning theory foundation for a Behavioral Ecological Model. We have tried to show the parallels between the BEM and natural, biological sciences, especially ecology. The BEM emphasizes environmental metacontingencies of reinforcement. Many interventions to date based on this model have been successful in changing contingencies for individual and group behavior. We believe this model to be more logically sound, efficacious, and efficient than models that rely on self-regulation and on unverifiable cognitive mediators of behavior, some of which may not be consistent with well-accepted scientific method. The California Tobacco Control Program employs many procedures that are consistent with the BEM, and results to date suggest efficacy. However, the BEM causes us to predict that tax support from tobacco sales may lead to inadvertent support of the tobacco industry. We attribute this to an incomplete understanding of contingencies that do not require support from tobacco sales. This example shows the potential for the BEM and that applications based on the BEM would be different and possibly more effective.

We believe this model to be more logically sound, efficacious, and efficient than models that rely on self-regulation.

Recent support by the Robert Wood Johnson Foundation for a major grants program aimed at the study of environmental interventions for promotion of physical activity in populations represents implicit recognition of the importance of the BEM (J. Sallis, personal communication, September 18, 2001). This also sets the stage for additional empirical support, to be forthcoming, from which the model might be verified and from which it will be refined. This can be expected to increase the understanding of physical activity among populations, as well as our societal means of affecting higher rates of physical activity among populations, with consequential health benefits.

The applications of an environmental model for the study of physical activity, if effective, may provide additional support for doing the same for behaviors that are more difficult to study, such as sexual practices. No doubt, such applications will be more difficult for many reasons, including the inability to measure sexual behavior objectively. However, one of the most important features of the BEM is that it is not necessarily dependent on information about individuals' sexual practices. Group contingency systems offer possibilities, albeit not without risk of side effects, but such side effects are not likely to be greater than existing ill effects of AIDS.

We hope that others will direct their empirical investigations toward both individual and cultural contingencies of reinforcement as key causal variables for health-related behavior of populations. This is critical for the development of large-scale prevention programs for numerous sources of morbidity and mortality. It will be difficult, as it requires a paradigm shift. The BEM requires the study and manipulation of variables normally so large as to be precluded from traditional medical or behavioral science. The study of large-scale contingencies, especially experiments, is difficult because of the magnitude of the independent variables. It is difficult to alter legal or communitywide social contingencies for driving behavior, for diet, exercise, and other important health-related behavior for defined populations.

The process is made all the more difficult if attempts to study metacontingencies are thwarted by alternative theoretical models and lay understandings of human behavior. The current popularity of cognitive models of health behavior, and preference for clinical, individual-based interventions for both treatment and prevention of health risk practices, compromises support for interventions based on BEM. The preference for clinical solutions to health-related behavior problems is driven both by the cognitive models that suggest individuals' thinking must be changed to change their behavior and also by the economic systems in place to compensate clinicians for attempting to change individuals' cognitions and behavior.

This chapter, other publications (Cohen et al., 2000), and programs such as the California Tobacco Control Program, provide support for, and maybe the critical mass, to establish a paradigm shift that will enable political and economic support of the BEM. We hope so; we believe this model is critical for making substantive and lasting changes to the uncontrolled epidemics in obesity, diabetes, AIDS, tuberculosis, and other diseases that are common worldwide.

References

Ader, R., Felten, D. L., & Cohen, N. (Eds.). (1991). *Psychoneuroimmunology.* Orlando, FL: Academic Press

Agras, W. S., Jacob, R. G., & Lebedeck, M. (1980). The California drought: A quasi-experimental analysis of social policy. *Journal of Applied Behavior Analysis, 13,* 561–570.

Baer, D. M., Peterson, R. F., & Sherman, J. A. (1967). The development of imitation by reinforcing behavioral similarity to a model. *Journal of the Experimental Analysis of Behavior, 10,* 405–416.

Balbach, E. D., Traynor, M. P., & Glantz, S. A. (2000). The implementation of California's tobacco tax initiative: The critical role of outsider strategies in protecting Proposition 99. *Journal of Health Politics, Policy and Law, 25,* 689–715.

Bandura, A. (1965). Influence of models' reinforcement contingencies on the acquisition of imitative responses. *Journal of Personality and Social Psychology, 1,* 589–595.

Bandura, A. (1986). *Social foundations of thought and action: A social cognitive theory.* Upper Saddle River NJ: Prentice Hall.

Bandura, A., & Walters, R. H. *Social learning and personality development.* New York: Holt, Rinehart, & Winston.

Bandura, A., Barbaranelli, C., Caprara, G. V., & Pastorelli, C. (1996). Mechanisms of moral disengagement in the exercise of moral agency. *Journal of Personality and Social Psychology, 71,* 364–374.

Baranowski, T., Thompson, W. O., DuRant, R. H., Baranowski, J., & Puhl, J. (1993). Observations on physical activity in physical locations: Age, gender, ethnicity, and month effects. *Research Quarterly for Exercise and Sport, 64,* 127–133.

Biglan, A. (1995). *Changing cultural practices: A contextualist framework for intervention research.* Reno, NV: Context Press.

Biglan, A., & Hayes, S. C. (1996). Should the behavioral sciences become more pragmatic? The case for functional contextualism in research on human behavior. *Applied and Preventive Psychology, 5,* 47–57.

Blamey, A., Mutrie, N., & Aitchison, T. (1995). Health promotion by encouraged use of stairs. *British Medical Journal, 311,* 289–290.

Borio, G. (2001). "Tobacco Timeline." Available: www.tobacco.org/History/Tobacco_History.html.

Breed, L. (2001). "Breed's Collection of Tobacco History Sites." Available: SmokingSides.com/docs/hist.html.

Brownell, K. D., Stunkard, A. J., & Albaum, J. M. (1980). Evaluation and modification of exercise patterns in the natural environment. *American Journal of Psychiatry, 137,* 1540–1545.

Cameron, J., Banko, K. M., & Pierce, W. D. (2001). Pervasive negative effects of rewards on intrinsic motivation: The myth continues. *Behavior Analyst, 24,* 1–44.

Cervero, R., & Gorham, R. (1995). Commuting in transit versus automobile neighborhoods. *Journal of the American Planning Association, 61,* 210–225.

Children and Families First. (2001). Available: www.prop10.org.

Cohen, D., Farley, T. A., Bedimo-Etome, J. R., Scribner, R., Ward, W., & Kendall, C. (1999). Implementation of condom social marketing in Lousiana, 1993 to 1998. *American Journal of Public Health, 89,* 204–208.

Cohen, D., Scribner, R., & Farley, T. A. (2000). A structural model of health behavior: A pragmatic approach to explain and influence health behavior at the population level. *Preventive Medicine, 30,* 146–154.

Darwin, C. (1936). *On the origin of species.* New York: Modern Library.

Eisenberger, R., & Cameron, J. (1996). Detrimental effects of reward: Reality or myth? *American Psychologist, 51,* 1153–1166.

Elder, J. P. (2001). *Behavior change and public health in the developing world.* Thousand Oaks, CA: Sage.

Elder, J. P., Geller, E. S., Hovell, M. F., & Mayer, J. A. (1994). *Motivating health behavior.* Albany, NY: Delmar Publishers.

Ferster, C. B., & Skinner, B. F. (1957). *Schedules of reinforcement.* New York: Appleton-Century-Croft.

Fichtenberg, C. M., & Glantz, S. A. (2000). Association of the California Tobacco Control Program with declines in the cigarette consumption and mortality from heart disease. *New England Journal of Medicine, 343,* 1772–1777.

Gewirtz, J. L., & Stingle, K. G. (1968). Learning of generalized imitation as the basis for identification. *Psychological Review, 75,* 374–397.

Givel, M. S., Dearlove, J., & Glantz, S. A. (2001). *Tobacco policy making in California 1999–2001: Stalled and adrift.* San Francisco: University of California, San Francisco, Institute for Health Policy Studies. Available: www.library.ucsf.edu/tobacco/ca2001.

Glantz, S. A., & Parmley, W. W. (1991). Passive smoking and heart disease: Epidemiology, physiology, and biochemistry. *Circulation, 83,* 1–12.

Glenn, S. S. (1988). Contingencies and metacontingencies: Toward a synthesis of behavior analysis and cultural materialism. *Behavior Analyst, 11,* 161–179.

Glenn, S. S. (1991). Contingencies and metacontingencies: Relation among behavioral, cultural, and biological evolution. In P. A. Lamal (Ed.), *Behavioral analysis of societies and cultural practices.* New York: Hemisphere.

Glenn, S. S., & Malagodi, E. F. (1991). Process and content in behavioral and cultural phenomena. *Behavior and Social Issues, 1,* 1–14.

Goldman, L. K., & Glantz, S. A. (1998). Evaluation of antismoking advertising campaigns. *Journal of the American Medical Association, 279,* 772–777.

Guerin, B. (1994). *Analyzing social behavior: Behavior analysis and the social sciences.* Reno, NV: Context Press.

Handy, S. (1995). Understanding the link between urban form and travel behavior. Paper presented at the Seventy-Fourth Annual Meeting of the Transportation Research Board.

Hanenberg, S., Ronanapithayakorn, W., Kunasol, P., & Sokal, D. (1994). Impact of Thailand's HIV-control programmes as indicated by decline of sexually transmitted disease. *Lancet, 344,* 243–245.

Hayes, S. C. (1989). *Rule-governed behavior: Cognition, contingencies, and instructional control.* New York: Plenum.

Hovell, M. F., Elder, J. P., Blanchard, J., & Sallis, J. F. (1986). Behavior analysis and public health perspectives: Combining paradigms to effect prevention. *Education and Treatment of Children, 9,* 287–306.

Hovell, M. F., Hillman, E. R., Blumberg, E., Sipan, C., Atkins, C., Hofstetter, C. R., & Myers, C. A. (1994). A behavioral-ecological model of adolescent sexual development: A template for AIDS prevention. *Journal of Sex Research, 31,* 267–281.

Hovell, M. F., Kaplan, R., & Hovell, F. (1991). Analysis of preventive medical services in the U.S. In P. A. Lamal (Ed.), *Behavior analysis of societies and cultural practices.* New York: Hemisphere.

Hovell, M. F., Wahlgren, D. R., & Russos, S. (1997). Preventive medicine and cultural contingencies: A natural experiment. In P. A. Lamal (Ed.), *Cultural contingencies: Behavior analytic perspectives on cultural practices.* New York: Praeger.

Ickovics, J., Morrill, A., Beren, S., Walsh, U., & Rodin, J. (1994). Limited effects of HIV counseling and testing for women: A prospective study of behavioral and psychological consequences. *Journal of the American Medical Association, 272,* 443–448.

Kaplan, R. M. (1990). Behavior as the central outcome in health care. *American Psychologist, 45,* 1211–1220.

Kaplan, R. M. (1994). The Ziggy theorem: Toward an outcomes-focused health psychology. *Health Psychology, 13,* 451–460.

Klesges, R. C., Eck, L. H., Hanson, C. L., Haddock, C. K., & Klesges, L. M. (1990). Effects of obesity, social interactions, and physical environment on physical activity in preschoolers. *Health Psychology, 9,* 435–449.

Lamal, P. A. (Ed.). (1991). *Behavioral analysis of societies and cultural practices.* New York: Hemisphere.

Lamal, P. A. (1997). *Cultural contingencies: Behavior analytic perspectives on cultural practices.* New York: Praeger.

Lavelle, J. M., Hovell, M. F., West, M. P., & Wahlgren, D. R. (1992). Promoting law enforcement for child protection: A community analysis. *Journal of Applied Behavior Analysis, 25,* 885–892.

Lloyd, J. W., Eberhardt, M. J., & Drake, G. P. (1996). Group versus individual reinforcement contingencies within the context of group study conditions. *Journal of Applied Behavior Analysis, 29,* 189–200.

Maiback, E., & Parrot, R. (Eds.). (1995). *Designing health messages: Approaches from communication theory and public health practice.* Thousand Oaks, CA: Sage.

Malagodi, E. F. (1986). On radicalizing behaviorism: A call for cultural analysis. *Behavior Analyst, 9,* 1–17.

Malagodi, E. F., & Jackson, K. (1989). Behavior analysts and cultural analysis: Troubles and issues. *Behavior Analyst, 12,* 17–33.

Martin, W. (2001, February). Message from the president (American Thoracic Society). *ATS News, 27*(3).

McGinnis, J. M., & Foege, W. H. (1993). Actual causes of death in the United States. *Journal of the American Medical Association, 270,* 2207–2212.

Murphy, S. L. (2000). *Deaths: Final data for 1998.* Hyattsville, MD: National Center for Health Statistics.

National Cancer Institute. (1994). *Tobacco and the clinician: Interventions for medical and dental practice.* NIH publication no. 94-3693. Bethesda, MD: Author. Available: rex.nci.nih.gov/NCI_MONOGRAPHS/MONO5/MONO5.HTM.

National Cancer Policy Board. (2000). *State programs can reduce tobacco use.* Washington, DC: Institute of Medicine, National Research Council. Available: www.nap.edu.

Orpinas, P., Kelder, S., Frankowski, R., Murray, N., Zhang, Q., & McAlister, A. (2000). Outcome evaluation of a multi-component violence-prevention program for middle schools: The Students for Peace project. *Health Education Research, 15,* 45–58.

Orpinas, P., Parcel, G. S., McAlister, A., & Frankowski, R. (1995). Violence prevention in middle schools: A pilot evaluation. *Journal of Adolescent Health, 17,* 360–371.

Otten, M., Zaidi, A., Wroten, J., Witte, J., & Peterman, T. (1993). Changes in sexually transmitted disease rates after HIV testing and posttest counseling. *American Journal of Public Health, 83,* 529–533.

Pavlov, I. P. (1927). *Conditioned reflexes.* (G. V. Anrep, Trans.) New York: Oxford University Press.

Perry, S., Card, C., Moffat, A., Ashman, T., Fishman, B., & Jacobsberg, L. (1994). Self-disclosure of HIV infection to sexual partners after repeated counseling. *AIDS Education and Prevention, 6,* 403–411.

Poulos, C. X., Hinson, R. E., & Siegel, S. (1981). The role of Pavlovian processes in drug tolerance and dependence: Implications for treatment. *Addictive Behaviors, 6,* 205–211.

Powell, K. E., & Blair, S. N. (1994). The public health burdens of sedentary living habits: Theoretical but realistic estimates. *Medicine and Science in Sports and Exercise, 26,* 851–856.

Replogle, M. (1995, July 20). Integrating pedestrian and bicycle factors into regional transportation planning models: Summary of state-of-the-art and suggested steps forward. In *Environmental Defense Fund Report.* Washington, DC: Government Printing Office.

Rugg, D., Hovell, M. F., & Franzini, L. (1989). Behavioral science and public health perspectives: Combining paradigms for the prevention and control of AIDS. In L. Temoshok & A. Baum (Eds.), *Psychological perspectives on AIDS: Etiology, prevention and treatment.* Hillsdale, NJ: Erlbaum.

Russos, S., Hovell, M. F., Keating, K. J., Jones, J. A., Burkham, S. M., Slymen, D. J., Hofstetter, C. R., & Rubin, B. (1997). Clinician compliance with primary prevention of tobacco use: The impact of social contingencies. *Preventive Medicine, 26,* 44–52.

Russos, S., Keating, K., Hovell, M. F., Jones, J. A., Slymen, D. J., Hofstetter, C. R., Rubin, B., & Morrison, T. (1999). Counseling youth in tobacco use prevention: Determinants of clinician compliance. *Preventive Medicine, 29,* 13–21.

Sallis, J. F., Bauman, A., & Pratt, M. (1998). Environmental and policy interventions to promote physical activity. *American Journal of Preventive Medicine, 15,* 379–397.

Sallis, J. F., Hovell, M. F., Hofstetter, C. R., Elder, J. P., Hackley, M., Caspersen, C. J., & Powell, K. E. (1990). Distance between homes and exercise facilities related to frequency of exercise among San Diego residents. *Public Health Reports, 105,* 179–185.

Sallis, J. F., Nader, P. R., Broyles, S. L., Berry, C. C., Elder, J. P., McKenzie, T. L., & Nelson, J. A. (1993). Correlates of physical activity at home in Mexican-American and Anglo-American preschool children. *Health Psychology, 12,* 390–398.

Sallis, J. F., & Owen, N. (1996). Ecological models. In K. Glanz, F. M. Lewis, & B. K. Rimer, (Eds.), *Health behavior and health education: Theory, research, and practice* (2nd ed., pp. 403–424). San Francisco: Jossey-Bass.

Sallis, J. F., & Owen, N. (1999). *Physical activity and behavioral medicine.* Thousand Oaks, CA: Sage.

Schroeder, S. T. (1999). *Effects of newsletters on promoting proenvironmental behaviors to improve ocean water quality.* Unpublished master's thesis, San Diego State University.

Schumaker, J., Hovell, M. F., & Sherman, J. A. (1977). An analysis of daily report cards and parent-managed privileges in the improvement of adolescents' classroom performance. *Journal of Applied Behavior Analysis, 10,* 449–464.

The shooting at Granite Hills High School. (2001, March 25). *San Diego Union-Tribune,* p. B-1.

Siegel, S. (1975). Evidence from rats that morphine tolerance is a learned response. *Journal of Comparative and Physiological Psychology, 89,* 498–506.

Siegel, S. (1982). Heroin "overdose" death: Contribution of drug-associated environmental cues. *Science, 216,* 436–437.

Skinner, B. F. (1953). *Science and human behavior.* New York: Free Press.

Skinner, B. F. (1957). *Verbal behavior.* Acton, MA: Copley.

Skinner, B. F. (1987). Why we are not acting to save the world. In B. F. Skinner (Ed.), *Upon further reflection.* Upper Saddle River, NJ: Prentice Hall.

Slavin, R. E. (1987). Cooperative learning: Where behavioral and humanistic approaches to classroom motivation meet. *Elementary School Journal, 88,* 29–37.

Tobacco Control Section. (1998). *A model for change: The California experience in tobacco control.* Sacramento: California Department of Health Services. Available: www.dhs.cahwnet.gov/ps/cdic/ccb/TCS/index.htm.

Tobacco Control Section. (2000). *California tobacco control update.* Sacramento: California Department of Health Services. Available: www.dhs.cahwnet.gov/ps/cdic/ccb/TCS/index.htm.

Traynor M. P., & Glantz S. A. (1996). California's tobacco tax initiative: The development and passage of Proposition 99. *Journal of Health Politics, Policy and Law, 21,* 543–585.

U.S. Department of Health, Education and Welfare. (1964). *Smoking and health: Report of the Advisory Committee to the Surgeon General of the Public Health Service.* Washington, DC: U.S. Department of Health, Education, and Welfare, Public Health Service.

U.S. Department of Health and Human Services. (1989). *Reducing the health consequences of smoking: Twenty-five years of progress. A report of the Surgeon General.* Washington, DC: U.S. Department of Health and Human Services, Public Health Service, Centers for Disease Control, Center for Chronic Disease Prevention and Health Promotion, Office on Smoking and Health.

U.S. Department of Health and Human Services. (2000). *Reducing tobacco use. A report of the Surgeon General.* Atlanta, Georgia: U.S. Department of Health and Human Services, Centers for Disease Control and Prevention, National Center for Chronic Disease Prevention and Health Promotion, Office on Smoking and Health.

U.S. Department of Health and Human Services. (2001). *Women and smoking. A report of the Surgeon General.* Atlanta, GA: U.S. Department of Health and Human Services, Centers for Disease Control and Prevention, National Center for Chronic Disease Prevention and Health Promotion, Office on Smoking and Health.

Vuori, I. M., Oja, P., & Paronen, O. (1994). Physically active commuting to work: Testing its potential for exercise promotion. *Medicine and Science in Sports and Exercise, 26,* 844–850.

Wenger, N., Greenberg, J., & Hillborne, L. (1992). Effect of HIV antibody testing and AIDS education on communication about HIV risk and sexual behavior. *Annals of Internal Medicine, 117,* 905–911.

Wilson, S. H., & Williams, R. L. (1973). The effects of group contingencies on first graders' academic and social behaviors. *Journal of School Psychology, 11,* 110–117.

CHAPTER FOURTEEN

REFLECTIONS ON EMERGING THEORIES IN HEALTH PROMOTION PRACTICE

Michelle C. Kegler
Richard A. Crosby
Ralph J. DiClemente

The chapters in this book provide a glimpse into the future of health promotion and disease prevention. Increasingly, theories in health promotion practice acknowledge the complex nature of attempting to change population health. Collectively, the emerging theories described in this book draw on a broad range of disciplines and conceptual orientations: political science, economics, psychology, ecology, and sociology. This diversity of new perspectives and insights constitutes a significant advance in our use of theory. Clearly, this multidisciplinary collection of theories can serve researchers and practitioners in their ongoing efforts to understand and promote health behavior across a spectrum of populations. In this final chapter, we reflect on overarching concepts and issues that are relevant to emerging theories in public health practice.

Development of Emerging Theories

The theories that dominate a field exert a powerful influence by shaping how problems are perceived and defined and how potential solutions are framed. Historically, a handful of theories have accounted for the majority of theory-based interventions in health promotion practice. Commonly applied theories include the Health Belief Model, Social Cognitive Theory, Diffusion of Innovations, the

Theory of Reasoned Action, the Theory of Planned Behavior, and the Trans-theoretical Model of Behavior Change (Glanz, Lewis, & Rimer, 1997). As noted in Chapter One, theory may become the lens used to understand and define the range of possible solutions to public health challenges. If, for example, we understand and define a problem using an individual-level theory, then we may develop intervention programs that focus on the individual at the expense of focusing on key contextual influences extrinsic to the individual. Thus, theory selection may properly be viewed as an integral step in the process of health promotion practice. In turn, effective theory selection demands that an elaborate continuum of theories is available, understandable, and logistically feasible to researchers and practitioners alike. The trajectory of theory development captured in this book reflects a common movement toward less reliance on individual-based approaches and greater use of theories that account for social and contextual influences. Thus, many of the chapters have provided a broad lens through which to understand and define health promotion practice.

One potentially useful way of reflecting on the theories described here is to consider four methods of theory development and application. One method adds new constructs to existing theory. A second refines existing theory to create a new and more parsimonious approach to public health practice. A related third method is the application of existing theory from other disciplines to health promotion practice. A final method is the development of theory based on approaches already accepted by practitioners. We discuss each method in turn in the following sections.

As theories are developed, they are applied to an increasing number of health issues, settings, and populations. Their robustness depends on the extent to which they retain parsimonious explanatory power in a variety of situations. Over time, new concepts may be designed to increase a theory's explanatory power, such as the refined stage model that Weinstein and Sandman describe in Chapter Two. Most notably, their description of the Precaution Adoption Process Model carefully delineates the initial stages of behavior change and provides a separate stage for those who decide not to act. This additional level of conceptual differentiation improves our ability to craft messages and strategies that are particularly meaningful to individuals and in turn may enhance the likelihood of individuals' progressing to the next stage in the process of behavior change.

Several theories presented here can be viewed as evolutions of existing theories through the addition or refinement of particular constructs. For example, Fisher and Fisher (Chapter Three) described the Information-Motivation-Behavioral Skills Model, which can be viewed as a refinement and extension of other well-known models, such as the Health Belief Model, the Theory of Reasoned Action, and the Theory of Planned Behavior. Fisher and Fisher reported empirical evidence suggesting that the IMB model is robust, explaining a substantial and significant proportion of the variance observed in HIV-associated risk behaviors. The extension of this model to health promotion behaviors such as breast self-examination and helmet use for those on motorcycles illustrates a potential trajectory that may culminate in a broader application of the model across health promotion practices. Similarly, Hobfall and Schumm (Chapter Eleven) built on empirical and theoretical work in the field of stress and coping in their Conservation of Resources Theory. The theory provides a model for preventing resource loss, maintaining existing resources, and gaining resources necessary for engaging in healthy behaviors.

Other theories presented in this book constitute new applications of theories previously established in other disciplines. For example in Chapter Four, Petty, Barden, and Wheeler provided examples of how the Elaboration Likelihood Model, originating from the discipline of social psychology, can be used in health promotion practice. In Chapter Five, Simons-Morton and Hartos built on theoretical work relevant to parenting styles and articulate how parenting goals, style, and practices may influence health outcomes among adolescents. Another example, the Theory of Gender and Power (Chapter Twelve), was originally developed to explain sexual inequality, gender, and power imbalance. Wingood and DiClemente refined the original theory to expand its applicability to health promotion practice, particularly in regard to reducing sexual risk behaviors among potentially vulnerable populations of women. Finally, Hovell, Wahlgren, and Gehrman (Chapter Thirteen) applied and extended basic propositions originally found in the field of operant conditioning; they suggest that interlocking reinforcement contingencies have significant potential to guide health promotion practices.

Although theories often emerge as a consequence of iterative cycles of empirical investigation and subsequent refinement, new theories can also emerge from the experience of practitioners. A recurring discussion in the academic literature centers on how practitioners use theory in developing programs. Public health practitioners design programs to achieve goals related to health outcomes, not to test theory. Based on semistructured interviews with practicing health educators, Burdine and McLeroy (1992) reported that practitioners did not describe themselves as using theories to develop interventions in any planned or explicit way. Rather, the practitioners they interviewed felt that theory was in fact largely common sense and believed that they did use theory in developing interventions, but not necessarily in a conscious way. For them, theories were often not sufficiently comprehensive to be of practical use. They spoke of the need for multiple theories in comprehensive projects, and much of their community-oriented practice was based on principles rather than theory.

In this book, several chapters advance theory by providing conceptual frameworks for health promotion approaches that are already widely accepted in practice. For example, coalition-based and natural helper approaches have been widely used in the field of health promotion but are typically considered models with loose ties to theory. In Chapter Six, Eng and Parker presented a natural helper intervention model that illustrates how these types of interventions lead to improved community competence, increased coordination of agency services, and improved health practices. Similarly, in Chapter Seven, Butterfoss and Kegler synthesized empirical findings with widely held assumptions about community coalitions into the Community Coalition Action Theory, complete with testable practice-proven propositions.

> *In this book, several chapters advance theory by providing conceptual frameworks for health promotion approaches that are already widely accepted in practice.*

All theories are originally based on observation. Interest in community capacity has grown out of the observation that communities vary significantly in their ability to mobilize to address their problems successfully. In Chapter Eight, Norton, McLeroy, Burdine, Felix, and Dorsey distilled several conceptualizations of community capacity into core dimensions of capacity. Similarly, interest in social capital as an important concept in community-based health promotion has grown out of the same observation but is empirically more advanced, with a growing body of evidence linking social capital to health outcomes. In Chapter Nine, Kreuter and Lezin described two types of social capital and illustrated how bridging social capital may be useful in understanding community-based health promotion processes and outcomes.

Challenges Countenanced by Emerging Theories

The theories described in this book span a tremendous range of approaches, health behaviors, and potential priority populations. Some provide new insights into why individuals behave as they do. Others elaborate on how interpersonal factors and social relationships influence health. Still others focus on community-level influences and provide models of community change. Several of these chapters deepen our understanding of models that have been used in health promotion practice for some time, such as natural helper models and community coalitions. Others present theoretical orientations that have recently emerged as important constructs in health promotion practice, such as social capital and community capacity.

Although the collective assets of emerging theories are appealing, these theories are not devoid of corresponding challenges. Here, we discuss three potential challenges countenanced by emerging theories. Issues presented relate to research design and analysis, necessary levels of empirical support, and theory selection.

Because many emerging theories focus on broad social and contextual influences, the constructs under examination can be complex. Thus, it will be difficult for these theories to evolve to the stage where interlocking propositions can be empirically tested. One important observation about emerging theories is that they tend to address multiple determinants of health behavior through a variety of strategies. Although this book has described a few theories that represent refinements of individual-level approaches to health promotion (Chapters Two, Three, and Four), the majority of theories have described focal points that go beyond the traditional reliance on individual cognition and skills as the sole mechanism of behavior change. A clear advantage of the traditional individual-level approach

A central challenge to emerging theories that address change produced through broader contextual approaches is to craft research design and analysis methods that are capable of determining program efficacy.

to health promotion is that existing research design and analytic techniques are highly compatible with evaluation of these theories; the same does not hold true for theories that depart from this approach. Thus, a central challenge to emerging theories that address change produced through broader contextual approaches is to craft research design and analysis methods that are capable of determining program efficacy. For example, the randomized controlled clinical trial is a problematic evaluation strategy for the testing of theories that target communities, focus on ecological strategies to health promotion practice, and include hypothesized outcomes that are often not amenable to evaluation at the individual level. For broad-level emerging theories to become firmly established among practitioners, researchers will need to define their objectives carefully and subsequently identify and create corresponding evaluation methodologies. These methods are likely to include multi-method designs that combine new types of quasi-experimental and observational research techniques.

With increasing theoretical complexity and the associated crossing of levels of analysis, empirical testing of theory becomes increasingly complex. For example, in Chapter Ten, Kennedy and Crosby described an emerging integrative framework consistent with the way practitioners use theory. The prevention marketing framework grew out of efforts of the Centers for Disease Control and Prevention to guide several human immunodeficiency virus prevention activities targeting youth. The approach integrates principles from three disciplines in an effort to provide an integrated, multilevel intervention framework. By building on behavioral science, community development, and social marketing, the model is comprehensive and has the potential to have a significant impact on health outcomes. However, because of its complexity, empirical testing of the framework presents a formidable challenge. Indeed, many of the complex and comprehensive theories presented in this book, such as the Theory of Gender and Power and the nascent theory of community capacity, face similar challenges.

Another challenge involves using appropriate methodologies for evaluating many of the emerging theories described here. In the absence of accepted evaluation strategies, one issue becomes whether these theories will become widely used. Thus, an important question for further evolution of these theories is how much and what level of empirical support is necessary before a theory is ready for widespread application. The current gold standard for testing theory effectiveness is the randomized controlled trial. Yet as we acknowledge the complexity of public health problems and the role of social networks, community capacity, gender and power relationships, and public policy in resolving them, the ease and, perhaps the applicability, appropriateness, and capacity to design or construct randomized controlled trials, diminishes. Qualitative methods are gaining respect, but their strengths lie in providing deep understandings of phenomena in specific settings and contexts. The usual definition of theory in public health practice is that of generalized propositions that parsimoniously explain and predict human behavior. Quite possibly, this current view may require further examination in light of emerging approaches that address systems rather than individuals and relational changes rather than propositions designed to change specific antecedents of health behaviors.

One apparent solution to the desire for evidence-based health promotion programs is adoption of a best practices approach to selecting programs for implementation. This approach involves presenting practitioners with a menu of programs considered as best or most promising. The literature discusses possible criteria for identifying best practices. One such system, developed by Cameron and colleagues (2001), includes three categories of criteria: effectiveness, plausibility, and practicality (Cameron, Jolin, Walker, McDermott, & Gough, 2001). The Task Force on Community Preventive Services engaged in a similar process and made recommendations based on evidence of effectiveness (Centers for Disease Control and Prevention, 2000). Consideration was given to the number of studies available, the suitability of the study designs, the quality of the execution of the studies, consistency of the results across studies, and the observed effect sizes.

Although the call for evidence-based programs and the accompanying reliance on programmatic activities identified as best may improve the practice of health promotion, the implications for theory development are less clear. Few of the proposed sets of criteria give significant weight to the use of theory. Theory is absent from some lists of criteria and grouped with beliefs in other sets of criteria (Cameron et al., 2001; Centers for Disease Control and Prevention, 2000; Kahan & Goodstadt, 2001). Although the need for evidence-based programs is obvious, we urge caution in adopting a best practices approach at the expense of interventions grounded in theory. As evidenced by many of the chapters in this book, we are still at an early stage in developing and understanding complex, eco- logical, theory-based approaches to influencing population health. Although our evaluation methods have not kept pace with these theoretical advances, method- ological strategies and statistical techniques are being developed to test these newer, contextually broader theories.

Another key challenge involves theory selection. The discipline of health pro- motion practice began to embrace a social ecological perspective in the late 1980s and the early 1990s (McLeroy, Bibeau, Steckler, & Glanz, 1988; Stokols, 1992). By conceptualizing multiple levels of influence such as organizational, commu- nity, and public policy, in addition to individual and interpersonal, the potential for understanding why people behave as they do is greatly expanded. However, with this broader perspective, we are confronted with a much more complex view of public health problems and how best to address them. Similarly, our interven- tion options are increasingly rich and diverse. The contents of this book make the richness and diversity of health promotion practices more salient than ever before. Clearly, no single theory can adequately explain all the variables and contexts that influence human behavior. Indeed, numerous theories exist at each of the levels of the social ecological framework. So how do we make decisions about which theories to use?

Published descriptions of interventions rarely provide adequate detail on how theory was used to inform and guide the design and implementation of inter- ventions. Usually there is a brief paragraph noting that the intervention was based on a particular model or theory. Similarly, advice on using theory in intervention design has typically been superficial. Fortunately, the situation has improved recently with intervention mapping, a new approach for engaging in theory-based program planning developed by Bartholomew, Parcel, Kok, and Gottlieb (2001). This approach is grounded in a problem-driven perspective. Problems are addressed by defining them carefully through iterative application of theory and empirical evidence, with the goal of solving the problem, not testing the theory. This problem-driven perspective often uses multiple theories, an approach incon- sistent with the traditional paradigm of theory testing. Finding the best theory or combination of theoretical constructs to solve a problem is described as one of the key challenges in intervention mapping, and the authors caution that reliance on any single theory may lead to a suboptimal solution.

Application Issues Relevant to Emerging Theories

Theories can be useful to researchers and practitioners by providing insights into the factors that influence behavior. By applying a particular theoretical framework, we can understand the genesis of long-term adoption of health-related behaviors among members of a given population. When this process begins with the goal of understanding a problem or behavior from various perspectives, it is sometimes referred to as the theory of the problem (Burdine & McLeroy, 1992). Regardless of the goal, the application of theory in health promotion is widely accepted as an important practice. As new theories emerge, one important question becomes whether new application issues will arise. We anticipate several.

One important application issue centers on measurement. A central challenge to the researcher or practitioner who applies emerging theory to health promotion practice is identifying and operationalizing the theory constructs. Clearly, measurement is inextricably linked to the operationalization and use of theory. Thus, the development of reliable and valid assessment measures designed to capture the desired theoretical constructs can be viewed as an important step in the use of the emerging theories described in this book. In addition, the availability of these measures can greatly facilitate the correct application of emerging theories. In turn, this fidelity to the intended application of theory sets the stage for more meaningful evaluation strategies that can subsequently inform researchers about the strengths and weaknesses of any given set of theoretical propositions. The eventual adoption of emerging theory by researchers and practitioners may be a function of how easily the theory can be understood and applied. This is not to say that implementation should necessarily be an easy process; health promotion practice is often a long, protracted, and labor-intensive process. Rather, the theory and the specific details for its application should be intuitively clear to provide practitioners and researchers with the vision necessary to plan and implement the desired theory-driven program.

Another important application issue involves the influence of cultural differences among people within the United States and the ability to apply these emerging theories in cultures outside the United States. For example the Theory of Gender and Power (see Chapter Twelve) posits that redressing inequalities between men and women can be an important strategy for promoting women's health. In highly paternalistic cultures and societies, interventions based on this theory may be difficult to implement or may not be feasible. Yet without addressing the broader entrenched societal norms that disenfranchise women and create power imbalances that favor men, it would be difficult to improve women's health status. Thus, understanding the cultural contexts and nuances allows practitioners and researchers to determine how best to translate and adapt a theory for their particular set of cultural constraints, thus maximizing the potential for achieving desired changes.

It is important to obtain empirical evidence of a theory's cross-cultural utility before proceeding with program design and implementation. Theories can and should be modified to be suitable for a particular cultural context (Airhihenbuwa, DiClemente, Wingood, & Lowe, 1992; Burdine & McLeroy, 1992). For instance, some constructs may differ in their meaning across cultures, and some cultures may not possess a particular theoretical construct. It is therefore important to determine the cultural equivalence and relevance of constructs across groups (Berry, 1996). Thus, theories should not constrain interventions through standardized application; rather, they should provide a foundation on which particular cultural elements and social-environmental constructs can be examined in a specific sociocultural context and appropriately integrated into the theoretical framework. It is this broad definition of theory, one that is capable of being tailored for different contexts, that is most appropriate for designing health promotion interventions.

Conclusion

Using broader-based contextual theories to understand and promote public health requires specification of a range of exposures and risk factors, a multilevel approach to intervention and prevention, and a broader conceptualization of the diversity and types of environmental and social contextual influences that could adversely or positively affect health. Employing these emerging theories marshals new kinds of data, asks new and broader questions regarding the factors that influence health, and creates new options for prevention.

References

Airhihenbuwa, C. O., DiClemente, R. J., Wingood, G. M., & Lowe, A. (1992). HIV/AIDS education and prevention among African-Americans: A focus on culture. *AIDS Education and Prevention, 4,* 251–260.

Bartholomew, L., Parcel, G., Kok, G., & Gottlieb, N. (2001) *Intervention mapping: Designing theory- and evidence-based health promotion programs.* Mountain View, CA: Mayfield.

Berry, J. (1996). On cross-cultural comparability. *International Journal of Psychology, 4,* 207–229.

Burdine, J. N., & McLeroy, K. (1992). Practitioners' use of theory: Examples from a workgroup. *Health Education Quarterly, 19,* 331–340.

Cameron, R., Jolin, M., Walker, R., McDermott, N., & Gough, M. (2001) Linking science and practice: Toward a system for enabling communities to adopt best practices for chronic disease prevention. *Health Promotion Practice, 2,* 35–42.

Centers for Disease Control and Prevention. (2000). Strategies for reducing exposure to environmental tobacco smoke, increasing tobacco-use cessation, and reducing initiation in communities and health-care systems. A report on recommendations of the Task Force on Community Preventive Services. *MMWR, 49,* 1–11.

Glanz, K., Lewis, F., & Rimer, B. (1997). *Health behavior and health education: Theory, research, and practice* (2nd ed.). San Francisco: Jossey-Bass.

Kahan, B., & Goodstadt, M. (2001) The interactive domain model of best practices in health promotion: Developing and implementing a best practices approach to health promotion. *Health Promotion Practice, 2,* 43–67.

McLeroy, K., Bibeau, D., Steckler, A., & Glanz, K. (1988). An ecological perspective on health promotion programs. *Health Education Quarterly, 15,* 351–377.

Stokols, D. (1992) Establishing and maintaining healthy environments: Toward a social ecology of health promotion. *American Psychologist, 47,* 6–22.

NAME INDEX

SUBJECT INDEX

A

Academy for Education Development (AED): BEHAVE logic model of, 274; and Prevention Marketing Initiative, 263, 264, 269, 271

Adolescent delinquency, and report card contingency system, 364–365

Adolescent health behavior: and alcohol/tobacco use, 108, 238–239; and Authoritative Parenting Model, 107–110; and driving risks, 110–120; HIV risk-reduction interventions, 263, 264–273

African American communities: case study of SISTA project in, 337–340; public health system and, 130–131, 332–333; and women's HIV risk exposures, 327, 323, 331, 332–333

AIDS (acquired immunodeficiency syndrome), 16–17, 338; and poverty, 322. *See also* HIV (human immunodeficiency virus)

Alcohol abuse interventions: and community coalitions, 185; and social capital, 238–239; for teens, 108

American Lung Association (ALA), 28

Applied behavioral analysis, and functional contextualism, 349–350

Attitudes: measurement of, 72; as theoretical construct of behavior, 71–72

Authoritative parenting, 101–106; and achievement orientation or motivation, 105; and adolescent outcomes, 109; and health-risk behaviors, 106; and instrumental competence, 104–106; measures for, 107; and school performance, 106; and teen driving risks, 113

Authoritative Parenting Model, 100–120; applied to adolescent health behavior, 107–110; applied to extensions of, 118–120; overview of, 9; and strategies for authoritative parenting,

115–118; and Young Drivers Intervention Study, 119, 120

Authoritative teaching concept, 119–120

B

Behavior analysis, and functional contextualism, 349–350

Behavior change: central and peripheral route cognitive processing in, 9, 73–75, 77–78, 79–80; and community change approach, 161–162; focused on general patterns versus specific acts, 43; and general model for health behavior change, 40; individual-focused, 161; traditional approach to 17–18. *See also specific interventions*

Behavior Decision Theory, 306

Behavioral and social science theory: and biomedical technology, 3; community-level approaches in, 6–7; development trajectory of, 5–8; expansion and refinement of, 4;